Dash Diet Cookbook for Beginners

1000+
Low-Sodium, Heart-Friendly Recipes to Make Every Meal of the Day Good for Your Heart

Abigail Castro

TABLE OF CONTENTS

INTRODUCTION 11
BREAKFAST 12
1. Quinoa Hashes 12
2. Artichoke Eggs 12
3. Quinoa Cakes 12
4. Bean Casserole 12
5. Grape Yogurt 12
6. Berry Pancakes 13
7. Western Omelet Quiche 13
8. Ginger French toast 13
9. Fruit Muffins 13
10. Omelet with Peppers 13
11. Vanilla Toasts 14
12. Raspberry Yogurt 14
13. Salsa Eggs 14
14. Fruit Scones 14
15. Cheese Omelet 14
16. Banana Pancakes 14
17. Aromatic Breakfast Granola 15
18. Morning Sweet Potatoes 15
19. Egg Toasts 15
20. Sweet Yogurt with Figs 15
21. Fruits and Rice Pudding 15
22. Asparagus Omelet 16
23. Bean Frittata 16
24. Peach Pancakes 16
25. Breakfast Splits 16
26. Whole Grain Pancakes 16
27. Granola Parfait 17
28. Curry Tofu Scramble 17
29. Scallions Omelet 17
30. Breakfast Almond Smoothie 17
31. Jack-o-Lantern Pancakes 17
32. Fruit Pizza 17
33. Flax Banana Yogurt Muffins 18
34. Apple Oats 18
35. Buckwheat Crepes 18
36. Spinach, Mushroom, and Feta Cheese Scramble 18
37. Red Velvet Pancakes with Cream Cheese Topping 19
38. Peanut Butter & Banana Breakfast Smoothie 19
39. No-Bake Breakfast Granola Bars 19
40. Mushroom Shallot Frittata 19
41. Very Berry Muesli 19
42. Veggie Quiche Muffins 20
43. Turkey Sausage and Mushroom Strata 20
44. Bacon Bits 20
45. Steel Cut Oat Blueberry Pancakes 20
46. Egg White Breakfast Mix 21
47. Pesto Omelet 21
48. Quinoa Bowls 21
49. Strawberry Sandwich 21
50. Apple Quinoa Muffins 21
51. Breakfast Fruits Bowls 22
52. Pumpkin Cookies 22
53. Veggie Scramble 22
54. Mushrooms and Turkey Breakfast 22
55. Mushrooms and Cheese Omelet 22
56. Easy Veggie Muffins 23
57. Carrot Muffins 23
58. Pineapple Oatmeal 23
59. Spinach Muffins 23
60. Chia Seeds Breakfast Mix 24
61. Salmon and Egg Scramble 24
62. Pumpkin Muffins 24
63. Sweet Berries Pancake 24
64. Zucchini Pancakes 24
65. Breakfast Banana Split 25
66. Mediterranean Toast 25
67. Instant Banana Oatmeal 25
68. Almond Butter-Banana Smoothie 25
69. Brown Sugar Cinnamon Oatmeal 25
70. Buckwheat Pancakes with Vanilla Almond Milk 25
71. Banana & Cinnamon Oatmeal 26
72. Bagels Made Healthy 26
73. Cereal with Cranberry-Orange Twist 26
74. No Cook Overnight Oats 26
75. Avocado Cup with Egg 26
76. French toast with Applesauce 27
77. Banana-Peanut Butter and Greens Smoothie 27
78. Baking Powder Biscuits 27
79. Oatmeal Banana Pancakes with Walnuts 27
80. Creamy Oats, Greens & Blueberry Smoothie 27
81. Stuffed Breakfast Peppers 28
82. Sweet Potato Toast Three Ways 28
83. Apple-Apricot Brown Rice Breakfast Porridge 28
84. Carrot Cake Overnight Oats 28
85. Steel-Cut Oatmeal with Plums and Pear 29
86. Creamy Apple-Avocado Smoothie 29
87. Strawberry, Orange, and Beet Smoothie 29
88. Blueberry-Vanilla Yogurt Smoothie 29
89. Greek Yogurt Oat Pancakes 29
90. Scrambled Egg and Veggie Breakfast Quesadillas 30
91. Spinach, Egg, and Cheese Breakfast Quesadillas 30
92. Simple Cheese and Broccoli Omelets 30
93. Creamy Avocado and Egg Salad Sandwiches 30
94. Breakfast Hash 31
95. Hearty Breakfast Casserole 31
96. Blueberry Waffles 31
97. Apple Pancakes 32
98. Super-Simple Granola 32
99. Savory Yogurt Bowls 32
100. Energy Sunrise Muffins 32
LUNCH 34
101. Pasta Primavera 34
102. Delicious Chicken Pasta 34
103. Flavorful Mac & Cheese 34
104. Flavors Herb Risotto 34
105. Delicious Pasta Primavera 35

106.	Tuscan Chicken Linguine	35
107.	Classic Beef Lasagna	35
108.	Spicy Veggie Pasta Bake	36
109.	Parmesan Spaghetti in Mushroom-Tomato Sauce	36
110.	Mustard Chicken Farfalle	36
111.	Italian Mushroom Pizza	37
112.	Chicken Bacon Ranch Pizza	37
113.	Fall Baked Vegetable with Rigatoni	37
114.	Walnut Pesto Pasta	38
115.	Beef Carbonara	38
116.	Coconut Flour Pizza	38
117.	Keto Pepperoni Pizza	38
118.	Fresh Bell Pepper Basil Pizza	39
119.	Basil & Artichoke Pizza	39
120.	Spanish-Style Pizza de Jarmon	39
121.	Curry Chicken Pockets	40
122.	Fajita Style Chili	40
123.	Fun Fajita Wraps	40
124.	Classic Chicken Noodle Soup	41
125.	Open Face Egg and Bacon Sandwich	41
126.	Tuscan Stew	41
127.	Tenderloin Fajitas	41
128.	Peanut Sauce Chicken Pasta	42
129.	Chicken Cherry Wraps	42
130.	Easy Barley Soup	42
131.	Cauliflower Lunch Salad	43
132.	Cheesy Black Bean Wraps	43
133.	Arugula Risotto	43
134.	Vegetarian Stuffed Eggplant	43
135.	Vegetable Tacos	44
136.	Lemongrass and Chicken Soup	44
137.	Easy Lunch Salmon Steaks	44
138.	Light Balsamic Salad	44
139.	Purple Potato Soup	45
140.	Leeks Soup	45
141.	Rice with Chicken	45
142.	Tomato Soup	45
143.	Cod Soup	46
144.	Sweet Potato Soup	46
145.	Sweet Potatoes and Zucchini Soup	46
146.	Hearty Chicken Fried Rice	46
147.	Creamy Chicken Breast	47
148.	Indian Chicken Stew	47
149.	Chicken, Bamboo, and Chestnuts Mix	47
150.	Salsa Chicken	47
151.	Hearty Roasted Cauliflower	47
152.	Cool Cabbage Fried Beef	48
153.	Fennel and Figs Lamb	48
154.	Black Berry Chicken Wings	48
155.	Mushroom and Olive "Mediterranean" Steak	48
156.	Generous Lemon Dredged Broccoli	49
157.	Tantalizing Almond butter Beans	49
158.	Healthy Chicken Cream Salad	49
159.	Generously Smothered Pork Chops	49
160.	Crazy Lamb Salad	50
161.	Chilled Chicken, Artichoke and Zucchini Platter	50
162.	Chicken and Carrot Stew	50
163.	Tasty Spinach Pie	50
164.	Mesmerizing Carrot and Pineapple Mix	51
165.	Blackberry Chicken Wings	51
166.	Secret Asian Green Beans	51
167.	Excellent Acorn Mix	51
168.	Crunchy Almond Chocolate Bars	51
169.	Lettuce and Chicken Platter	52
170.	Greek Lemon Chicken Bowl	52
171.	Garden Salad	52
172.	Spicy Cabbage Dish	52
173.	Extreme Balsamic Chicken	53
174.	Enjoyable Spinach and Bean Medley	53
175.	Tantalizing Cauliflower and Dill Mash	53
176.	Traditional Black Bean Chili	53
177.	Very Wild Mushroom Pilaf	54
178.	Green Palak Paneer	54
179.	Sporty Baby Carrots	54
180.	Saucy Garlic Greens	54
181.	Parmesan Baked Chicken	55
182.	Buffalo Chicken Lettuce Wraps	55
183.	Crazy Japanese Potato and Beef Croquettes	55
184.	Spicy Chili Crackers	55
185.	Golden Eggplant Fries	56
186.	Chicken and Carrot Stew	56
187.	The Delish Turkey Wrap	56
188.	Almond butternut Chicken	56
189.	Zucchini Zoodles with Chicken and Basil	57
190.	Duck with Cucumber and Carrots	57
191.	Epic Mango Chicken	57
192.	Chicken and Cabbage Platter	57
193.	Hearty Chicken Liver Stew	58
194.	Chicken Quesadilla	58
195.	Mustard Chicken	58
196.	Fascinating Spinach and Beef Meatballs	58
197.	Juicy and Peppery Tenderloin	58
198.	Healthy Avocado Beef Patties	59
199.	Ravaging Beef Pot Roast	59
200.	Lovely Faux Mac and Cheese	59

DINNER — 59

201.	The Almond Breaded Chicken Goodness	60
202.	Almond butter Pork Chops	60
203.	Healthy Mediterranean Lamb Chops	60
204.	Brown Butter Duck Breast	60
205.	Chipotle Lettuce Chicken	61
206.	Zucchini Beef Sauté with Coriander Greens	61
207.	Walnuts and Asparagus Delight	61
208.	Beef Soup	61
209.	Clean Chicken and Mushroom Stew	62
210.	Zucchini Zoodles with Chicken and Basil	62
211.	Pan-Seared Lamb Chops	62
212.	Lamb & Pineapple Kebabs	62
213.	Spiced Pork One	63
214.	Pork chops in Creamy Sauce	63
215.	Decent Beef and Onion Stew	63
216.	Ground Beef with Cabbage	64
217.	Beef & Veggies Chili	64
218.	Beef Meatballs in Tomato Gravy	64
219.	Spicy Lamb Curry	65
220.	Ground Lamb with Harissa	65
221.	Roasted Lamb Chops	65
222.	Baked Meatballs & Scallions	66

223.	Pork Chili	66
224.	Baked Pork & Mushroom Meatballs	66
225.	Citrus Beef with Bok Choy	67
226.	Ground Beef with Greens & Tomatoes	67
227.	Curried Beef Meatballs	67
228.	Grilled Skirt Steak Coconut	68
229.	Lamb with Prunes	68
230.	Ground Lamb with Peas	68
231.	Basil Halibut	69
232.	Beef with Mushroom & Broccoli	69
233.	Beef with Zucchini Noodles	69
234.	Spiced Ground Beef	70
235.	Ground Beef with Veggies	70
236.	Shrimp & Corn Chowder	70
237.	Leek & Cauliflower Soup	71
238.	Easy Beef Brisket	71
239.	Coconut Shrimp	71
240.	Asian Salmon	71
241.	Fennel Sauce Tenderloin	72
242.	Beefy Fennel Stew	72
243.	Currant Pork Chops	72
244.	Spicy Tomato Shrimp	72
245.	Beef Stir Fry	73
246.	Grilled Chicken with Lemon and Fennel	73
247.	Caramelized Pork Chops and Onion	73
248.	Hearty Pork Belly Casserole	73
249.	Apple Pie Crackers	74
250.	Paprika Lamb Chops	74
251.	Sweet and Sour Cabbage and Apples	74
252.	Delicious Aloo Palak	74
253.	Orange and Chili Garlic Sauce	75
254.	Tantalizing Mushroom Gravy	75
255.	Everyday Vegetable Stock	75
256.	The Vegan Lovers Refried Beans	75
257.	Cool Apple and Carrot Harmony	76
258.	Mac and Chokes	76
259.	Black Eyed Peas and Spinach Platter	76
260.	Humble Mushroom Rice	76
261.	Chipotle Lettuce Chicken	76
262.	Balsamic Chicken and Vegetables	77
263.	Cream Dredged Corn Platter	77
264.	Exuberant Sweet Potatoes	77
265.	Ethiopian Cabbage Delight	77
266.	Amazing Sesame Breadsticks	78
267.	Brown Butter Duck Breast	78
268.	Generous Garlic Bread Stick	78
269.	Cauliflower Bread Stick	78
270.	Bacon and Chicken Garlic Wrap	79
271.	The Almond Breaded Chicken Goodness	79
272.	South-Western Pork Chops	79
273.	Almond butter Pork Chops	79
274.	Chicken Salsa	80
275.	Healthy Mediterranean Lamb Chops	80
276.	Amazing Grilled Chicken and Blueberry Salad	80
277.	Clean Chicken and Mushroom Stew	80
278.	Elegant Pumpkin Chili Dish	81
279.	Zucchini Zoodles with Chicken and Basil	81
280.	Tasty Roasted Broccoli	81
281.	Zucchini Beef Sauté with Coriander Greens	81
282.	Hearty Lemon and Pepper Chicken	82
283.	Walnuts and Asparagus Delight	82
284.	Healthy Carrot Chips	82
285.	Beef Soup	82
286.	Lime Shrimp and Kale	82
287.	Parsley Cod Mix	83
288.	Salmon and Cabbage Mix	83
289.	Decent Beef and Onion Stew	83
290.	Clean Parsley and Chicken Breast	83
291.	Fruit Shrimp Soup	84
292.	Mussels and Chickpea Soup	84
293.	Fish Stew	84
294.	Shrimp and Broccoli Soup	84
295.	Coconut Turkey Mix	85
296.	Shrimp Cocktail	85
297.	Quinoa and Scallops Salad	85
298.	Squid and Shrimp Salad	85
299.	Parsley Seafood Cocktail	86
300.	Shrimp and Onion Ginger Dressing	86

MAINS 86

301.	Cauliflower Tabbouleh	86
302.	Stuffed Artichoke	87
303.	Beef Salpicao	87
304.	Cream Dredged Corn Platter	87
305.	Ethiopian Cabbage Delight	87
306.	Mushroom Soup	87
307.	Stuffed Portobello Mushrooms	88
308.	Lettuce Salad	88
309.	Onion Soup	88
310.	Asparagus Salad	88
311.	Prosciutto-Wrapped Asparagus	89
312.	Stuffed Bell Peppers	89
313.	Stuffed Eggplants with Goat Cheese	89
314.	Korma Curry	89
315.	Zucchini Bars	90
316.	Tuna Tartare	90
317.	Clam Chowder	90
318.	Asian Beef Salad	90
319.	Carbonara	91
320.	Cauliflower Soup with Seeds	91
321.	Crepe Pie	91
322.	Coconut Soup	91
323.	Fish Tacos	92
324.	Cobb Salad	92
325.	Cheese Soup	92
326.	Veggie Wrap	92
327.	Salmon Wrap	92
328.	Dill Chicken Salad	93
329.	Spinach Rolls	93
330.	Goat Cheese Fold-Overs	93
331.	Sweet and Sour Vegetable Noodles	93
332.	Tuna Sandwich	94
333.	Fruited Quinoa Salad	94
334.	Turkey Wrap	94
335.	Chicken Wrap	94
336.	Veggie Variety	94
337.	Vegetable Pasta	95
338.	Vegetable Noodles with Bolognese	95
339.	Harissa Bolognese with Vegetable Noodles	95
340.	Curry Vegetable Noodles with Chicken	96
341.	Mushroom Cakes	96

342.	Glazed Eggplant Rings	96
343.	Sweet Potato Balls	96
344.	Chickpea Curry	96
345.	Pan-Fried Salmon with Salad	97
346.	Vegan Chili	97
347.	Aromatic Whole Grain Spaghetti	97
348.	Chunky Tomatoes	97
349.	Baked Falafel	97
350.	Paella	98
351.	Hassel back Eggplant	98
352.	Vegetarian Kebabs	98
353.	White Beans Stew	98
354.	Vegetarian Lasagna	98
355.	Carrot Cakes	99
356.	Gnocchi with Tomato Basil Sauce	99
357.	Creamy Pumpkin Pasta	99
358.	Mexican-Style Potato Casserole	99
359.	Black Bean Stew with Cornbread	100
360.	Mushroom Florentine	100
361.	Eggplant Parmesan Stacks	100
362.	Roasted Vegetable Enchiladas	101
363.	Lentil Avocado Tacos	101
364.	Tomato & Olive Orecchiette with Basil Pesto	101
365.	Italian Stuffed Portobello Mushroom Burgers	102
366.	Tofu & Green Bean Stir-Fry	102
367.	Peanut Vegetable Pad Thai	102
368.	Spicy Tofu Burrito Bowls with Cilantro Avocado Sauce	103
369.	Sweet Potato Cakes with Classic Guacamole	103
370.	Chickpea Cauliflower Tikka Masala	103
371.	Roasted Sweet Potato and Red Beets	104
372.	Sichuan Style Baked Chioggia Beets and Broccoli Florets	104
373.	Baked Enoki and Mini Cabbage	104
374.	Roasted Triple Mushrooms	104
375.	Roasted Mini Cabbage and Sweet Potato	105
376.	Roasted Soy Beans and Winter Squash	105
377.	Roasted Button Mushrooms and Squash	105
378.	Roasted Tomatoes Rutabaga and Kohlrabi Main	105
379.	Roasted Brussels sprouts and Broccoli	106
380.	Roasted Broccoli Sweet Potatoes & Bean Sprouts	106
381.	Thai Roasted Spicy Black Beans and Choy Sum	106
382.	Simple Roasted Broccoli and Cauliflower	107
383.	Roasted Napa Cabbage and Turnips Extra	107
384.	Simple Roasted Kale Artichoke Heart and Choy Sum Extra	107
385.	Roasted Kale and Bok Choy Extra	107
386.	Very Wild Mushroom Pilaf	108
387.	Sporty Baby Carrots	108
388.	Garden Salad	108
389.	Baked Smoky Broccoli and Garlic	108
390.	Roasted Cauliflower and Lima Beans	109
391.	The Delish Turkey Wrap	109
392.	Zucchini Zoodles with Chicken and Basil	109
393.	Parmesan Baked Chicken	109
394.	Crazy Japanese Potato and Beef Croquettes	110
395.	Golden Eggplant Fries	110
396.	Juicy and Peppery Tenderloin	110
397.	Ravaging Beef Pot Roast	110
398.	Epic Mango Chicken	111
399.	Hearty Chicken Liver Stew	111
400.	Mustard Chicken	111

SIDES & APPETIZERS — **111**

401.	Mediterranean Pop Corn Bites	111
402.	Hearty Buttery Walnuts	111
403.	Refreshing Watermelon Sorbet	112
404.	Lovely Faux Mac and Cheese	112
405.	Beautiful Banana Custard	112
406.	Pumpkin Pie Fat Bombs	112
407.	Sensational Lemonade Fat Bomb	112
408.	Sweet Almond and Coconut Fat Bombs	113
409.	Almond and Tomato Balls	113
410.	Avocado Tuna Bites	113
411.	Juicy Simple Lemon Fat Bombs	113
412.	Chocolate Coconut Bombs	113
413.	Terrific Jalapeno Bacon Bombs	114
414.	Yummy Espresso Fat Bombs	114
415.	Crispy Coconut Bombs	114
416.	Spiced Up Pumpkin Seeds Bowls	114
417.	Mozzarella Cauliflower Bars	114
418.	Tomato Pesto Crackers	115
419.	Garlic Cottage Cheese Crispy	115
420.	Tasty Cucumber Bites	115
421.	Hearty Almond Crackers	115
422.	Black Bean Salsa	115
423.	Corn Spread	116
424.	Moroccan Leeks Snack	116
425.	The Bell Pepper Fiesta	116
426.	Hearty Cashew and Almond Butter	116
427.	Red Coleslaw	116
428.	Avocado Mayo Medley	116
429.	Amazing Garlic Aioli	117
430.	Easy Seed Crackers	117
431.	Chickpeas and Curried Veggies	117
432.	Brussels sprouts Casserole	117
433.	Tasty Cauliflower	117
434.	Artichoke and Spinach Dip	118
435.	Apple Salsa	118
436.	Quinoa Curry	118
437.	Lemon and Cilantro Rice	118
438.	Chili Beans	118
439.	Bean Spread	119
440.	Stir-Fried Steak, Shiitake, and Asparagus	119
441.	Jalapeno Black-Eyed Peas Mix	119
442.	Sour Cream Green Beans	119
443.	Cumin Brussels sprouts	120
444.	Peach and Carrots	120
445.	Baby Spinach and Grains Mix	120
446.	Pilaf with Bella Mushrooms	120
447.	Parsley Fennel	120
448.	Sweet Butternut	120
449.	Mushroom Sausages	121
450.	Parsley Red Potatoes	121
451.	Spiced Broccoli Florets	121
452.	Lima Beans Dish	121
453.	Soy Sauce Green Beans	122
454.	Butter Corn	122

455.	Stevia Peas with Marjoram	122
456.	Colored Iceberg Salad	122
457.	Fennel Salad with Arugula	122
458.	Corn Mix	123
459.	Persimmon Salad	123
460.	Avocado Side Salad	123
461.	Spicy Brussels sprouts	123
462.	Baked Cauliflower with Chili	123
463.	Baked Broccoli	124
464.	Slow Cooked Potatoes with Cheddar	124
465.	Squash Salad with Orange	124
466.	Easy Carrots Mix	124
467.	Tasty Grilled Asparagus	124
468.	Roasted Carrots	125
469.	Oven Roasted Asparagus	125
470.	Baked Potato with Thyme	125
471.	Italian Roasted Cabbage	125
472.	Tex-Mex Cole Slaw	125
473.	Roasted Okra	126
474.	Brown Sugar Glazed Carrots	126
475.	Oven-Roasted Beets with Honey Ricotta	126
476.	Creamy Broccoli Cheddar Rice	126
477.	Smashed Brussels sprouts	127
478.	Cilantro Lime Rice	127
479.	Corn Salad with Lime Vinaigrette	127
480.	Mediterranean Chickpea Salad	127
481.	Spanish rice	128
482.	Sweet Potatoes and Apples	128
483.	Roasted Turnips	128
484.	No-Mayo Potato Salad	128
485.	Zucchini Tomato Bake	129
486.	Avocado, Tomato, and Olives Salad	129
487.	Radish and Olives Salad	129
488.	Spinach and Endives Salad	129
489.	Basil Olives Mix	129
490.	Arugula Salad	130
491.	Balsamic Cabbage	130
492.	Chili Broccoli	130
493.	Hot Brussels sprouts	130
494.	Paprika Brussels sprouts	130
495.	Creamy Cauliflower Mash	131
496.	Turmeric Endives	131
497.	Parmesan Endives	131
498.	Lemon Asparagus	131
499.	Lime Carrots	131
500.	Garlic Potato Pan	131

SEAFOOD — 132

501.	Lemon Garlic Shrimp	132
502.	Shrimp Fra Diavolo	132
503.	Fish Amandine	132
504.	Air-Fryer Fish Cakes	132
505.	Pesto Shrimp Pasta	133
506.	Monkfish with Sautéed Leeks, Fennel, and Tomatoes	133
507.	Caramelized Fennel and Sardines with Penne	133
508.	Coppin	134
509.	Green Goddess Crab Salad with Endive	134
510.	Seared Scallops with Blood Orange Glaze	134
511.	Flounder with Tomatoes and Basil	134
512.	Grilled Mahi-Mahi with Artichoke Caponata	135
513.	Cod and Cauliflower Chowder	135
514.	Sardine Bruschetta with Fennel and Lemon Cream	135
515.	Chopped Tuna Salad	136
516.	Shrimp, Snow Peas and Bamboo Soup	136
517.	Lemony Mussels	136
518.	Citrus-Glazed Salmon with Zucchini Noodles	136
519.	Salmon Cakes with Bell Pepper plus Lemon Yogurt	136
520.	Halibut in Parchment with Zucchini, Shallots, and Herbs	137
521.	Basil Tilapia	137
522.	Salmon Meatballs with Garlic	137
523.	Tuna Cakes	137
524.	Spiced Cod Mix	138
525.	Italian Shrimp	138
526.	Salmon with Mushroom	138
527.	Cod Sweet Potato Chowder	138
528.	Salmon with Cinnamon	139
529.	Scallops and Strawberry Mix	139
530.	Baked Haddock with Avocado Mayonnaise	139
531.	Salmon Casserole	139
532.	Scallops, Sweet Potatoes and Cauliflower Mix	139
533.	Spiced Salmon	140
534.	Salmon and Tomatoes Salad	140
535.	Coconut Cream Shrimp	140
536.	Tuna Pate	140
537.	Shrimp and Avocado Salad	140
538.	Shrimp with Cilantro Sauce	141
539.	Citrus Calamari	141
540.	Mussels Curry with Lime	141
541.	Spanish Mussels Mix	141
542.	Quinoa and Scallops Salad	141
543.	Salmon and Veggies Soup	142
544.	Salmon Salsa	142
545.	Salmon and Easy Cucumber Salad	142
546.	Inspiring Cajun Snow Crab	142
547.	Grilled Lime Shrimp	142
548.	Calamari Citrus	143
549.	Spiced Up Salmon	143
550.	Coconut Cream Shrimp	143
551.	Salmon and Orange Dish	143
552.	Mesmerizing Coconut Haddock	143
553.	Asparagus and Lemon Salmon Dish	144
554.	Ecstatic "Foiled" Fish	144
555.	Brazilian Shrimp Stew	144
556.	Simple Sautéed Garlic and Parsley Scallops	144
557.	Salmon and Cucumber Platter	145
558.	Tuna Pate	145
559.	Cinnamon Salmon	145
560.	Scallop and Strawberry Mix	145
561.	Salmon with Peas and Parsley Dressing	145
562.	Mackerel and Orange Medley	146
563.	Spicy Chili Salmon	146
564.	Simple One Pot Mussels	146
565.	Lemon Pepper and Salmon	146
566.	Roasted Lemon Swordfish	146
567.	Especial Glazed Salmon	147
568.	Generous Stuffed Salmon Avocado	147
569.	Spanish Mussels	147

570.	Tilapia Broccoli Platter	147
571.	Saffron Shrimp	148
572.	Crab, Zucchini and Watermelon Soup	148
573.	Shrimp and Orzo	148
574.	Lemon and Garlic Scallops	148
575.	Walnut Encrusted Salmon	149
576.	Smoked Salmon with Capers and Radishes	149
577.	Trout Spread	149
578.	Easy Shrimp and Mango	149
579.	Spring Salmon Mix	149
580.	Smoked Salmon and Green Beans	149
581.	Aromatic Salmon with Fennel Seeds	150
582.	Shrimp Quesadillas	150
583.	The OG Tuna Sandwich	150
584.	Easy to Understand Mussels	150
585.	Cheesy Shrimp Mix	151
586.	Cod Salad with Mustard	151
587.	Broccoli and Cod Mash	151
588.	Greek Style Salmon	151
589.	Spicy Ginger Sea bass	151
590.	Yogurt Shrimps	152
591.	Creamy Salmon and Asparagus Mix	152
592.	Salmon and Brussels sprouts	152
593.	Salmon and Beets Mix	152
594.	Garlic Shrimp Mix	152
595.	Salmon and Potatoes Mix	153
596.	Balsamic Salmon and Peaches Mix	153
597.	Salmon and Bean s Mix	153
598.	Lemony Salmon and Pomegranate Mix	153
599.	Salmon and Veggie Mix	154
600.	Greek Salmon with Yogurt	154

POULTRY ... 154

601.	Chicken Sliders	154
602.	White Chicken Chili	154
603.	Sweet Potato-Turkey Meatloaf	155
604.	Oaxacan Chicken	155
605.	Spicy Chicken with Minty Couscous	155
606.	Chicken, Pasta and Snow Peas	156
607.	Chicken with Noodles	156
608.	Honey Crusted Chicken	156
609.	Paella with Chicken, Leeks, and Tarragon	156
610.	Southwestern Chicken and Pasta	156
611.	Stuffed Chicken Breasts	157
612.	Buffalo Chicken Salad Wrap	157
613.	Chicken with Mushrooms	157
614.	Baked Chicken	157
615.	Garlic Pepper Chicken	158
616.	Mustard Chicken Tenders	158
617.	Salsa Chicken Chili	158
618.	Lemon Garlic Chicken	158
619.	Simple Mediterranean Chicken	159
620.	Roasted Chicken Thighs	159
621.	Mediterranean Turkey Breast	159
622.	Olive Capers Chicken	159
623.	Chicken with Potatoes Olives & Sprouts	159
624.	Garlic Mushroom Chicken	160
625.	Grilled Chicken	160
626.	Delicious Lemon Chicken Salad	160
627.	Healthy Chicken Orzo	160
628.	The Ultimate Faux-Tisserie Chicken	161

629.	Oregano Chicken Thighs	161
630.	Pesto Chicken Breasts with Summer Squash	161
631.	Chicken, Tomato and Green Beans	161
632.	Chicken Tortillas	162
633.	Pumpkin and Black Beans Chicken	162
634.	Chicken Thighs and Apples Mix	162
635.	Thai Chicken Thighs	162
636.	Falling "Off" The Bone Chicken	162
637.	Feisty Chicken Porridge	163
638.	Parmesan and Chicken Spaghetti Squash	163
639.	Apricot Chicken	163
640.	Oven-Fried Chicken Breasts	163
641.	Rosemary Roasted Chicken	163
642.	Artichoke and Spinach Chicken	164
643.	Creamy Chicken Fried Rice	164
644.	Chicken Tikka	164
645.	Honey Spiced Cajun Chicken	164
646.	Italian Chicken	165
647.	Lemon-Parsley Chicken Breast	165
648.	Teriyaki Chicken Wings	165
649.	Hot Chicken Wings	165
650.	Crispy Cashew Chicken	165
651.	Chicken Tortellini Soup	166
652.	Chicken Divan	166
653.	Sweet Potato-Turkey Meatloaf	166
654.	Oaxacan Chicken	167
655.	Spicy Chicken with Minty Couscous	167
656.	Chicken, Pasta and Snow Peas	167
657.	Chicken with Noodles	167
658.	Southwestern Chicken and Pasta	168
659.	Stuffed Chicken Breasts	168
660.	Buffalo Chicken Salad Wrap	168
661.	Chicken Sliders	168
662.	White Chicken Chili	169
663.	Salsa Chicken Chili	169
664.	Honey Crusted Chicken	169
665.	Paella with Chicken, Leeks, and Tarragon	169
666.	Olive Capers Chicken	170
667.	Chicken with Mushrooms	170
668.	Baked Chicken	170
669.	Garlic Pepper Chicken	170
670.	Mustard Chicken Tenders	170
671.	Healthy Chicken Orzo	171
672.	Lemon Garlic Chicken	171
673.	Simple Mediterranean Chicken	171
674.	Roasted Chicken Thighs	171
675.	Mediterranean Turkey Breast	172
676.	Fruity Chicken Salad	172
677.	Chicken Corn Chili	172
678.	Chicken Noodles Soup	172
679.	Sweet Chicken and Peaches	173
680.	Pineapple Glazed Chicken	173
681.	Salsa Chicken	173
682.	Pear Chicken Casserole	173
683.	Poached Chicken with Rice	174
684.	Hawaiian Chicken	174
685.	Fruity Chicken Bites	174
686.	Chicken Tortillas	174
687.	Chicken with Potatoes Olives & Sprouts	175
688.	Garlic Mushroom Chicken	175

689.	Grilled Chicken	175
690.	Delicious Lemon Chicken Salad	175
691.	Feisty Chicken Porridge	176
692.	The Ultimate Faux-Tisserie Chicken	176
693.	Oregano Chicken Thighs	176
694.	Pesto Chicken Breasts with Summer Squash	176
695.	Chicken, Tomato and Green Beans	176
696.	Artichoke and Spinach Chicken	177
697.	Pumpkin and Black Beans Chicken	177
698.	Chicken Thighs and Apples Mix	177
699.	Thai Chicken Thighs	177
700.	Falling "Off" The Bone Chicken	177

MEAT **178**

701.	Pork Tenderloin with Apples and Balsamic Vinegar	178
702.	Pork Tenderloin with Apples and Blue Cheese	178
703.	Pork Tenderloin with Fennel Sauce	178
704.	Spicy Beef Kebabs	179
705.	Spicy Beef Curry	179
706.	Pork Tenderloin with Apples and Sweet Potatoes	179
707.	Pork Medallions with Five Spice Powder	179
708.	Grilled Pork Fajitas	180
709.	New York Strip Steak with Mushroom Sauce	180
710.	Pork Chops with Black Currant Jam	180
711.	Pork Medallion with Herbes de Provence	180
712.	Simple Beef Brisket and Tomato Soup	181
713.	Beef Stew with Fennel and Shallots	181
714.	Rustic Beef and Barley Soup	181
715.	Beef Stroganoff	181
716.	Curried Pork Tenderloin in Apple Cider	182
717.	Pork and Roasted Tomatoes Mix	182
718.	Provence Pork Medallions	182
719.	Garlic Pork Shoulder	182
720.	Grilled Flank Steak with Lime Vinaigrette	183
721.	Asian Pork Tenderloin	183
722.	Roast and Mushrooms	183
723.	Pork and Celery Mix	183
724.	Pork and Dates Sauce	184
725.	Pork Roast and Cranberry Roast	184
726.	Easy Pork Chops	184
727.	Beef & Vegetable Stir-Fry	184
728.	Simple Veal Chops	184
729.	Beef and Barley Farmers Soup	185
730.	Simple Pork and Capers	185
731.	A "Boney" Pork Chop	185
732.	Beef Pot	185
733.	Beef with Cucumber Raito	186
734.	Bistro Beef Tenderloin	186
735.	The Surprising No "Noodle" Lasagna	186
736.	Lamb Chops with Kale	186
737.	Beef with Mushrooms	187
738.	Lemony Braised Beef Roast	187
739.	Grilled Fennel-Cumin Lamb Chops	187
740.	Beef Heart	187
741.	Jerk Beef and Plantain Kabobs	187
742.	Authentic Pepper Steak	188
743.	Lamb Chops with Rosemary	188
744.	Cane Wrapped Around In Prosciutto	188
745.	Beef Veggie Pot Meal	188

746.	Braised Beef Shanks	189
747.	Pork and Capers	189
748.	Pork and Red Peppers Mix	189
749.	Garlic Pork and Kale	189
750.	Italian Pork Soup	189
751.	Pork, Shallots and Watercress Soup	190
752.	Pork and Fennel Mix	190
753.	Pork Casserole with Cabbage	190
754.	French Pork Mix	190
755.	Easy Pork and Okra Stew	190
756.	Burgundy Stew	191
757.	Pork Roast with Mushrooms	191
758.	Pork Meatloaf	191
759.	Garlic Meatballs Salad	191
760.	Meatballs and Sauce	192
761.	Stir Fry Ground Pork	192
762.	Citrus Pork	192
763.	Pork Chops with Nutmeg	192
764.	Italian Parmesan Pork	193
765.	Pork Roast with Cranberry	193
766.	Pork Patties	193
767.	Pork, Water Chestnuts and Cabbage Salad	193
768.	Pork and Zucchini Stew	194
769.	Pork Roast, Leeks and Carrots	194
770.	Easy Veal Chops	194
771.	Pork with Apple Sauce	194
772.	Pork with Mushrooms Bowls	194
773.	Pork and salsa	195
774.	Pork Stew with Shallots	195
775.	Pork Chops with Thyme and Apples	195
776.	Pork and Roasted Tomatoes Mix	195
777.	Balsamic Chili Roast	196
778.	Spiced Winter Pork Roast	196
779.	Creamy Smoky Pork Chops	196
780.	Pork with Dates Sauce	196
781.	Pork Chops and Apples	196
782.	Spiced Beef	197
783.	Tomato Beef	197
784.	Hoisin Pork	197
785.	Sage Beef Loin	197
786.	Beef Chili	197
787.	Ground Pork and Kale Soup	198
788.	Peaches and Kale Steak Salad	198
789.	Garlic Pork Meatballs	198
790.	Fajita Pork Strips	198
791.	Pepper Pork Tenderloins	198
792.	Pork and Veggies Mix	198
793.	Pork Chili	199
794.	Pork and Sweet Potatoes with Chili	199
795.	Pork and Pumpkin Chili	199
796.	Spiced Pork Soup	200
797.	Tarragon Pork Steak with Tomatoes	200
798.	Pork Meatballs	200
799.	Pork with Scallions and Peanuts	200
800.	Mediterranean Lamb Mix	200

VEGETABLES **201**

801.	Loaded Baked Sweet Potatoes	201
802.	White Beans with Spinach and Pan-Roasted Tomatoes	201
803.	Black-Eyed Peas and Greens Power Salad	201

804.	Butternut-Squash Macaroni and Cheese	202
805.	Pasta with Tomatoes and Peas	202
806.	Quinoa Bowl	202
807.	Vegan Meatloaf	202
808.	Red Beans and Rice	203
809.	Hearty Lentil Soup	203
810.	Black-Bean Soup	203
811.	Paella	203
812.	Mushroom Cakes	203
813.	Glazed Eggplant Rings	204
814.	Sweet Potato Balls	204
815.	Chickpea Curry	204
816.	Tofu Turkey	204
817.	Cauliflower Tots	205
818.	Aromatic Whole Grain Spaghetti	205
819.	Chunky Tomatoes	205
820.	Baked Falafel	205
821.	Stuffed Portobello	205
822.	Chile Relents	206
823.	Carrot Cakes	206
824.	Vegan Chili	206
825.	Spinach Casserole	206
826.	Mac Stuffed Sweet Potatoes	206
827.	Tofu Tikka Masala	207
828.	Tofu Parmigiana	207
829.	Mushroom Stroganoff	207
830.	Eggplant Croquettes	207
831.	Baked Eggs in Avocado	207
832.	Vegetarian Lasagna	208
833.	Lentil Quiche	208
834.	Corn Patties	208
835.	Tofu Stir Fry	208
836.	Greek Flatbread with Spinach, Tomatoes & Feta	208
837.	Mushroom Risotto with Peas	209
838.	Loaded Tofu Burrito with Black Beans	209
839.	Southwest Tofu Scramble	209
840.	Black-Bean and Vegetable Burrito	209
841.	Tomato & Olive Orecchiette with Basil Pesto	210
842.	Italian Stuffed Portobello Mushroom Burgers	210
843.	Gnocchi with Tomato Basil Sauce	210
844.	Creamy Pumpkin Pasta	211
845.	Quinoa-Stuffed Peppers	211
846.	Sweet Potato Cakes with Classic Guacamole	211
847.	Chickpea Cauliflower Tikka Masala	212
848.	Eggplant Parmesan Stacks	212
849.	Roasted Vegetable Enchiladas	212
850.	Lentil Avocado Tacos	213
851.	Stuffed Eggplant Shells	213
852.	Southwestern Vegetables Tacos	213
853.	Tofu & Green Bean Stir-Fry	213
854.	Peanut Vegetable Pad Thai	214
855.	Spicy Tofu Burrito Bowls with Cilantro Avocado Sauce	214
856.	Vegetable Cheese Calzone	214
857.	Mixed Vegetarian Chili	215
858.	Zucchini Pepper Kebabs	215
859.	Asparagus Cheese Vermicelli	215
860.	Corn Stuffed Peppers	215
861.	Chunky Black-Bean Dip	216
862.	Classic Hummus	216
863.	Crispy Potato Skins	216
864.	Roasted Chickpeas	216
865.	Carrot-Cake Smoothie	216
866.	Southwestern Bean-And-Pepper Salad	217
867.	Cauliflower Mashed Potatoes	217
868.	Roasted Brussels sprouts	217
869.	Broccoli with Garlic and Lemon	217
870.	Brown Rice Pilaf	217
871.	Pasta with Tomatoes and Peas	218
872.	Healthy Vegetable Fried Rice	218
873.	Portobello-Mushroom Cheeseburgers	218
874.	And-Rosemary Omelet	218
875.	Chilled Cucumber-And-Avocado Soup with Dill	219
876.	Black-Bean Soup	219
877.	Loaded Baked Sweet Potatoes	219
878.	White Beans with Spinach and Pan-Roasted Tomatoes	219
879.	Black-Eyed Peas and Greens Power Salad	220
880.	Butternut-Squash Macaroni and Cheese	220
881.	Southwest Tofu Scramble	220
882.	Black-Bean and Vegetable Burrito	220
883.	Baked Eggs in Avocado	221
884.	Red Beans and Rice	221
885.	Hearty Lentil Soup	221
886.	Brown Rice Casserole with Cottage Cheese	221
887.	Quinoa-Stuffed Peppers	222
888.	Greek Flatbread with Spinach, Tomatoes & Feta	222
889.	Mushroom Risotto with Peas	222
890.	Loaded Tofu Burrito with Black Beans	222
891.	Sweet Potato Rice with Spicy Peanut Sauce	223
892.	Vegetable Red Curry	223
893.	Black Bean Burgers	223
894.	Summer Barley Pilaf with Yogurt Dill Sauce	224
895.	Lentil Quinoa Gratin with Butternut Squash	224
896.	Moroccan-Inspired Tagine with Chickpeas & Vegetables	224
897.	Spaghetti Squash with Maple Glaze & Tofu Crumbles	225
898.	Stuffed Tex-Mex Baked Potatoes	225
899.	Lentil-Stuffed Zucchini Boats	225
900.	Baked Eggplant Parmesan	226

SNACK AND DESSERTS — 226

901.	The Mean Green Smoothie	226
902.	Mint Flavored Pear Smoothie	226
903.	Chilled Watermelon Smoothie	227
904.	Banana Ginger Medley	227
905.	Banana and Almond Flax Glass	227
906.	Sensational Strawberry Medley	227
907.	Sweet Almond and Coconut Fat Bombs	227
908.	Almond and Tomato Balls	227
909.	Avocado Tuna Bites	228
910.	Mediterranean Pop Corn Bites	228
911.	Hearty Buttery Walnuts	228
912.	Refreshing Watermelon Sorbet	228
913.	Refreshing Mango and Pear Smoothie	228
914.	Epic Pineapple Juice	228
915.	Choco Lovers Strawberry Shake	229

916.	Healthy Coffee Smoothie	229
917.	Blackberry and Apple Smoothie	229
918.	Tasty Mediterranean Peanut Almond butter Popcorns	229
919.	Just a Minute worth Muffin	229
920.	Hearty Almond Bread	229
921.	Mixed Berries Smoothie	230
922.	Satisfying Berry and Almond Smoothie	230
923.	Decisive Lime and Strawberry Popsicle	230
924.	Ravaging Blueberry Muffin	230
925.	The Coconut Loaf	230
926.	Fresh Figs with Walnuts and Ricotta	231
927.	Authentic Medjool Date Truffles	231
928.	Fennel and Almond Bites	231
929.	Feisty Coconut Fudge	231
930.	No Bake Cheesecake	231
931.	Easy Chia Seed Pumpkin Pudding	232
932.	Lovely Blueberry Pudding	232
933.	Heart Warming Cinnamon Rice Pudding	232
934.	Pure Avocado Pudding	232
935.	Sweet Almond and Coconut Fat Bombs	232
936.	Spicy Popper Mug Cake	232
937.	The Most Elegant Parsley Soufflé Ever	233
938.	Mesmerizing Avocado and Chocolate Pudding	233
939.	Hearty Pineapple Pudding	233
940.	Healthy Berry Cobbler	233
941.	Tasty Poached Apples	233
942.	Home Made Trail Mix for the Trip	234
943.	Mini Teriyaki Turkey Sandwiches	234
944.	Elegant Cranberry Muffins	234
945.	Apple and Almond Muffins	234
946.	Stylish Chocolate Parfait	235
947.	Supreme Matcha Bomb	235
948.	Pork Beef Bean Nachos	235
949.	Pressure Cooker Cranberry Hot Wings	235
950.	Bacon hot Dog Bites	236
951.	Instant Pot cocktail Wieners	236
952.	Pressure Cooker Braised Pulled Ham	236
953.	Ginger and Cinnamon Pudding	236
954.	Honey Compote	236
955.	Dark Cherry and Stevia Compote	236
956.	Vanilla Grapes Bowls	237
957.	Pears Mix	237
958.	Mandarin Pudding	237
959.	Cherry Stew	237
960.	Walnut Apple Mix	237
961.	Vanilla and Grapes Compote	238
962.	Soft Pudding	238
963.	Green Pudding	238
964.	Lemony Plum Cake	238
965.	Lentils Sweet Bars	238
966.	Lentils and Dates Brownies	239
967.	Rose Lentils Ice Cream	239
968.	Coconut Figs	239
969.	Lemony Banana Mix	239
970.	Cocoa Banana Dessert Smoothie	239
971.	Kiwi Bars	239
972.	Black Tea Bars	240
973.	Lovely Faux Mac and Cheese	240
974.	Beautiful Banana Custard	240
975.	Summer Jam	240
976.	Cinnamon Pudding	240
977.	Orange Compote	241
978.	Chocolate Bars	241
979.	Lemon Zest Pudding	241
980.	Maple Syrup Poached Pears	241
981.	Ginger and Pumpkin Pie	241
982.	Cashew and Carrot Muffins	242
983.	Lemon Custard	242
984.	Rhubarb Dip	242
985.	Resilient Chocolate Cream	242
986.	Vanilla Poached Strawberries	242
987.	Lemon Bananas	242
988.	Pecans Cake	243
989.	Coconut Cream and Plums Cake	243
990.	Pumpkin Pudding	243
991.	Cashew Lemon Fudge	243
992.	Brown Cake	243
993.	Delicious Berry Pie	244
994.	Cinnamon Peach Cobbler	244
995.	Cherry Stew	244
996.	Rice Pudding	244
997.	Apple Loaf	244
998.	Cauliflower Cinnamon Pudding	245
999.	Rhubarb Stew	245
1000.	Plum Cake	245
1001.	Lentils Sweet Bars	245
1002.	Dates Brownies	245
1003.	Rose Lentils Ice Cream	246
1004.	Mandarin Almond Pudding	246
1005.	Green tea and Banana Sweetening Mix	246
1006.	Cheesecake Made Easy!	246
1007.	Grapefruit Compote	247
1008.	Instant Pot Applesauce	247
1009.	Green Pudding	247
1010.	Healthy Tahini Buns	247
1011.	Spicy Pecan Bowl	247
CONCLUSION		**248**

INTRODUCTION

The Dash Diet Cookbook is a revolutionary diet plan created by dietitians and nutritional experts. The Dash Diet Cookbook provides invaluable insights into following the program and offers helpful tips and tricks to keep you on track. At Dash Diet, we believe that everyone should live a healthy lifestyle without detaching themselves from the lifestyle they love. That's why we created the Dash Diet Cookbook.

We also believe that dietary changes shouldn't have to be complicated or tedious. That's why we created the Dash Diet Cookbook. Compiled is a collection of some of our favorite recipes, and we've made them so easy to follow and understand that anyone can cook great-tasting meals while losing weight at the same time.

The Dash Diet Dash Diet Cookbook is a step-by-step guide to help you achieve your next health and wellness level.

This easy-to-use cookbook offers you quick, healthy, and delicious meals for breakfast, lunch, dinner, snacks, and desserts. It provides you the recipes needed to achieve optimum health without sacrificing flavor or convenience. Use this cookbook to help you meet your goals by using the principles of the Dash Diet.

The Dash Diet Dash Diet Cookbook was created using the latest software technology and printed on high-quality glossy paper. It was designed for ease of use while offering you complete information online about the Dash Diet. This cookbook has specifically created a useful tool to help anyone interested in the Dash Diet's benefits.

The Dash Diet Dash Diet Cookbook contains everything that you need to know about the Dash Diet from an ex-model's viewpoint, as well as advice from some of today's top physicians and nutritionists. This cookbook provides all of the information that you will need to follow this healthy lifestyle with ease and efficiency.

The Dash Diet Cookbook has all the information you need. Many dieters struggle with portion control, but that doesn't have to be a problem when using the easy-to-follow recipes in this cookbook.

If you're ready to start losing weight, the Dash Diet Cookbook will guide you through every step of the process. This easy-to-use guide teaches you how to shop for healthier foods, how to prepare them properly, and how to eat them. The Dash Diet Cookbook also includes advice on using smaller plates, avoiding added sugar and salt, and making healthier swaps in your favorite recipes.

With all the tools and information provided in the Dash Diet Cookbook, it's easy to get started on your weight loss journey today. All it takes is one cookbook purchase, and you'll have access to this comprehensive guide for life!

The Dash Diet Cookbook is the perfect book for anyone who wants to start a new and healthy lifestyle. Inside, you'll find all the information that will help you stick to the Dash Diet. We've included tricks and tips that will make each day more comfortable. We've even included our best-selling recipes so that you can start your NEW lifestyle with ease!

Have you tried to lose weight on a crash diet? If so, you know how hard it can be to stick to that plan. You might encounter problems like hunger, fatigue, and cravings.

If you've never tried one of those kinds of diets, you might be surprised to learn that they're not as effective as they used to be. Experts say that diets designed today need more attention to diet quality than their predecessors. That's because they tend to be quite restrictive and prescribed with several fad diets and lifestyle changes.

Besides, people today are more open about what they eat thanks to technology like the Internet and social media. Other people can see what you're eating or drinking when you post pictures and videos on Facebook, Twitter, or Instagram. There's also the whole realm of online health forums where people share their "healthy" recipes and meals that are not good for your body long term. All this, combined with our hectic lifestyles, can make it challenging to stay on track with healthy eating habits.

So what is a better solution? Some experts recommend incorporating more healthy foods into your diet, even if you think your current diet plan works for you. A new book called "Dash Diet Cookbook" by Dr. Alexandra Levit has come up with an excellent answer for people who want some ways to make their healthy eating plan more comfortable and more convenient: Dash Diet Cookbook!

In this book, the Dash Diet creator has created 35 delicious recipes for various meals in 5 different dietary styles, including the Dash Diet, Blood Type Diet, South Beach Diet, Whole30 compliant diet, and Paleo Diet! The recipes cover essential meals such as breakfast, lunch, dinner, snacks, drinks, desserts, side dishes, and condiments with full nutritional facts included!

BREAKFAST

1. Quinoa Hashes

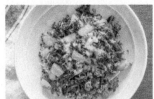

Preparation time: 10 minutes
Cooking time: 25 minutes
Servings: 2
Ingredients:
- 3 oz. quinoa
- 6 oz. water
- 2 potatoes, grated
- 1 egg, beaten
- 1 tablespoon avocado oil
- 1 teaspoon chives, chopped

Directions:
1. Cook quinoa in water for 15 minutes.
2. Heat up avocado oil in the skillet.
3. Then mix up all remaining ingredients in the bowl. Add quinoa and mix up well.
4. Add quinoa hash browns, cook for 5 minutes on each side.

Nutrition: 344 Calories, 12.5g Protein, 61.3g Carbohydrates, 5.9g Fat, 8.4g Fiber, 82mg Cholesterol, 49mg Sodium, 1160mg Potassium.

2. Artichoke Eggs

Preparation time: 5 minutes
Cooking time: 20 minutes
Servings: 4
Ingredients:
- 5 eggs, beaten
- 2 oz. low-fat feta, chopped
- 1 yellow onion, chopped
- 1 tablespoon canola oil
- 1 tablespoon cilantro, chopped
- 1 cup artichoke hearts, canned, chopped

Directions:
1. Grease 4 ramekins with the oil.
2. Mix up all remaining ingredients and divide the mixture between prepared ramekins.
3. Bake the meal at 380F for 20 minutes.

Nutrition: 177 Calories, 10.6 Protein, 7.4g Carbohydrates, 12.2g Fat, 2.5g Fiber, 217mg Cholesterol, 259mg Sodium, 235mg Potassium.

3. Quinoa Cakes

Preparation time: 25 minutes
Cooking time: 10 minutes
Servings: 4

Ingredients:
- 7 oz. quinoa
- 1 cup cauliflower, shredded
- 1 cup of water
- ½ cup vegan parmesan, grated
- 1 egg, beaten
- 1 tablespoon olive oil
- ½ teaspoon ground black pepper

Directions:
1. Mix up the quinoa with the cauliflower, water, and ground black pepper, stir, bring to a simmer over medium heat and cook for 15 minutes/
2. Cool the mixture and add parmesan and the eggs, stir well, shape medium cakes out of this mix.
3. Heat up a pan with the oil over medium-high heat, add the quinoa cakes. Cook them for 4-5 minutes per side.

Nutrition: 280 Calories, 14.9g Protein, 36.4g Carbohydrates, 7.6g Fat, 4.2g Fiber, 41mg Cholesterol, 222mg Sodium, 374mg Potassium.

4. Bean Casserole

Preparation time: 10 minutes
Cooking time: 30 minutes
Servings: 8
Ingredients:
- 5 eggs, beaten
- ½ cup bell pepper, chopped
- 1 cup red kidney beans, cooked
- ½ cup white onions, chopped
- 1 cup low-fat mozzarella cheese, shredded

Directions:
1. Spread the beans over the casserole mold. Add onions and bell pepper.
2. Add the eggs mixed with the cheese.
3. Bake the casserole 380 F for 30 minutes.

Nutrition: 142 Calories, 12.8g Protein, 16g Carbohydrates, 3g Fat, 4.3g Fiber, 105mg Cholesterol, 162mg Sodium, 374mg Potassium.

5. Grape Yogurt

Preparation time: 10 minutes
Cooking time: 0 minutes
Servings: 3
Ingredients:
- 1 ½ cup low-fat yogurt
- ½ cup grapes, chopped
- 1 oz. walnuts, chopped

Directions:
1. Mix up all ingredients together and transfer them in the serving glasses.

Nutrition: 156 Calories, 9.4g Protein, 12.2g Carbohydrates, 7.1g Fat, 0.8g Fiber, 7mg Cholesterol, 86mg Sodium, 365mg Potassium.

6. Berry Pancakes

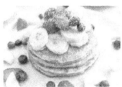

Preparation time: 10 minutes
Cooking time: 8 minutes
Servings: 12
Ingredients:
- 2 eggs, whisked
- 4 tablespoons almond milk
- 1 cup low-fat yogurt
- 3 tablespoons margarine, melted
- ½ teaspoon vanilla extract
- 1 cup almond flour
- 1 cup strawberries

Directions:
1. Pour the margarine in the skillet.
2. Mix up all remaining ingredients and blend with the help of the mixer.
3. Then pour the dough in the hot skillet in the shape of the pancakes and cook for 1.5 minutes from each side.

Nutrition: 80 Calories, 2.8g Protein, 3.3g Carbohydrates, 6.2g Fat, 0.6g Fiber, 29mg Cholesterol, 60mg Sodium, 91mg Potassium.

7. Western Omelet Quiche

Preparation time: 10 minutes
Cooking Time: 30 minutes
Servings: 4-6
Ingredients:
- 6 beaten eggs
- 1/8 teaspoon of mineral salt and black pepper
- ¾ cup diced peppers
- ¾ spring onions, sliced
- ¾ cup shredded cheese
- ½ cup half and half
- 8 oz., chopped Canadian bacon
- ¼ cup shredded cheddar cheese to garnish

Directions:
1. Add two cups of water to bottom of instant pot and then add trivet.
2. Spray a soufflé dish with butter or cooking spray, and then in a mixing bowl add the eggs, salt, milk, and pepper together.
3. Add the rest of the ingredients to the dish and mix it well.
4. Put it in soufflé dish, and from there, add to instant pot, cooking on high pressure for 30 minutes cook time.
5. Open up lid and sprinkle the top of it with more cheese.

Nutrition: Calories: 365, Fat: 15g, Carbs: 6g, Net Carbs: 4g, Protein: 24g, Fiber: 2g

8. Ginger French toast

Preparation time: 10 minutes
Cooking time: 5 minutes
Servings: 2
Ingredients:
- 4 whole-wheat bread slices

- ½ cup low-fat milk
- 2 eggs, whisked
- 1 teaspoon ground ginger
- Cooking spray

Directions:
1. Spray the skillet with cooking spray.
2. In the mixing bowl mix up milk and eggs.
3. Then add ginger and dip the bread in the liquid.
4. Roast the bread in the preheated skillet for 2 minutes from each side.

Nutrition: 229 Calories, 15.6g Protein, 29.4g Carbohydrates, 8g Fat, 4g Fiber, 167mg Cholesterol, 388mg Sodium, 150mg Potassium.

9. Fruit Muffins

Preparation time: 35 minutes
Cooking time: 10 minutes
Servings: 6
Ingredients:
- 1 cup apple, grated
- 1 cup quinoa
- 2 cups oatmeal
- ½ cup of coconut milk
- 1 tablespoon liquid honey
- 1 teaspoon vanilla extract
- 1 tablespoon olive oil
- 1 cup of water
- 1 teaspoon ground nutmeg

Directions:
1. Mix up water and quinoa and the mixture for 15 minutes, fluff with a fork and transfer to a bowl.
2. Add all remaining ingredients and mix up well.
3. Transfer the batter in the muffin molds and bake them at 375F for 20 minutes.

Nutrition: 308 Calories, 8.2g Protein, 46g Carbohydrates, 10.8g Fat, 6.2g Fiber, 0mg Cholesterol, 7mg Sodium, 355mg Potassium.

10. Omelet with Peppers

Preparation time: 10 minutes
Cooking time: 15 minutes
Servings: 4
Ingredients:
- 4 eggs, beaten
- 1 tablespoon margarine
- 1 cup bell peppers, chopped
- 2 oz. scallions, chopped

Directions:
1. Toss the margarine in the skillet and melt it.
2. In the mixing bowl mix up eggs and bell peppers. Add scallions.
3. Pour the egg mixture in the hot skillet and roast the omelet for 12 minutes.

Nutrition: 102 Calories, 6.1g Protein, 3.7g Carbohydrates, 7.3g Fat, 0.8g Fiber, 164mg Cholesterol, 98mg Sodium, 156mg Potassium.

11. Vanilla Toasts

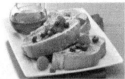

Preparation time: 10 minutes
Cooking time: 5 minutes
Servings: 3
Ingredients:

- 3 whole-grain bread slices
- 1 teaspoon vanilla extract
- 1 egg, beaten
- 2 tablespoons low-fat sour cream
- 1 tablespoon margarine

Directions:
1. Melt the butter in the skillet.
2. Meanwhile, in the bowl mix up vanilla extract, eggs, and low-fat sour cream.
3. Dip the bread slices in the egg mixture well.
4. Then transfer them in the melted margarine and roast for 2 minutes from each side.

Nutrition: 166 Calories,5.1g Protein, 18.7g Carbohydrates, 7.9g Fat, 2g Fiber, 58mg Cholesterol, 229mg Sodium, 39mg Potassium.

12. Raspberry Yogurt

Preparation time: 5 minutes
Cooking time: 0 minutes
Servings: 2
Ingredients:

- 1/2 cup low-fat yogurt
- 1/2 cup raspberries
- 1 teaspoon almond flakes

Directions:
1. Mix up yogurt and raspberries and transfer them in the serving glasses.
2. Top yogurt with almond flakes.

Nutrition: 77 Calories,3.9g Protein, 8.6g Carbohydrates, 3.4g Fat, 2.6g Fiber, 4mg Cholesterol, 32mg Sodium, 192mg Potassium.

13. Salsa Eggs

Preparation time: 10 minutes
Cooking time: 10 minutes
Servings: 4
Ingredients:

- 2 tomatoes, chopped
- 1 chili pepper, chopped
- 2 cucumbers, chopped
- 1 red onion, chopped
- 2 tablespoons parsley, chopped
- 1 tablespoon olive oil
- 1 tablespoon lemon juice
- 4 eggs
- 1 cup water, for cooking eggs

Directions:
1. Put eggs in the water and boil them for 7 minutes. Cool the cooked eggs in the cold water and peel.
2. After this, make salsa salad: mix up tomatoes, chili pepper, cucumbers, red onion, parsley, olive oil, and lemon juice.
3. Cut the eggs into the halves and sprinkle generously with cooked salsa salad.

Nutrition: 140 Calories,7.5g Protein, 11.1g Carbohydrates, 8.3g Fat, 2.2g Fiber, 164mg Cholesterol, 71mg Sodium, 484mg Potassium.

14. Fruit Scones

Preparation time: 10 minutes
Cooking time: 12 minutes
Servings: 8
Ingredients:

- 2 cups whole-grain wheat flour
- ½ teaspoon baking powder
- ¼ cup cranberries, dried
- ¼ cup chia seeds
- ¼ cup apricots, chopped
- ¼ cup almonds, chopped
- 1 tablespoon liquid honey
- 1 egg, whisked

Directions:
1. In the bowl mix up all the ingredients and knead the dough.
2. Cut the dough into 16 pieces (scones)
3. Bake them at 350 degrees F for 12 minutes in the lined with baking paper tray.
4. Cool the scones well.

Nutrition: 156 Calories, 6.1g Protein, 27.1g Carbohydrates, 3.7g Fat, 5.5g Fiber, 20mg Cholesterol, 10mg Sodium, 216mg Potassium.

15. Cheese Omelet

Preparation time: 10 minutes
Cooking time: 10 minutes
Servings: 4
Ingredients:

- 1 tablespoon olive oil
- ½ teaspoon ground black pepper
- 1 cup baby spinach, chopped
- 3 eggs, beaten
- 2 oz. low-fat Low-fat feta cheese, crumbled
- 1 tablespoons cilantro, chopped

Directions:
1. Heat up a pan with the oil over the medium-high heat, add spinach and sauté for 3 minutes.
2. Then add all remaining ingredients and stir gently. Close the lid and cook an omelet for 7 minutes on low heat or until it is solid.

Nutrition: 117 Calories, 6.4g Protein, 1.3g Carbohydrates, 9.8g Fat, 0.3g Fiber, 135mg Cholesterol, 211mg Sodium, 99mg Potassium.

16. Banana Pancakes

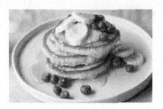

Preparation time: 10 minutes
Cooking time: 15 minutes
Servings: 5

Ingredients:
- 2 bananas, mashed
- 1/2 cup 1% milk
- 1 1/2 cup whole-grain flour
- 1 teaspoon liquid honey
- 1 teaspoon vanilla extract
- 1 teaspoon baking powder
- 1 tablespoon lemon juice
- 1 tablespoon olive oil

Directions:
1. Mix up mashed bananas and milk.
2. Then add flour, liquid honey, vanilla extract, baking powder, and lemon juice.
3. Whisk the mixture until you get a smooth batter.
4. After this, heat up olive oil in the skillet.
5. When the oil is hot, pour the pancake mixture in the skillet and flatten in the shape of pancakes.
6. Cook them for 1 minute and then flip on another side. Cook the pancakes for 1 minute more.

Nutrition: 207 Calories, 6.3g Protein, 39.9g Carbohydrates, 3.9g Fat, 5.7g Fiber, 1mg Cholesterol, 15mg Sodium, 458mg Potassium.

17. Aromatic Breakfast Granola

Preparation time: 10 minutes
Cooking time: 25 minutes
Servings: 2

Ingredients:
- 2 tablespoons avocado oil
- 1 tablespoon liquid honey
- 1/4 teaspoon ground cinnamon
- 1/4 cup almonds, chopped
- 1 tablespoon chia seeds
- 1 teaspoon sesame seeds
- 2 tablespoons cut oats
- Cooking spray

Directions:
1. Heat up avocado oil and liquid honey until you get a homogenous mixture.
2. Then add ground cinnamon, almonds, chia seeds, sesame seeds, and cut oats.
3. Stir until homogenous.
4. Spray the baking tray with cooking spray and place the almond mixture inside.
5. Flatten it in the shape of a square.
6. Bake the granola at 345F for 20 minutes.
7. Cut it into servings.

Nutrition: 203 calories, 5.7g protein, 22.3g carbohydrates, 11.4g fat, 5.9g fiber, 0mg cholesterol, 2mg sodium, 211mg potassium.

18. Morning Sweet Potatoes

Preparation time: 5 minutes
Cooking time: 20 minutes
Servings: 2

Ingredients:
- 2 sweet potatoes
- 1 tablespoon chives, chopped

- 2 teaspoons margarine
- 1/4 teaspoon chili flakes

Directions:
1. Preheat the oven to 400F.
2. Put the sweet potatoes in the oven and cook them for 20 minutes or until the vegetables are soft.
3. Then cut the sweet potato into halves and top with margarine, chives, and chili flakes. Wait till margarine starts to melt.

Nutrition: 35 Calories, 0.1g Protein, 0.4g Carbohydrates, 3.8g Fat, 0.1g Fiber, 0mg Cholesterol, 45mg Sodium, 15mg Potassium.

19. Egg Toasts

Preparation time: 5 minutes
Cooking time: 5 minutes
Servings: 3

Ingredients:
- 3 eggs
- 3 whole-grain bread slices
- 1 teaspoon olive oil
- 1/4 teaspoon minced garlic
- 1/4 teaspoon ground black pepper

Directions:
1. Heat up olive oil in the skillet.
2. Crack the eggs inside and cook them for 4 minutes.
3. Meanwhile, rub the bread slices with minced garlic.
4. Top the bread with cooked eggs and sprinkle with ground black pepper.

Nutrition: 157 Calories, 8.6g Protein, 13.5g Carbohydrates, 7.4g Fat, 2.1g Fiber, 164mg Cholesterol, 182mg Sodium, 62mg Potassium.

20. Sweet Yogurt with Figs

Preparation time: 5 minutes
Cooking time: 0 minutes
Servings: 1

Ingredients:
- 1/3 cup low-fat yogurt
- 1 teaspoon almond flakes
- 1 fresh fig, chopped
- 1 teaspoon liquid honey
- 1/4 teaspoon sesame seeds

Directions:
1. Mix up yogurt and honey and pour the mixture in the serving glass.
2. Top it with chopped fig, almond flakes, and sesame seeds.

Nutrition: 178 Calories, 6.2g Protein, 24.4g Carbohydrates, 6.8g Fat, 3.1g Fiber, 5mg Cholesterol, 44mg Sodium, 283mg Potassium.

21. Fruits and Rice Pudding

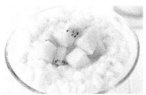

Preparation time: 10 minutes
Cooking time: 10 minutes
Servings: 3

Ingredients:

- 1/2 cup long-grain rice
- 1 1/2 cup low-fat milk
- 1 teaspoon vanilla extract
- 2 oz. apricots, chopped

Directions:

1. Pour milk and add rice in the saucepan.
2. Close the lid and cook the rice on the medium-high heat for 10 minutes.
3. Then add vanilla extract and stir the rice well.
4. Transfer the pudding in the bowls and top with apricots.

Nutrition: 171 Calories, 6.4g Protein, 32.9g Carbohydrates, 0.3g Fat, 0.8g Fiber, 2mg Cholesterol, 67mg Sodium, 276mg Potassium.

22. Asparagus Omelet

Preparation time: 5 minutes
Cooking time: 10 minutes
Servings: 2

Ingredients:

- 3 oz. asparagus, boiled, chopped
- 1/4 teaspoon ground paprika
- 1/2 teaspoon ground cumin
- 3 eggs, beaten
- 2 tablespoons low-fat milk
- 1 teaspoon avocado oil

Directions:

1. Heat up avocado oil in the skillet.
2. Meanwhile, mix up ground paprika, ground cumin. Eggs, and milk.
3. Pour the liquid in the hot skillet and cook it for 2 minutes.
4. Then add chopped asparagus and close the lid.
5. Cook the omelet for 5 minutes on low heat.

Nutrition: 115 Calories, 9.9g Protein, 3.4g Carbohydrates, 7.2g Fat, 1.2g Fiber, 246mg Cholesterol, 101mg Sodium, 220mg Potassium.

23. Bean Frittata

Preparation time: 5 minutes
Cooking time: 12 minutes
Servings: 4

Ingredients:

- 4 eggs, beaten
- 1/2 cup red kidney beans, canned
- 1/2 onion, diced
- 1 tablespoon margarine
- 1 teaspoon dried dill

Directions:

1. Toss the margarine in the skillet. Add onion and sauté it for 4 minutes or until it is soft.
2. Then add red kidney beans and dried dill. Mix the mixture up.
3. Pour the eggs over it and close the lid.
4. Cook the frittata on medium-low heat for 7 minutes or until it is set or bake it in the oven at 390F for 5 minutes.

Nutrition: 172 Calories, 11g Protein, 15.9g Carbohydrates, 7.5g Fat, 3.8g Fiber, 164mg Cholesterol, 99mg Sodium, 401mg Potassium.

24. Peach Pancakes

Preparation time: 10 minutes

Cooking time: 10 minutes
Servings: 6

Ingredients:

- 1 cup whole-wheat flour
- 1 egg, beaten
- 1 teaspoon vanilla extract
- 2 peaches, chopped
- 1 tablespoon margarine
- 1/2 teaspoon baking powder
- 1 teaspoon apple cider vinegar
- 1/4 cup skim milk

Directions:

1. Make the pancake batter: in the mixing bowl mix up eggs, whole-wheat flour, vanilla extract, baking powder, apple cider vinegar, and skim milk.
2. Then melt the margarine in the skillet.
3. Pour the prepared batter in the skillet with the help of the ladle and flatten in the shape of the pancake.
4. Cook the pancakes for 2 minutes from each side over the medium-low heat.
5. Top the cooked pancakes with peaches.

Nutrition: 129 Calories, 3.9g Protein, 21.5g Carbohydrates, 3g Fat, 1.3g Fiber, 27mg Cholesterol, 39mg Sodium, 188mg Potassium.

25. Breakfast Splits

Preparation time: 15 minutes
Cooking time: 0 minutes
Servings: 2

Ingredients:

- 2 bananas, peeled
- 4 tablespoons granola
- 2 tablespoons low-fat yogurt
- 1/2 teaspoon ground cinnamon
- 1 strawberry, chopped

Directions:

1. In the mixing bowl, mix up yogurt with ground cinnamon, and strawberries.
2. Then make the lengthwise cuts in bananas and fill with the yogurt mass.
3. Top the fruits with granola.

Nutrition: 154 Calories, 6.8g Protein, 45.2g Carbohydrates, 8g Fat, 6.3g Fiber, 1mg Cholesterol, 20mg Sodium, 635mg Potassium.

26. Whole Grain Pancakes

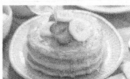

Preparation time: 10 minutes
Cooking time: 5 minutes
Servings: 4

Ingredients:

- 1/2 teaspoon baking powder
- 1/4 cup skim milk
- 1 cup whole-grain wheat flour
- 2 teaspoons liquid honey
- 1 teaspoon olive oil

Directions:

1. Mix up baking powder and flour in the bowl.

2. Add skim milk and olive oil. Whisk the mixture well.
3. Preheat the non-stick skillet and pour the small amount of dough inside in the shape of the pancake. Cook it for 2 minutes from each side or until the pancake is golden brown.
4. Top the cooked pancakes with liquid honey.

Nutrition: 129 Calories,4.6g Protein, 25.7g Carbohydrates, 1.7g Fat, 3.7g Fiber, 0mg Cholesterol, 10mg Sodium, 211mg Potassium.

27. Granola Parfait

Preparation time: 10 minutes
Cooking time: 0 minutes
Servings: 2
Ingredients:
- ½ cup low-fat yogurt
- 4 tablespoons granola

Directions:
1. Put ½ tablespoon of granola in every glass.
2. Then add 2 tablespoons of low-fat yogurt.
3. Repeat the steps till you use all ingredients.
4. Store the parfait in the fridge for up to 2 hours.

Nutrition: 79 Calories, 8g Protein, 20.6g Carbohydrates, 8.1g Fat, 2.8g Fiber, 4mg Cholesterol, 51mg Sodium, 308mg Potassium.

28. Curry Tofu Scramble

Preparation time: 10 minutes
Cooking time: 5 minutes
Servings: 3
Ingredients:
- 12 oz. tofu, crumbled
- 1 teaspoon curry powder
- 1/4 cup skim milk
- 1 teaspoon olive oil
- 1/4 teaspoon chili flakes

Directions:
1. Heat up olive oil in the skillet.
2. Add crumbled tofu and chili flakes.
3. In the bowl mix up curry powder and skim milk.
4. Pour the liquid over the crumbled tofu and stir well.
5. Cook the scrambled tofu for 3 minutes on the medium-high heat.

Nutrition: 102 Calories, 10g Protein, 3.3g Carbohydrates, 6.4g Fat, 1.2g Fiber, 0mg Cholesterol, 25mg Sodium, 210mg Potassium.

29. Scallions Omelet

Preparation time: 10 minutes
Cooking time: 10 minutes
Servings: 2
Ingredients:
- 1 oz. scallions, chopped
- 2 eggs, beaten
- 1 tablespoon low-fat low-fat sour cream
- 1/4 teaspoon ground black pepper
- 1 teaspoon olive oil

Directions:
1. Heat up olive oil in the skillet.
2. Meanwhile, in the mixing bowl mix up all remaining ingredients.
3. Pour the egg mixture in the hot skillet, flatten well and cook for 7 minutes over the medium-low heat.
4. The omelet is cooked when it is set.

Nutrition: 101 Calories, 6g Protein, 1.8g Carbohydrates, 8g Fat, 0.4g Fiber, 166mg Cholesterol, 67mg Sodium, 110mg Potassium.

30. Breakfast Almond Smoothie

Preparation time: 5 minutes
Cooking time: 2 minutes
Servings: 3
Ingredients:
- 1/2 cup almonds, chopped
- 1 cup low-fat milk
- 1 banana, peeled, chopped

Directions:
1. Put all ingredients in the blender and blend until smooth.
2. Pour the smoothie in the serving glasses.

Nutrition: 161 Calories,6.5g Protein, 16.4g Carbohydrates, 8.8g Fat, 3g Fiber, 4mg Cholesterol, 36mg Sodium, 379mg Potassium.

31. Jack-o-Lantern Pancakes

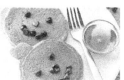

Preparation time: 15 minutes
Cooking time: 5 minutes
Servings: 8
Ingredients:
- 1 Egg
- 1/2 c. Canned pumpkin
- 1 3/4 c. Low-fat milk
- 2 tbsps. Vegetable oil
- 2 c. Flour
- 2 tbsps. Brown sugar
- 1 tbsp. Baking powder
- 1 tsp. Pumpkin pie spice
- 1 tsp. Salt

Directions:
1. In a mixing bowl, mix milk, pumpkin, eggs, and oil. Add dry ingredients to egg mixture. Stir gently. Coat skillet lightly with cooking spray and heat on medium.
2. When the skillet is hot, spoon (using a dessert spoon) batter onto the skillet. When bubbles start bursting, flip pancakes over and cook until it's a nice golden-brown color.

Nutrition: Calories: 313, Protein 15g, Carbs 28g, Fat 16g, Sodium 1 mg

32. Fruit Pizza

Preparation time: 15 minutes
Cooking time: 0 minutes
Servings: 2
Ingredients:

- 1 English muffin
- 2 tbsps. Fat-free cream cheese
- 2 tbsps. sliced strawberries
- 2 tbsps. blueberries
- 2 tbsps. crushed pineapple

Directions:
1. Cut English muffin in half and toast halves until slightly browned. Coat both halves with cream cheese. Arrange fruits atop cream cheese on muffin halves. Serve soon after preparation. Any leftovers refrigerate within 2 hours.

Nutrition: Calories: 119, Protein 6g, Carbs 23g, Fat 1g, Sodium 288 mg

33. Flax Banana Yogurt Muffins

Preparation time: 15 minutes
Cooking time: 20 minutes
Servings: 12
Ingredients:
- 1 c. Whole wheat flour
- 1 c. Old-fashioned rolled oats
- 1 tsp. Baking soda
- 2 tbsps. Ground flaxseed
- 3 large ripe bananas
- 1/2 c. Greek yogurt
- 1/4 c. Unsweetened applesauce
- 1/4 c. Brown sugar
- 2 tsp. Vanilla extract

Directions:
1. Set oven at 355 0F and preheat. Prepare muffin tin, or you can use cooking spray or cupcake liners. Combine dry ingredients in a mixing bowl.
2. In a separate bowl, mix yogurt, banana, sugar, vanilla, and applesauce. Combine both mixtures and mix. Do not over mix. The batter should not be smooth but lumpy. Bake for 20 mins, or when inserted, toothpick comes out clean.

Nutrition: Calories: 136, Protein 4g, Carbs 30g, Fat 2g, Sodium 242 mg

34. Apple Oats

Preparation time: 5 minutes
Cooking time: 5 minutes
Servings: 2
Ingredients:
- 1/2 cup oats
- 1 cup of water
- 1 apple, chopped
- 1 teaspoon olive oil
- 1/2 teaspoon vanilla extract

Directions:
1. Pour olive oil in the saucepan and add oats. Cook them for 2 minutes, stir constantly.
2. After this, add water and mix up.
3. Close the lid and cook oats on low heat for 5 minutes.
4. After this, add chopped apples and vanilla extract. Stir the meal.

Nutrition: 159 Calories, 3g Protein, 29.4g Carbohydrates, 3.9g Fat, 4.8g Fiber, 0mg Cholesterol, 6mg Sodium, 196mg Potassium.

35. Buckwheat Crepes

Preparation time: 8 minutes
Cooking time: 15 minutes
Servings: 6
Ingredients:
- 1 cup buckwheat flour
- 1/3 cup whole grain flour
- 1 egg, beaten
- 1 cup skim milk
- 1 teaspoon olive oil
- 1/2 teaspoon ground cinnamon

Directions:
1. In the mixing bowl, mix up all ingredients and whisk until you get a smooth batter.
2. Heat up the non-stick skillet on high heat for 3 minutes.
3. With the help of the ladle pour the small amount of batter in the skillet and flatten it in the shape of crepe.
4. Cook it for 1 minute and flip on another side. Cook it for 30 seconds more.
5. Repeat the same steps with the remaining batter.

Nutrition: 122 Calories, 5.7g Protein, 211.G Carbohydrates, 2.2g Fat, 2g Fiber, 28mg Cholesterol, 34mg Sodium, 216mg Potassium.

36. Spinach, Mushroom, and Feta Cheese Scramble

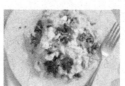

Preparation time: 15 minutes
Cooking time: 4 minutes
Servings: 1
Ingredients:
- Olive oil cooking spray
- ½ c. sliced Mushroom
- 1 c. chopped Spinach
- 3 Eggs
- 2 tbsps. Feta cheese
- Pepper

Directions:
1. Set a lightly greased, medium skillet over medium heat. Add spinach and mushrooms, and cook until spinach wilts.
2. Combine egg whites, cheese, pepper, and whole egg in a medium bowl, whisk to combine. Pour into your skillet and cook, while stirring, until set (about 4 minutes). Serve.

Nutrition: Calories: 236.5, Protein 22.2g, Carbs 12.9g, Fat 11.4g, Sodium 405 mg

37. Red Velvet Pancakes with Cream Cheese Topping

Preparation time: 15 minutes
Cooking time: 10 minutes
Servings: 2
Ingredients:
- Cream Cheese Topping:
- 2 oz. Cream cheese
- 3 tbsps. Yogurt
- 3 tbsps. Honey
- 1 tbsp. Milk
- Pancakes:
- 1/2 c. Whole wheat Flour
- 1/2 c. all-purpose flour
- 2 1/4tsps. Baking powder
- 1/2 tsp. Unsweetened Cocoa powder
- 1/4 tsp. Salt
- 1/4 c. Sugar
- 1 large Egg
- 1 c. + 2 tbsps. Milk
- 1 tsp. Vanilla
- 1 tsp. Red paste food coloring

Directions:
1. Combine all your topping ingredients in a medium bowl, and set aside. Add all your pancake ingredients in a large bowl and fold until combined. Set a greased skillet over medium heat to get hot.
2. Add ¼ cup of pancake batter onto the hot skillet and cook until bubbles begin to form on the top. Flip and cook until set. Repeat until your batter is done well. Add your toppings and serve.

Nutrition: Calories: 231, Protein 7g, Carbs 43g, Fat 4g, Sodium 0mg

38. Peanut Butter & Banana Breakfast Smoothie

Preparation time: 15 minutes
Cooking time: 0 minutes
Servings: 1
Ingredients:
- 1 c. Non-fat milk
- 1 tbsp. Peanut butter
- 1 Banana
- 1/2 tsp. Vanilla

Directions:
1. Place non-fat milk, peanut butter, and banana in a blender. Blend until smooth.

Nutrition: Calories: 295, Protein 133g, Carbs 42g, Fat 8.4g, Sodium 100 mg

39. No-Bake Breakfast Granola Bars

Preparation time: 15 minutes
Cooking time: 0 minutes
Servings: 18
Ingredients:

- 2 c. Old fashioned oatmeal
- 1/2 c. Raisins
- 1/2 c. Brown sugar
- 2 1/2 c. Corn rice cereal
- 1/2 c. Syrup
- 1/2 c. Peanut butter
- 1/2 tsp. Vanilla

Directions:
1. In a suitable size mixing bowl, mix using a wooden spoon, rice cereal, oatmeal, and raisins. In a saucepan, combine corn syrup and brown sugar. On a medium-high flame, continuously stir the mixture and bring to a boil.
2. On boiling, take away from heat. In a saucepan, stir vanilla and peanut into the sugar mixture. Stir until very smooth.
3. Spoon peanut butter mixture on the cereal and raisins into the mixing bowl and combine — shape mixture into a 9 x 13 baking tin. Allow to cool properly, then cut into bars (18 pcs).

Nutrition: Calories: 152, Protein 4g, Carbs 26g, Fat 4.3g, Sodium 160 mg

40. Mushroom Shallot Frittata

Preparation time: 15 minutes
Cooking time: 25 minutes
Servings: 4
Ingredients:
- 1 tsp. butter
- 4 chopped shallots
- ½ lb. chopped mushrooms
- 2 tsp. chopped parsley
- 1 tsp. dried thyme
- Black pepper
- 3 medium Eggs
- 5 large Egg whites
- 1 tbsp. Milk
- ¼ c. grated parmesan cheese

Directions:
1. Heat oven to 350 0F. In a suitable size oven-proof skillet, heat butter over medium flame. Add shallots and sauté for about 5 mins. Or until golden brown. Add to pot, thyme, parsley, chopped mushroom, and black pepper to taste.
2. Whisk milk, egg whites, parmesan, and eggs into a bowl. Pour mixture into the skillet, ensuring the mushroom is covered completely. Transfer the skillet to the oven as soon as the edges begin to set.
3. Bake until frittata is cooked (15-20 mins). Should be served warm, cut into equal wedges (4 pcs).

Nutrition: Calories: 346, Protein 19.1g, Carbs 48.3g, Fat 12g, Sodium 218 mg

41. Very Berry Muesli

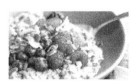

Preparation time: 15 minutes
Cooking time: 0 minutes
Servings: 2
Ingredients:
- 1 c. Oats
- 1 c. Fruit flavored Yogurt
- ½ c. Milk
- 1/8 tsp. Salt
- ½ c dried Raisins
- ½ c. Chopped Apple
- ½ c. Frozen Blueberries
- ¼ c. chopped Walnuts

Directions:
1. Combine your yogurt, salt, and oats in a medium bowl, mix well, and then cover it tightly. Fridge for at least 6 hours. Add your raisins and apples the gently fold. Top with walnuts and serve. Enjoy!

Nutrition: Calories: 195, Protein 6g, Carbs 31g, Fat 4g, Sodium 0mg

42. Veggie Quiche Muffins

Preparation time: 15 minutes
Cooking time: 40 minutes
Servings: 12
Ingredients:
- 3/4 c. shredded Cheddar
- 1 c. chopped Green Onion
- 1 c. chopped Broccoli
- 1 c. diced Tomatoes
- 2 c. Milk
- 4 Eggs
- 1 c. Pancake mix
- 1 tsp. Oregano
- 1/2 tsp. Salt
- 1/2 tsp. Pepper

Directions:
1. Preheat your oven to 375 0F, and lightly grease a 12-cup muffin tin with oil. Sprinkle your tomatoes, broccoli, onions, and cheddar into your muffin cups.
2. Combine your remaining ingredients in a medium, whisk to combine, then pour evenly on top of your veggies.
3. Set to bake in your preheated oven for about 40 minutes or until golden brown. Allow to cool slightly (about 5 minutes), then serve. Enjoy!

Nutrition: Calories: 58.5, Protein 5.1 g, Carbs 2.9 g, Fat 3.2 g, Sodium 340 mg

43. Turkey Sausage and Mushroom Strata

Preparation time: 15 minutes
Cooking time: 8 minutes
Servings: 12
Ingredients:
- 8 oz. cubed Ciabatta bread
- 12 oz. chopped turkey sausage
- 2 c. Milk
- 4 oz. shredded Cheddar
- 3 large Eggs
- 12 oz. Egg substitute

- ½ c. chopped Green onion
- 1 c. diced Mushroom
- ½ tsp. Paprika
- ½ tsp. Pepper
- 2 tbsps. grated Parmesan cheese

Directions:
1. Set oven to preheat to 400 0F. Lay your bread cubes flat on a baking tray and set it to toast for about 8 min. Meanwhile, add a skillet over medium heat with sausage and cook while stirring, until fully brown and crumbled.
2. Mix salt, pepper, paprika, parmesan cheese, egg substitute, eggs, cheddar cheese, and milk in a large bowl. Add in your remaining ingredients and toss well to incorporate.
3. Transfer mixture to a large baking dish (preferably a 9x13-inch), then tightly cover and allow to rest in the refrigerator overnight. Set your oven to preheat to 3500F, remove the cover from your casserole, and set to bake until golden brown and cooked through. Slice and serve.

Nutrition: Calories: 288.2, Protein 24.3g, Carbs 18.2g, Fat. 12.4g, Sodium 355 mg

44. Bacon Bits

Preparation time: 15 minutes
Cooking time: 60 minutes
Servings: 4
Ingredients:
- 1 c. Millet
- 5 c. Water
- 1 c. diced Sweet potato
- 1 tsp. ground Cinnamon
- 2 tbsps. Brown sugar
- 1 medium diced Apple
- 1/4 c. Honey

Directions:
1. In a deep pot, add your sugar, sweet potato, cinnamon, water, and millet, then stir to combine, then boil on high heat. After that, simmer on low.
2. Cook like this for about an hour, until your water is fully absorbed and millet is cooked. Stir in your remaining ingredients and serve.

Nutrition: Calories: 136, Protein 3.1g, Carbs 28.5g, Fat 1.0g, Sodium 120 mg

45. Steel Cut Oat Blueberry Pancakes

Preparation time: 15 minutes
Cooking time: 15 minutes
Servings: 4
Ingredients:
- 11/2 c. Water
- 1/2 c. steel-cut oats
- 1/8 tsp. Salt
- 1 c. Whole wheat Flour
- 1/2 tsp. Baking powder
- 1/2 tsp. Baking soda
- 1 Egg
- 1 c. Milk
- 1/2 c. Greek yogurt

- 1 c. Frozen Blueberries
- 3/4 c. Agave Nectar

Directions:
1. Combine your oats, salt, and water in a medium saucepan, stir, and allow to come to a boil over high heat. Adjust the heat to low, and allow to simmer for about 10 min, or until oats get tender. Set aside.
2. Combine all your remaining ingredients, except agave nectar, in a medium bowl, then fold in oats. Preheat your skillet, and lightly grease it. Cook ¼ cup of milk batter at a time for about 3 minutes per side. Garnish with Agave Nectar.

Nutrition: Calories: 257, Protein 14g, Carbs 46g, Fat 7g, Sodium 123 mg

46. Egg White Breakfast Mix

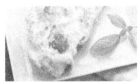

Preparation time: 10 minutes
Cooking time: 10 minutes
Servings: 4
Ingredients:
- 1 yellow onion, chopped
- 3 plum tomatoes, chopped
- 10 ounces spinach, chopped
- A pinch of black pepper
- 2 tablespoons water
- 12 egg whites
- Cooking spray

Directions:
1. Mix the egg whites with water and pepper in a bowl. Grease a pan with cooking spray, heat up over medium heat, add ¼ of the egg whites, spread into the pan, and cook for 2 minutes.
2. Spoon ¼ of the spinach, tomatoes, and onion, fold, and add to a plate. 4. Serve for breakfast. Enjoy!

Nutrition: Calories: 31, Carbs: 0g, Fat: 2g, Protein: 3g, Sodium: 55 mg

47. Pesto Omelet

Preparation time: 10 minutes
Cooking time: 6 minutes
Servings: 2
Ingredients:
- 2 teaspoons olive oil
- Handful cherry tomatoes, chopped
- 3 tablespoons pistachio pesto
- A pinch of black pepper
- 4 eggs

Directions:
1. In a bowl, combine the eggs with cherry tomatoes, black pepper, and pistachio pesto and whisk well. Add eggs mix, spread into the pan, cook for 3 minutes, flip, cook for 3 minutes more, divide between 2 plates, and serve on a heated pan with the oil over medium-high heat.

Nutrition: Calories: 240, Carbs: 23g, Fat: 9g, Protein: 17g, Sodium: 292 mg

48. Quinoa Bowls

Preparation time: 10 minutes
Cooking time: 20 minutes
Servings: 2
Ingredients:
- 1 peach, sliced
- 1/3 cup quinoa, rinsed
- 2/3 cup low-fat milk
- ½ teaspoon vanilla extract
- 2 teaspoons brown sugar
- 12 raspberries
- 14 blueberries

Directions:
1. Mix the quinoa with the milk, sugar, and vanilla in a small pan, simmer over medium heat, cover the pan, cook for 20 minutes and flip with a fork. Divide this mix into 2 bowls, top each with raspberries and blueberries and serve for breakfast.

Nutrition: Calories: 170, Carbs: 31g, Fat: 3g, Protein: 6g, Sodium: 120 mg

49. Strawberry Sandwich

Preparation time: 10 minutes
Cooking time: 0 minutes
Servings: 4
Ingredients:
- 8 ounces low-fat cream cheese, soft
- 1 tablespoon stevia
- 1 teaspoon lemon zest, grated
- 4 whole-wheat English muffins, toasted
- 2 cups strawberries, sliced

Directions:
1. In your food processor, combine the cream cheese with the stevia and lemon zest and pulse well. Spread 1 tablespoon of this mix on 1 muffin half and top with some of the sliced strawberries. Repeat with the rest of the muffin halves and serve for breakfast. Enjoy!

Nutrition: Calories: 150, Carbs: 23g, Fat: 7g, Protein: 2g, Sodium: 70 mg

50. Apple Quinoa Muffins

Preparation time: 10 minutes
Cooking time: 35 minutes
Servings: 4
Ingredients:
- ½ cup natural, unsweetened applesauce
- 1 cup banana, peeled and mashed
- 1 cup quinoa
- 2 and ½ cups old-fashioned oats
- ½ cup almond milk
- 2 tablespoons stevia
- 1 teaspoon vanilla extract
- 1 cup of water
- Cooking spray
- 1 teaspoon cinnamon powder
- 1 apple, cored, peeled, and chopped

Directions:

1. Put the water in a small pan, bring to a simmer over medium heat, add quinoa, cook within 15 minutes, and fluff with a fork, and transfer to a bowl.
2. Add all ingredients, stir, divide into a muffin pan greases with cooking spray, introduce in the oven, and bake within 20 minutes at 375 degrees F. Serve for breakfast.

Nutrition: Calories: 241, Carbs: 31g, Fat: 11g, Protein: 5g, Sodium: 251 mg

51. Breakfast Fruits Bowls

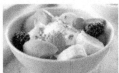

Preparation time: 10 minutes
Cooking time: 0 minutes
Servings: 2
Ingredients:
- 1 cup mango, chopped
- 1 banana, sliced
- 1 cup pineapple, chopped
- 1 cup almond milk

Directions:
1. Mix the mango with the banana, pineapple, and almond milk in a bowl, stir, divide into smaller bowls, and serve.

Nutrition: Calories: 10, Carbs: 0g, Fat: 1g, Protein: 0g, Sodium: 0mg

52. Pumpkin Cookies

Preparation time: 10 minutes
Cooking time: 25 minutes
Servings: 6
Ingredients:
- 2 cups whole wheat flour
- 1 cup old-fashioned oats
- 1 teaspoon baking soda
- 1 teaspoon pumpkin pie spice
- 15 ounces pumpkin puree
- 1 cup coconut oil, melted
- 1 cup of coconut sugar
- 1 egg
- ½ cup pepitas, roasted
- ½ cup cherries, dried

Directions:
1. Mix the flour the oats, baking soda, pumpkin spice, pumpkin puree, oil, sugar, egg, pepitas, and cherries in a bowl, stir well, shape medium cookies out of this mix, arrange them all on a baking sheet, then bake within 25 minutes at 350 degrees F. Serve the cookies for breakfast.

Nutrition: Calories: 150, Carbs: 24g, Fat: 8g, Protein: 1g, Sodium: 220 mg

53. Veggie Scramble

Preparation time: 10 minutes
Cooking time: 2 minutes
Servings: 1
Ingredients:

- 1 egg
- 1 tablespoon water
- ¼ cup broccoli, chopped
- ¼ cup mushrooms, chopped
- A pinch of black pepper
- 1 tablespoon low-fat mozzarella, shredded
- 1 tablespoon walnuts, chopped
- Cooking spray

Directions:
1. Grease a ramekin with cooking spray, add the egg, water, pepper, mushrooms, and broccoli, and whisk well. Introduce in the microwave and cook for 2 minutes. Add mozzarella and walnuts on top and serve for breakfast.

Nutrition: Calories: 128, Carbs: 24g, Fat: 0g, Protein: 9g, Sodium: 86 mg

54. Mushrooms and Turkey Breakfast

Preparation time: 10 minutes
Cooking time: 1 hour and 5 minutes
Servings: 12
Ingredients:
- 8 ounces whole-wheat bread, cubed
- 12 ounces turkey sausage, chopped
- 2 cups fat-free milk
- 5 ounces low-fat cheddar, shredded
- 3 eggs
- ½ cup green onions, chopped
- 1 cup mushrooms, chopped
- ½ teaspoon sweet paprika
- A pinch of black pepper
- 2 tablespoons low-fat parmesan, grated

Directions:
1. Put the bread cubes on a prepared lined baking sheet, bake at 400 degrees F for 8 minutes. Meanwhile, heat a pan over medium-high heat, add turkey sausage, stir, and brown for 7 minutes.
2. In a bowl, combine the milk with the cheddar, eggs, parmesan, black pepper, and paprika and whisk well.
3. Add mushrooms, sausage, bread cubes, and green onions stir, pour into a baking dish, and bake at 350 degrees F within 50 minutes. 5. Slice, divide between plates and serve for breakfast.

Nutrition: Calories: 88, Carbs: 1g, Fat: 9g, Protein: 1g, Sodium: 74 mg

55. Mushrooms and Cheese Omelet

Preparation time: 10 minutes
Cooking time: 15 minutes
Servings: 4
Ingredients:
- 2 tablespoons olive oil
- A pinch of black pepper
- 3 ounces mushrooms, sliced
- 1 cup baby spinach, chopped
- 3 eggs, whisked
- 2 tablespoons low-fat cheese, grated

- 1 small avocado, peeled, pitted, and cubed
- 1 tablespoons parsley, chopped

Directions:
1. Add mushrooms, stir, cook them for 5 minutes and transfer to a bowl on a heated pan with the oil over medium-high heat.
2. Heat-up the same pan over medium-high heat, add eggs and black pepper, spread into the pan, cook within 7 minutes, and transfer to a plate.
3. Spread mushrooms, spinach, avocado, and cheese on half of the omelet, fold the other half over this mix, sprinkle parsley on top, and serve.

Nutrition: Calories: 136, Carbs: 5g, Fat: 5g, Protein: 16g, Sodium: 192 mg

56. Easy Veggie Muffins

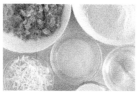

Preparation time: 10 minutes
Cooking time: 40 minutes
Servings: 4
Ingredients:
- 3/4 cup cheddar cheese, shredded
- 1 cup green onion, chopped
- 1 cup tomatoes, chopped
- 1 cup broccoli, chopped
- 2 cups non-fat milk
- 1 cup biscuit mix
- 4 eggs
- Cooking spray
- 1 teaspoon Italian seasoning
- A pinch of black pepper

Directions:
1. Grease a muffin tray with cooking spray and divide broccoli, tomatoes, cheese, and onions in each muffin cup.
2. In a bowl, combine green onions with milk, biscuit mix, eggs, pepper, and Italian seasoning, whisk well and pour into the muffin tray as well.
3. Cook the muffins in the oven at 375 degrees F for 40 minutes, divide them between plates, and serve.

Nutrition: Calories: 80, Carbs: 3g, Fat: 5g, Protein: 7g, Sodium: 25 mg

57. Carrot Muffins

Preparation time: 10 minutes
Cooking time: 30 minutes
Servings: 5
Ingredients:
- 1 and ½ cups whole wheat flour
- ½ cup stevia
- 1 teaspoon baking powder
- ½ teaspoon cinnamon powder
- ½ teaspoon baking soda
- ¼ cup natural apple juice
- ¼ cup olive oil

- 1 egg
- 1 cup fresh cranberries
- 2 carrots, grated
- 2 teaspoons ginger, grated
- ¼ cup pecans, chopped
- Cooking spray

Directions:
1. Mix the flour with the stevia, baking powder, cinnamon, and baking soda in a large bowl. Add apple juice, oil, egg, cranberries, carrots, ginger, and pecans and stir well.
2. Oiled a muffin tray with cooking spray, divide the muffin mix, put in the oven, and cook at 375 degrees F within 30 minutes. Divide the muffins between plates and serve for breakfast.

Nutrition: Calories: 34, Carbs: 6g, Fat: 1g, Protein: 0g, Sodium: 52 mg

58. Pineapple Oatmeal

Preparation time: 10 minutes
Cooking time: 25 minutes
Servings: 4
Ingredients:
- 2 cups old-fashioned oats
- 1 cup walnuts, chopped
- 2 cups pineapple, cubed
- 1 tablespoon ginger, grated
- 2 cups non-fat milk
- 2 eggs
- 2 tablespoons stevia
- 2 teaspoons vanilla extract

Directions:
1. In a bowl, combine the oats with the pineapple, walnuts, and ginger, stir and divide into 4 ramekins. Mix the milk with the eggs, stevia, and vanilla in a bowl and pour over the oats mix. Bake at 400 degrees F within 25 minutes. 4. Serve for breakfast.

Nutrition: Calories: 200, Carbs: 40g, Fat: 1g, Protein: 3g, Sodium: 275 mg

59. Spinach Muffins

Preparation time: 10 minutes
Cooking time: 30 minutes
Servings: 6
Ingredients:
- 6 eggs
- ½ cup non-fat milk
- 1 cup low-fat cheese, crumbled
- 4 ounces spinach
- ½ cup roasted red pepper, chopped
- 2 ounces prosciutto, chopped
- Cooking spray

Directions:
1. Mix the eggs with the milk, cheese, spinach, red pepper, and prosciutto in a bowl. Grease a muffin tray with cooking spray, divide the muffin mix, introduce in the oven, and bake at 350 degrees F within 30 minutes. Divide between plates and serve for breakfast.

Nutrition: Calories: 112, Carbs: 19g, Fat: 3g, Protein: 2g, Sodium: 274 mg

60. Chia Seeds Breakfast Mix

Preparation time: 8 hours
Cooking time: 0 minutes
Servings: 4
Ingredients:
- 2 cups old-fashioned oats
- 4 tablespoons chia seeds
- 4 tablespoons coconut sugar
- 3 cups of coconut milk
- 1 teaspoon lemon zest, grated
- 1 cup blueberries

Directions:
1. In a bowl, combine the oats with chia seeds, sugar, milk, lemon zest, and blueberries, stir, divide into cups and keep in the fridge for 8 hours. 2. Serve for breakfast.

Nutrition: Calories: 69, Carbs: 0g, Fat: 5g, Protein: 3g, Sodium: 0 mg

61. Salmon and Egg Scramble

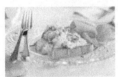

Preparation time: 15 minutes
Cooking time: 4 minutes
Servings: 4
Ingredients:
- 1 teaspoon of olive oil
- 3 organic whole eggs
- 3 tablespoons of water
- 1 minced garlic
- 6 Oz. Smoked salmon, sliced
- 2 avocados, sliced
- Black pepper to taste
- 1 green onion, chopped

Directions:
1. Warm-up olive oil in a large skillet and sauté onion in it. Take a medium bowl and whisk eggs in it, add water and make a scramble with the help of a fork. Add to the skillet the smoked salmon along with garlic and black pepper.
2. Stir for about 4 minutes until all ingredients get fluffy. At this stage, add the egg mixture. Once the eggs get firm, serve on a plate with a garnish of avocados.

Nutrition: Calories: 120, Carbs: 3g, Fat: 4g, Protein: 19g, Sodium: 898 mg, Potassium: 129mg

62. Pumpkin Muffins

Preparation time: 15 minutes
Cooking time: 20 minutes
Servings: 4
Ingredients:
- 4 cups of almond flour
- 2 cups of pumpkin, cooked and pureed
- 2 large whole organic eggs
- 3 teaspoons of baking powder

- 2 teaspoons of ground cinnamon
- 1/2 cup raw honey
- 4 teaspoons almond butter

Directions:
1. Preheat the oven at 400-degree F. Line the muffin paper on the muffin tray. Mix almond flour, pumpkin puree, eggs, baking powder, cinnamon, almond butter, and honey in a large bowl.
2. Put the prepared batter into a muffin tray and bake within 20 minutes. Once golden-brown, serve, and enjoy.

Nutrition: Calories: 136, Carbs: 22g, Fat: 5g, Protein: 2g, Sodium: 11 mg, Potassium: 699 mg

63. Sweet Berries Pancake

Preparation time: 15 minutes
Cooking time: 15 minutes
Servings: 4
Ingredients:
- 4 cups of almond flour
- Pinch of sea salt
- 2 organic eggs
- 4 teaspoons of walnut oil
- 1 cup of strawberries, mashed
- 1 cup of blueberries, mashed
- 1 teaspoon baking powder
- Honey for topping, optional

Directions:
1. Take a bowl and add almond flour, baking powder, and sea salt. Take another bowl and add eggs, walnut oil, strawberries, and blueberries mash. Combine ingredients of both bowls.
2. Heat a bit of walnut oil in a cooking pan and pour the spoonful mixture to make pancakes. Once the bubble comes on the top, flip the pancake to cook from the other side. Once done, serve with the glaze of honey on top.

Nutrition: Calories: 161, Carbs: 23g, Fat: 6g, Protein: 3g, Cholesterol: 82 mg, Sodium: 91 mg, Potassium: 252mg

64. Zucchini Pancakes

Preparation time: 15 minutes
Cooking time: 10 minutes
Servings: 4
Ingredients:
- 4 large zucchinis
- 4 green onions, diced
- 1/3 cup of milk
- 1 organic egg
- Sea Salt, just a pinch
- Black pepper, grated
- 2 tablespoons of olive oil

Directions:
1. First, wash the zucchinis and grate it with a cheese grater. Mix the egg and add in the grated zucchinis and milk in a large bowl. Warm oil in a skillet and sauté onions in it.
2. Put the egg batter into the skillet and make pancakes. Once cooked from both sides. Serve by sprinkling salt and pepper on top.

Nutrition: Calories: 70, Carbs: 8g, Fat: 3g, Protein: 2g, Cholesterol: 43 mg, Sodium: 60 mg, Potassium: 914mg

65. Breakfast Banana Split

Preparation time: 15 minutes
Cooking time: 0 minutes
Servings: 3
Ingredients:
- 2 bananas, peeled
- 1 cup oats, cooked
- 1/2 cup low-fat strawberry yogurt
- 1/3 teaspoon honey, optional
- 1/2 cup pineapple, chunks

Directions:
1. Peel the bananas and cut lengthwise. Place half of the banana in each separate bowl. Spoon strawberry yogurt on top and pour cooked oats with pineapple chunks on each banana. Serve immediately with a glaze of honey of liked.

Nutrition: Calories: 145, Carbs: 18g, Fat: 7g, Protein: 3g, Sodium: 2 mg, Potassium: 380 mg

66. Mediterranean Toast

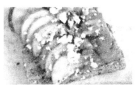

Preparation time: 10 minutes
Cooking time: 0 minutes
Servings: 2
Ingredients:
- 1 ½ tsp. reduced Fat crumbled feta
- 3 sliced Greek olives
- ¼ mashed avocado
- 1 slice good whole wheat bread
- 1 tbsp. roasted red pepper hummus
- 3 sliced cherry tomatoes
- 1 sliced hardboiled egg

Directions:
1. First, toast the bread and top it with ¼ mashed avocado and 1 tablespoon hummus. Add the cherry tomatoes, olives, hardboiled egg, and feta. To taste, season with salt and pepper.

Nutrition: Calories: 333.7, Fat: 17 g, Carbs: 33.3 g, Protein: 16.3 g, Sugars: 1 g, Sodium: 19 mg

67. Instant Banana Oatmeal

Preparation time: 1 minute
Cooking time: 2 minutes
Servings: 1
Ingredients:
- 1 mashed ripe banana
- ½ c. water
- ½ c. quick oats

Directions:
1. Measure the oats and water into a microwave-safe bowl and stir to combine. Place bowl in microwave and heat on high for 2 minutes. Remove the bowl, then stir in the mashed banana and serve.

Nutrition: Calories: 243, Fat: 3 g, Carbs: 50 g, Protein: 6 g, Sugars: 20 g, Sodium: 30 mg

68. Almond Butter-Banana Smoothie

Preparation time: 5 minutes
Cooking time: 0 minutes
Servings: 1
Ingredients:
- 1 tbsp. Almond butter
- ½ c. ice cubes
- ½ c. packed spinach
- 1 peeled and a frozen medium banana
- 1 c. Fat-free milk

Directions:
1. Blend all the listed fixing above in a powerful blender until smooth and creamy. Serve and enjoy.

Nutrition: Calories: 293, Fat: 9.8 g, Carbs: 42.5 g, Protein: 13.5 g, Sugars: 12 g, Sodium: 40 mg

69. Brown Sugar Cinnamon Oatmeal

Preparation time: 1 minute
Cooking time: 3 minutes
Servings: 4
Ingredients:
- ½ tsp. ground cinnamon
- 1 ½ tsp. pure vanilla extract
- ¼ c. light brown sugar
- 2 c. low- Fat milk
- 1 1/3 c. quick oats

Directions:
1. Put the milk plus vanilla into a medium saucepan and boil over medium-high heat.
2. Lower the heat to medium once it boils. Mix in oats, brown sugar, plus cinnamon, and cook, stirring 2–3 minutes. Serve immediately.

Nutrition: Calories: 208, Fat: 3 g, Carbs: 38 g, Protein: 8 g, Sugars: 15 g, Sodium: 33 mg

70. Buckwheat Pancakes with Vanilla Almond Milk

Preparation time: 10 minutes
Cooking time: 10 minutes
Servings: 1
Ingredients:
- ½ c. unsweetened vanilla almond milk
- 2-4 packets natural sweetener
- 1/8 tsp. salt
- ½ cup buckwheat flour
- ½ tsp. double-acting baking powder

Directions:
1. Prepare a nonstick pancake griddle and spray with the cooking spray, place over medium heat. Whisk the

buckwheat flour, salt, baking powder, and stevia in a small bowl and stir in the almond milk after.

2. Onto the pan, scoop a large spoonful of batter, cook until bubbles no longer pop on the surface and the entire surface looks dry and (2-4 minutes). Flip and cook for another 2-4 minutes. Repeat with all the remaining batter.

Nutrition: Calories: 240, Fat: 4.5 g, Carbs: 2 g, Protein: 11 g, Sugars: 17 g, Sodium: 38 mg

71. Banana & Cinnamon Oatmeal

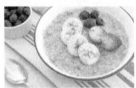

Preparation time: 5 minutes
Cooking time: 0 minutes
Servings: 6
Ingredients:
- 2 c. quick-cooking oats
- 4 c. Fat-free milk
- 1 tsp. ground cinnamon
- 2 chopped large ripe banana
- 4 tsp. Brown sugar
- Extra ground cinnamon

Directions:
1. Place milk in a skillet and bring to boil. Add oats and cook over medium heat until thickened, for two to four minutes.
2. Stir intermittently. Add cinnamon, brown sugar, and banana and stir to combine. If you want, serve with the extra cinnamon and milk. Enjoy!

Nutrition: Calories: 215, Fat: 2 g, Carbs: 42 g, Protein: 10 g, Sugars: 1 g, Sodium: 40 mg

72. Bagels Made Healthy

Preparation time: 5 minutes
Cooking time: 40 minutes
Servings: 8
Ingredients:
- 1 ½ c. warm water
- 1 ¼ c. bread flour
- 2 tbsps. Honey
- 2 c. whole wheat flour
- 2 tsp. Yeast
- 1 ½ tbsps. Olive oil
- 1 tbsp. vinegar

Directions:
1. In a bread machine, mix all ingredients, and then process on dough cycle. Once done, create 8 pieces shaped like a flattened ball. Create a donut shape using your thumb to make a hole at the center of each ball.
2. Place donut-shaped dough on a greased baking sheet then covers and let it rise about ½ hour. Prepare about 2 inches of water to boil in a large pan.

3. 3 In boiling water, drop one at a time the bagels and boil for 1 minute, then turn them once. Remove them and return to the baking sheet and bake at 350oF for about 20 to 25 minutes until golden brown.

Nutrition: Calories: 228, Fat: 3.7 g, Carbs: 41.8 g, Protein: 6.9 g, Sugars: 0 g, Sodium: 15 mg

73. Cereal with Cranberry-Orange Twist

Preparation time: 5 minutes
Cooking time: 0 minutes
Servings: 1
Ingredients:
- ½ c. water
- ½ c. orange juice
- 1/3 c. oat bran
- ¼ c. dried cranberries
- Sugar
- Milk

Directions:
1. In a bowl, combine all ingredients. For about 2 minutes, microwave the bowl, then serve with sugar and milk. Enjoy!

Nutrition: Calories: 220, Fat: 2.4 g, Carbs: 43.5 g, Protein: 6.2 g, Sugars: 8 g, Sodium: 1 mg

74. No Cook Overnight Oats

Preparation time: 5 minutes
Cooking time: 0 minutes
Servings: 1
Ingredients:
- 1 ½ c. low-fat milk
- 5 whole almond pieces
- 1 tsp. chia seeds
- 2 tbsps. Oats
- 1 tsp. sunflower seeds
- 1 tbsp. Craisins

Directions:
1. In a jar or mason bottle with a cap, mix all ingredients. Refrigerate overnight. Enjoy for breakfast.

Nutrition: Calories: 271, Fat: 9.8 g, Carbs: 35.4 g, Protein: 16.7 g, Sugars: 9, Sodium: 103 mg

75. Avocado Cup with Egg

Preparation time: 5 minutes
Cooking time: 0 minutes
Servings: 4
Ingredients:
- 4 tsp. parmesan cheese
- 1 chopped stalk scallion
- 4 dashes pepper
- 4 dashes paprika
- 2 ripe avocados
- 4 medium eggs

Directions:

1. Preheat oven to 375 0F. Slice avocadoes in half and discard the seed. Slice the rounded portions of the avocado to make it level and sit well on a baking sheet.
2. Place avocadoes on a baking sheet and crack one egg in each hole of the avocado. Season each egg evenly with pepper and paprika. Bake within 25 minutes or until eggs is cooked to your liking. Serve with a sprinkle of parmesan.

Nutrition: Calories: 206, Fat: 15.4 g, Carbs: 11.3 g, Protein: 8.5 g, Sugars: 0.4 g, Sodium: 21 mg

76. French toast with Applesauce

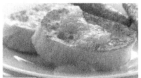

Preparation time: 5 minutes
Cooking time: 5 minutes
Servings: 6

Ingredients:
- ¼ c. unsweetened applesauce
- ½ c. skim milk
- 2 packets Stevia
- 2 eggs
- 6 slices whole-wheat bread
- 1 tsp. ground cinnamon

Directions:
1. Mix well applesauce, sugar, cinnamon, milk, and eggs in a mixing bowl. Soak the bread into the applesauce mixture until wet. On medium fire, heat a large nonstick skillet.
2. Add soaked bread on one side and another on the other side. Cook in a single layer within 2-3 minutes per side on medium-low fire or until lightly browned. Serve and enjoy.

Nutrition: Calories: 122.6, Fat: 2.6 g, Carbs: 18.3 g, Protein: 6.5 g, Sugars: 14.8 g, Sodium: 11mg

77. Banana-Peanut Butter and Greens Smoothie

Preparation time: 5 minutes
Cooking time: 0 minutes
Servings: 1

Ingredients:
- 1 c. chopped and packed Romaine lettuce
- 1 frozen medium banana
- 1 tbsp. all-natural peanut butter
- 1 c. cold almond milk

Directions:
1. In a heavy-duty blender, add all ingredients. Puree until smooth and creamy. Serve and enjoy.

Nutrition: Calories: 349.3, Fat: 9.7 g, Carbs: 57.4 g, Protein: 8.1 g, Sugars: 4.3 g, Sodium: 18 mg

78. Baking Powder Biscuits

Preparation time: 5 minutes
Cooking time: 5 minutes
Servings: 1

Ingredients:
- 1 egg white
- 1 c. white whole-wheat flour
- 4 tbsps. Non-hydrogenated vegetable shortening
- 1 tbsp. sugar
- 2/3 c. low-Fat milk
- 1 c. unbleached all-purpose flour
- 4 tsp.
- Sodium-free baking powder

Directions:
1. Warm oven to 450°F. Put the flour, sugar, plus baking powder into a mixing bowl and mix. Split the shortening into the batter using your fingers until it resembles coarse crumbs. Put the egg white plus milk and stir to combine.
2. Put the dough out onto a lightly floured surface and knead 1 minute. Roll dough to ¾ inch thickness and cut into 12 rounds. Place rounds on the baking sheet. Bake 10 minutes, then remove the baking sheet and place biscuits on a wire rack to cool.

Nutrition: Calories: 118, Fat: 4 g, Carbs: 16 g, Protein: 3 g, Sugars: 0.2 g, Sodium: 6 mg

79. Oatmeal Banana Pancakes with Walnuts

Preparation time: 15 minutes
Cooking time: 5 minutes
Servings: 8

Ingredients:
- 1 finely diced firm banana
- 1 c. whole wheat pancake mix
- 1/8 c. chopped walnuts
- ¼ c. old-fashioned oats

Directions:
1. Make the pancake mix, as stated in the directions on the package. Add walnuts, oats, and chopped banana. Coat a griddle with cooking spray. Add about ¼ cup of the pancake batter onto the griddle when hot.
2. Turn pancake over when bubbles form on top. Cook until golden brown. Serve immediately.

Nutrition: Calories: 155, Fat: 4 g, Carbs: 28 g, Protein: 7 g, Sugars: 2.2 g, Sodium: 16 mg

80. Creamy Oats, Greens & Blueberry Smoothie

Preparation time: 4 minutes
Cooking time: 0 minutes
Servings: 1

Ingredients:
- 1 c. cold
- Fat-free milk
- 1 c. salad greens
- ½ c. fresh frozen blueberries

- ½ c. frozen cooked oatmeal
- 1 tbsp. sunflower seeds

Directions:
1. Blend all ingredients using a powerful blender until smooth and creamy. Serve and enjoy.

Nutrition: Calories: 280, Fat: 6.8 g, Carbs: 44.0 g, Protein: 14.0 g, Sugars: 32 g, Sodium: 141 mg

81. Stuffed Breakfast Peppers

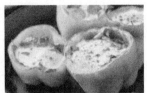

Preparation time: 15 minutes
Cooking time: 45 minutes
Servings: 4
Ingredients:
- 4 bell peppers (any color)
- 1 (16-ounce) bag frozen spinach
- 4 eggs
- ¼ cup shredded low-fat cheese (optional)
- Freshly ground black pepper

Directions:
1. Preheat the oven to 400°F. Line a baking dish with aluminum foil. Cut the tops off the pepper, then discard the seeds. Discard the tops and seeds. Put the peppers in the baking dish, and bake for about 15 minutes.
2. While the peppers bake, defrost the spinach and drain off the excess moisture. Remove the peppers, then stuff the bottoms evenly with the defrosted spinach.
3. Crack an egg over the spinach inside each pepper. Top each egg with a tablespoon of the cheese (if using) and season with black pepper to taste. Bake within 15 to 20 minutes, or until the egg whites are set and opaque.

Nutrition: Calories: 136, Fat: 5g, Sodium: 131mg, Potassium: 576mg, Carbohydrates: 15g, Protein: 11g

82. Sweet Potato Toast Three Ways

Preparation time: 15 minutes
Cooking time: 25 minutes
Servings:
Ingredients:
- 1 large sweet potato, unpeeled
- Topping Choice #1:
- 4 tablespoons peanut butter
- 1 ripe banana, sliced
- Dash ground cinnamon
- Topping Choice #2:
- ½ avocado, peeled, pitted, and mashed
- 2 eggs (1 per slice)
- Topping Choice #3:
- 4 tablespoons nonfat or low-fat ricotta cheese
- 1 tomato, sliced

- Dash black pepper

Directions:
1. Slice the sweet potato lengthwise into ¼-inch thick slices. Place the sweet potato slices in a toaster on high for about 5 minutes or until cooked through.
2. Repeat multiple times, if necessary, depending on your toaster settings. Top with your desired topping choices and enjoy.

Nutrition: Calories: 137, Fat: 0g, Sodium: 17mg, Potassium: 265mg, Carbohydrates: 32g, Fiber: 4g, Sugars: 0g, Protein: 2g

83. Apple-Apricot Brown Rice Breakfast Porridge

Preparation time: 15 minutes
Cooking time: 8 minutes
Servings: 4
Ingredients:
- 3 cups cooked brown rice
- 1¾ cups nonfat or low-fat milk
- 2 tablespoons lightly packed brown sugar
- 4 dried apricots, chopped
- 1 medium apple, cored and diced
- ¾ teaspoon ground cinnamon
- ¾ teaspoon vanilla extract

Directions:
1. Combine the rice, milk, sugar, apricots, apple, and cinnamon in a medium saucepan. Boil it on medium heat, lower the heat down slightly and cook within 2 to 3 minutes. Turn it off, then stir in the vanilla extract. Serve warm.

Nutrition: Calories: 260, Fat: 2g, Sodium: 50mg, Potassium: 421mg, Carbohydrates: 57g, Fiber: 4g, Sugars: 22g, Protein: 7g

84. Carrot Cake Overnight Oats

Preparation time: overnight
Cooking time: 2 minutes
Servings: 1
Ingredients:
- ½ cup rolled oats
- ½ cup plain nonfat or low-fat Greek yogurt
- ½ cup nonfat or low-fat milk
- ¼ cup shredded carrot
- 2 tablespoons raisins
- ½ teaspoon ground cinnamon
- 1 to 2 tablespoons chopped walnuts (optional)

Directions:
1. Mix all of the fixings in a lidded jar, shake well, and refrigerate overnight. Serve.

Nutrition: Calories: 331, Fat: 3g, Sodium: 141mg, Carbohydrates: 59g, Fiber: 8g, Sugars: 26g, Protein: 22g

85. Steel-Cut Oatmeal with Plums and Pear

Preparation time: 15 minutes
Cooking time: 25 minutes
Servings: 4
Ingredients:
- 2 cups of water
- 1 cup nonfat or low-fat milk
- 1 cup steel-cut oats
- 1 cup dried plums, chopped
- 1 medium pear, cored, and skin removed, diced
- 4 tablespoons almonds, roughly chopped

Directions:
1. Mix the water, milk, plus oats in a medium pot and bring to a boil over high heat. Reduce the heat and cover. Simmer for about 10 minutes, stirring occasionally.
2. Add the plums and pear, and cover. Simmer for another 10 minutes. Turn off the heat and let stand within 5 minutes until all of the liquid is absorbed. To serve, top each portion with a sprinkling of almonds.

Nutrition: Calories: 307, Fat: 6g, Sodium: 132mg, Potassium: 640mg, Carbohydrates: 58g, Fiber: 9g, Sugars: 24g, Protein: 9g

86. Creamy Apple-Avocado Smoothie

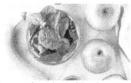

Preparation time: 15 minutes
Cooking time: 0 minutes
Servings: 2
Ingredients:
- ½ medium avocado, peeled and pitted
- 1 medium apple, chopped
- 1 cup baby spinach leaves
- 1 cup nonfat vanilla Greek yogurt
- ½ to 1 cup of water
- 1 cup ice
- Freshly squeezed lemon juice (optional)

Directions:
1. Blend all of the fixing using a blender, and blend until smooth and creamy. Put a squeeze of lemon juice on top if desired, and serve immediately.

Nutrition: Calories: 200, Fat: 7g, Sodium: 56mg, Potassium: 378mg. Carbohydrates: 27g, Fiber: 5g, Sugars: 20g, Protein: 10g

87. Strawberry, Orange, and Beet Smoothie

Preparation time: 5 minutes
Cooking time: 0 minutes
Servings: 2
Ingredients:
- 1 cup nonfat milk
- 1 cup of frozen strawberries
- 1 medium beet, cooked, peeled, and cubed
- 1 orange, peeled and quartered
- 1 frozen banana, peeled and chopped
- 1 cup nonfat vanilla Greek yogurt
- 1 cup ice

Directions:
1. In a blender, combine all of the fixings, and blend until smooth. Serve immediately.

Nutrition: Calories: 266, Fat: 0g, Cholesterol: 7mg, Sodium: 104mg, Carbohydrates: 51g, Fiber: 6g, Sugars: 34g, Protein: 15g

88. Blueberry-Vanilla Yogurt Smoothie

Preparation time: 5 minutes
Cooking time: 0 minutes
Servings: 2
Ingredients:
- 1½ cups frozen blueberries
- 1 cup nonfat vanilla Greek yogurt
- 1 frozen banana, peeled and sliced
- ½ cup nonfat or low-fat milk
- 1 cup ice

Directions:
1. In a blender, combine all of the fixing listed, and blend until smooth and creamy. Serve immediately.

Nutrition: Calories: 228, Fat: 1g, Sodium: 63mg, Potassium: 470mg, Carbohydrates: 45g, Fiber: 5g, Sugars: 34g, Protein: 12g

89. Greek Yogurt Oat Pancakes

Preparation time: 15 minutes
Cooking time: 10 minutes
Servings: 2
Ingredients:
- 6 egg whites (or ¾ cup liquid egg whites)
- 1 cup rolled oats
- 1 cup plain nonfat Greek yogurt
- 1 medium banana, peeled and sliced
- 1 teaspoon ground cinnamon
- 1 teaspoon baking powder

Directions:
1. Blend all of the listed fixing using a blender. Warm a griddle over medium heat. Spray the skillet with nonstick cooking spray.
2. Put 1/3 cup of the mixture or batter onto the griddle. Allow to cook and flip when bubbles on the top burst, about 5 minutes. Cook again within a minute until golden brown. Repeat with the remaining batter. Divide between two serving plates and enjoy.

Nutrition: Calories: 318, Fat: 4g, Sodium: 467mg, Potassium: 634mg, Carbohydrates: 47g, Fiber: 6g, Sugars: 13g, Protein: 28g

90. Scrambled Egg and Veggie Breakfast Quesadillas

Preparation time: 15 minutes
Cooking time: 15 minutes
Servings: 2
Ingredients:

- 2 eggs
- 2 egg whites
- 2 to 4 tablespoons nonfat or low-fat milk
- ¼ teaspoon freshly ground black pepper
- 1 large tomato, chopped
- 2 tablespoons chopped cilantro
- ½ cup canned black beans, rinsed and drained
- 1½ tablespoons olive oil, divided
- 4 corn tortillas
- ½ avocado, peeled, pitted, and thinly sliced

Directions:

1. Mix the eggs, egg whites, milk, and black pepper in a bowl. Using an electric mixer, beat until smooth. To the same bowl, add the tomato, cilantro, and black beans, and fold into the eggs with a spoon.
2. Warm-up half of the olive oil in a medium pan over medium heat. Add the scrambled egg mixture and cook for a few minutes, stirring, until cooked through. Remove from the pan.
3. Divide the scrambled-egg mixture between the tortillas, layering only on one half of the tortilla. Top with avocado slices and fold the tortillas in half.
4. Heat the remaining oil over medium heat, and add one of the folded tortillas to the pan. Cook within 1 to 2 minutes on each side or until browned. Repeat with remaining tortillas. Serve immediately.

Nutrition: Calories: 445, Fat: 24g, Sodium: 228mg, Potassium: 614mg, Carbohydrates: 42g, Fiber: 11g, Sugars: 2g, Protein: 19g

91. Spinach, Egg, and Cheese Breakfast Quesadillas

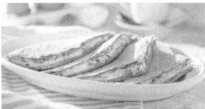

Preparation time: 15 minutes
Cooking time: 15 minutes
Servings: 4
Ingredients:

- 1½ tablespoons extra-virgin olive oil
- ½ medium onion, diced
- 1 medium red bell pepper, diced
- 4 large eggs
- 1/8 teaspoon salt
- 1/8 teaspoon freshly ground black pepper
- 4 cups baby spinach
- ½ cup crumbled feta cheese

- Nonstick cooking spray
- 4 (6-inch) whole-wheat tortillas, divided
- 1 cup shredded part-skim low-moisture mozzarella cheese, divided

Directions:

1. Warm-up oil over medium heat in a large skillet. Add the onion and bell pepper and sauté for about 5 minutes, or until soft.
2. Mix the eggs, salt, and black pepper in a medium bowl. Stir in the spinach and feta cheese. Put the egg batter in the skillet and scramble for about 2 minutes, or until the eggs are cooked. Remove from the heat.
3. Coat a clean skillet with cooking spray and add 2 tortillas. Place one-quarter of the spinach-egg mixture on one side of each tortilla. Sprinkle each with ¼ cup of mozzarella cheese. Fold the other halves of the tortillas down to close the quesadillas and brown for about 1 minute.
4. Turnover and cook again in a minute on the other side. Repeat with the remaining 2 tortillas and ½ cup of mozzarella cheese. Cut each quesadilla in half or wedges. Divide among 4 storage containers or reusable bags.

Nutrition: Calories: 453, Fat: 28g, Carbohydrates: 28g, Fiber: 4.5g, Protein: 23g, Potassium: 205mg. Sodium: 837mg

92. Simple Cheese and Broccoli Omelets

Preparation time: 15 minutes
Cooking time: 10 minutes
Servings: 4
Ingredients:

- 3 tablespoons extra-virgin olive oil, divided
- 2 cups chopped broccoli
- 8 large eggs
- ¼ cup 1% milk
- ½ teaspoon freshly ground black pepper
- 8 tablespoons shredded reduced-fat Monterey Jack cheese, divided

Directions:

1. In a nonstick skillet, heat 1 tablespoon of oil over medium-high heat. Add the broccoli and sauté, occasionally stirring, for 3 to 5 minutes, or until the broccoli turns bright green. Scrape into a bowl.
2. Mix the eggs, milk, plus pepper in a small bowl. Wipe out the skillet and heat ½ tablespoon of oil. Add one-quarter of the egg mixture and tilt the skillet to ensure an even layer. Cook for 2 minutes and then add 2 tablespoons of cheese and one-quarter of the broccoli. Use a spatula to fold into an omelet.
3. Repeat step 3 with the remaining 1½ tablespoons of oil, remaining egg mixture, 6 tablespoons of cheese, and remaining broccoli to make a total of 4 omelets. Divide into 4 storage containers.

Nutrition: Calories: 292, Fat: 23g, Carbohydrates: 4g, Fiber: 1g, Protein: 18g, Potassium: 308mg, Sodium: 282mg

93. Creamy Avocado and Egg Salad Sandwiches

Preparation time: 15 minutes

Cooking time: 15 minutes
Servings: 4
Ingredients:
- 2 small avocados, halved and pitted
- 2 tablespoons nonfat plain Greek yogurt
- Juice of 1 large lemon
- ¼ teaspoon salt
- ½ teaspoon freshly ground black pepper
- 8 large eggs, hardboiled, peeled, and chopped
- 3 tablespoons finely chopped fresh dill
- 3 tablespoons finely chopped fresh parsley
- 8 whole wheat bread slices (or your choice)

Directions:
1. Scoop the avocados into a large bowl and mash. Mix in the yogurt, lemon juice, salt, and pepper. Add the eggs, dill, and parsley and combine.
2. Store the bread and salad separately in 4 reusable storage bags and 4 containers and assemble the night before or serving. To serve, divide the mixture evenly among 4 of the bread slices and top with the other slices to make sandwiches.

Nutrition: Calories: 488, Fat: 22g, Carbohydrates: 48g, Fiber: 8g, Protein: 23g, Potassium: 469mg, Sodium: 597mg

94. Breakfast Hash

Preparation time: 15 minutes
Cooking time: 25 minutes
Servings: 4
Ingredients:
- Nonstick cooking spray
- 2 large sweet potatoes, ½-inch cubes
- 1 scallion, finely chopped
- ¼ teaspoon salt
- ½ teaspoon freshly ground black pepper
- 8 ounces extra-lean ground beef (96% or leaner)
- 1 medium onion, diced
- 2 garlic cloves, minced
- 1 red bell pepper, diced
- ¼ teaspoon ground cumin
- ¼ teaspoon paprika
- 2 cups coarsely chopped kale leaves
- ¾ cup shredded reduced-fat Cheddar cheese
- 4 large eggs

Directions:
1. Oiled a large skillet with cooking spray and heat over medium heat. Add the sweet potatoes, scallion, salt, and pepper. Sauté for 10 minutes, stirring often.
2. Add the beef, onion, garlic, bell pepper, cumin, and paprika. Sauté, frequently stirring, for about 4 minutes, or until the meat browns. Add the kale to the skillet and stir until wilted. Sprinkle with the Cheddar cheese.
3. Make four wells in the hash batter and crack an egg into each. Cover and let the eggs cook until the white is fully cooked and the yolk is to your liking. Divide into 4 storage containers.

Nutrition: Calories: 323, Fat: 15g, Carbohydrates: 23g, Fiber: 4g, Protein: 25g, Potassium: 676mg, Sodium: 587mg

95. Hearty Breakfast Casserole

Preparation time: 15 minutes
Cooking time: 30 minutes
Servings: 4
Ingredients:
- Nonstick cooking spray
- 1 large green bell pepper, diced
- 8 ounces Cremini mushrooms, diced
- ½ medium onion, diced
- 3 garlic cloves, minced
- 1 large sweet potato, grated
- 1 cup baby spinach
- 12 large eggs
- 3 tablespoons 1% milk
- 1 teaspoon mustard powder
- 1 teaspoon paprika
- 1 teaspoon freshly ground black pepper
- ½ teaspoon salt
- ½ cup shredded reduced-fat Colby-Jack cheese

Directions:
1. Preheat the oven to 350°F. Oiled at a 9-by-13-inch baking dish with cooking spray. Coat a large skillet with cooking spray and heat over medium heat. Add the bell pepper, mushrooms, onion, garlic, and sweet potato.
2. Sauté, frequently stirring, for 3 to 4 minutes, or until the onion is translucent. Add the spinach and continue to sauté while stirring, until the spinach has wilted. Remove, then set aside to cool slightly.
3. Mix the eggs, milk, mustard powder, paprika, black pepper, and salt in a large bowl. Add the sautéed vegetables. Put the batter into the prepared baking dish.
4. Bake for 30 minutes. Remove from the oven, sprinkle with the Colby-Jack cheese, return to the oven, and bake again within 5 minutes to melt the cheese. Divide into 4 storage containers.

Nutrition: Calories: 378, Fat: 25g, Carbohydrates: 17g, Fiber: 3g, Protein: 26g, Potassium: 717mg, Sodium: 658mg

96. Blueberry Waffles

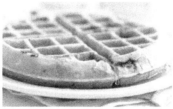

Preparation time: 15 minutes
Cooking time: 15 minutes
Servings: 8
Ingredients:
- 2 cups whole wheat flour
- 1 tablespoon baking powder
- 1 teaspoon ground cinnamon
- 2 tablespoons sugar
- 2 large eggs
- 3 tablespoons unsalted butter, melted
- 3 tablespoons nonfat plain Greek yogurt

- 1½ cups 1% milk
- 2 teaspoons vanilla extract
- 4 ounces blueberries
- Nonstick cooking spray
- ½ cup maple almond butter

Directions:
1. Preheat waffle iron. Mix the flour, baking powder, cinnamon, plus sugar in a large bowl. Mix the eggs, melted butter, yogurt, milk, and vanilla in a small bowl. Combine well.
2. Put the wet fixing to the dry mix and whisk until well combined. Do not over whisk; it's okay if the mixture has some lumps. Fold in the blueberries.
3. Oiled the waffle iron with cooking spray, then cook 1/3 cup of the batter until the waffles are lightly browned and slightly crisp. Repeat with the rest of the batter.
4. Place 2 waffles in each of 4 storage containers. Store the almond butter in 4 condiment cups. To serve, top each warm waffle with 1 tablespoon of maple almond butter.

Nutrition: Calories: 647, Fat: 37g, Carbohydrates: 67g, Protein: 22g, Sodium: 156mg

97. Apple Pancakes

Preparation time: 15 minutes
Cooking time: 5 minutes
Servings: 16
Ingredients:
- ¼ cup extra-virgin olive oil, divided
- 1 cup whole wheat flour
- 2 teaspoons baking powder
- 1 teaspoon baking soda
- 1 teaspoon ground cinnamon
- 1 cup 1% milk
- 2 large eggs
- 1 medium Gala apple, diced
- 2 tablespoons maple syrup
- ¼ cup chopped walnuts

Directions:
1. Set aside 1 teaspoon of oil to use for greasing a griddle or skillet. In a large bowl, stir the flour, baking powder, baking soda, cinnamon, milk, eggs, apple, and the remaining oil.
2. Warm griddle or skillet on medium-high heat and coat with the reserved oil. Working in batches, pour in about ¼ cup of the batter for each pancake. Cook until browned on both sides.
3. Place 4 pancakes into each of 4 medium storage containers and the maple syrup in 4 small containers. Put each serving with 1 tablespoon of walnuts and drizzle with ½ tablespoon of maple syrup.

Nutrition: Calories: 378, Fat: 22g, Carbohydrates: 39g, Protein: 10g, Sodium: 65mg

98. Super-Simple Granola

Preparation time: 15 minutes
Cooking time: 25 minutes
Servings: 8
Ingredients:
- ¼ cup extra-virgin olive oil

- ¼ cup honey
- ½ teaspoon ground cinnamon
- ½ teaspoon vanilla extract
- ¼ teaspoon salt
- 2 cups rolled oats
- ½ cup chopped walnuts
- ½ cup slivered almonds

Directions:
1. Preheat the oven to 350°F. Mix the oil, honey, cinnamon, vanilla, and salt in a large bowl. Add the oats, walnuts, and almonds. Stir to coat. Put the batter out onto the prepared sheet pan. Bake for 20 minutes. Let cool.

Nutrition: Calories: 254, Fat: 16g, Carbohydrates: 25g, Fiber: 3.5g, Protein: 5g, Potassium: 163mg, Sodium: 73mg

99. Savory Yogurt Bowls

Preparation time: 15 minutes
Cooking time: 0 minutes
Servings: 4
Ingredients:
- 1 medium cucumber, diced
- ½ cup pitted Kalamata olives, halved
- 2 tablespoons fresh lemon juice
- 1 tablespoon extra-virgin olive oil
- 1 teaspoon dried oregano
- ¼ teaspoon freshly ground black pepper
- 2 cups nonfat plain Greek yogurt
- ½ cup slivered almonds

Directions:
1. In a small bowl, mix the cucumber, olives, lemon juice, oil, oregano, and pepper. Divide the yogurt evenly among 4 storage containers. Top with the cucumber-olive mix and almonds.

Nutrition: Calories: 240, Fat: 16g, Carbohydrates: 10gm, Protein: 16g, Potassium: 353mg, Sodium: 350mg

100. Energy Sunrise Muffins

Preparation time: 15 minutes
Cooking time: 25 minutes
Servings: 16
Ingredients:
- Nonstick cooking spray
- 2 cups whole wheat flour
- 2 teaspoons baking soda
- 2 teaspoons ground cinnamon
- 1 teaspoon ground ginger
- ¼ teaspoon salt
- 3 large eggs
- ½ cup packed brown sugar
- 1/3 cup unsweetened applesauce
- ¼ cup honey
- ¼ cup vegetable or canola oil
- 1 teaspoon grated orange zest
- Juice of 1 medium orange
- 2 teaspoons vanilla extract
- 2 cups shredded carrots
- 1 large apple, peeled and grated

- ½ cup golden raisins
- ½ cup chopped pecans
- ½ cup unsweetened coconut flakes

Directions:

1. If you can fit two 12-cup muffin tins side by side in your oven, then leave a rack in the middle, then preheat the oven to 350°F.
2. Coat 16 cups of the muffin tins with cooking spray or line with paper liners. Mix the flour, baking soda, cinnamon, ginger, and salt in a large bowl. Set aside.
3. Mix the eggs, brown sugar, applesauce, honey, oil, orange zest, orange juice, and vanilla until combined in a medium bowl. Add the carrots and apple and whisk again.
4. Mix the dry and wet ingredients with a spatula. Fold in the raisins, pecans, and coconut. Mix everything once again, just until well combined. Put the batter into the prepared muffin cups, filling them to the top.
5. Bake within 20 to 25 minutes, or until a wooden toothpick inserted into the middle of the center muffin comes out clean (switching racks halfway through if baking on 2 racks). Cool for 5 minutes in the tins, then transfers to a wire rack to cool for an additional 5 minutes. Cool completely before storing in containers.

Nutrition: Calories: 292, Fat: 14g, Carbohydrates: 42g, Protein: 5g, Sodium: 84mg

101. Pasta Primavera

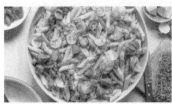

Preparation time: 10 minutes
Cooking time: 25 minutes
Servings: 4
Ingredients:
- 2 cups cauliflower florets, cut into matchsticks
- 16 oz. tortiglioni
- ¼ cup olive oil
- ½ cup chopped fresh green onions
- 1 red bell pepper, thinly sliced
- 4 garlic cloves, minced
- 1 cup grape tomatoes, halved
- 2 tsp. dried Italian seasoning
- ½ lemon, juiced
- ½ cup grated Pecorino Romano cheese

Directions:
2. In a pot of boiling water, cook the tortiglioni pasta for 8-10 minutes until al dente. Drain and set aside.
3. Heat olive oil in a skillet and sauté onion, cauliflower, and bell pepper for 7 minutes. Mix in garlic and cook until fragrant, 30 seconds.
4. Stir in the tomatoes and Italian seasoning; cook until the tomatoes soften, 5 minutes. Mix in the lemon juice and tortiglioni and adjust the taste with salt and black pepper.
5. Garnish with the Pecorino Romano cheese.

Nutrition: Calories: 381; Protein: 25.3 Grams; Fat: 12.9 Grams; Carbs: 9.7 Grams; Sodium: 480 mg; Cholesterol: 37 mg

102. Delicious Chicken Pasta

Preparation Time: 10 minutes
Cooking Time: 17 minutes
Servings: 4
Ingredients:
- 3 chicken breasts, skinless, boneless, cut into pieces
- 9 oz. whole-grain pasta
- 1/2 cup olives, sliced
- 1/2 cup sun-dried tomatoes
- 1 tbsp. roasted red peppers, chopped
- 14 oz. can tomatoes, diced
- 2 cups marinara sauce
- 1 cup chicken broth
- Pepper
- Salt

Directions:
1. Add all ingredients except whole-grain pasta into the instant pot and stir well. Seal pot with lid and cook on high for 12 minutes.

2. Once done, allow to release pressure naturally. Remove lid. Add pasta and stir well. Seal pot again and select manual and set timer for 5 minutes.
3. Once done, allow to release pressure naturally for 5 minutes then release remaining using quick release. Remove lid. Stir well and serve.

Nutrition: Calories: 381; Protein: 25.3 Grams; Fat: 12.9 Grams; Carbs: 9.7 Grams; Sodium: 480 mg; Cholesterol: 37 mg

103. Flavorful Mac & Cheese

Preparation Time: 10 minutes
Cooking Time: 10 minutes
Servings: 6
Ingredients:
- 16 oz. whole-grain elbow pasta
- 4 cups of water
- 1 cup can tomatoes, diced
- 1 tsp. garlic, chopped
- 2 tbsp. olive oil
- 1/4 cup green onions, chopped
- 1/2 cup parmesan cheese, grated
- 1/2 cup mozzarella cheese, grated
- 1 cup cheddar cheese, grated
- 1/4 cup passata
- 1 cup unsweetened almond milk
- 1 cup marinated artichoke, diced
- 1/2 cup sun-dried tomatoes, sliced
- 1/2 cup olives, sliced
- 1 tsp. salt

Directions
2. Add pasta, water, tomatoes, garlic, oil, and salt into the instant pot and stir well. Seal pot with lid and cook on high for 4 minutes.
3. Once done, allow to release pressure naturally for 5 minutes then release remaining using quick release. Remove lid. Set pot on sauté mode.
4. Add green onion, parmesan cheese, mozzarella cheese, cheddar cheese, passata, almond milk, artichoke, sun-dried tomatoes, and olive. Mix well. Stir well and cook until cheese is melted. Serve and enjoy.

Nutrition: Calories: 381; Protein: 25.3 Grams; Fat: 12.9 Grams; Carbs: 9.7 Grams; Sodium: 480 mg; Cholesterol: 37 mg

104. Flavors Herb Risotto

Preparation Time: 10 minutes
Cooking Time: 15 minutes
Servings: 4
Ingredients:
- 2 cups of rice
- 2 tbsp. parmesan cheese, grated
- oz. heavy cream
- 1 tbsp. fresh oregano, chopped
- 1 tbsp. fresh basil, chopped

- 1/2 tbsp. sage, chopped
- 1 onion, chopped
- 2 tbsp. olive oil
- 1 tsp. garlic, minced
- 4 cups vegetable stock
- Pepper
- Salt

Directions:

3. Add oil into the inner pot of instant pot and set the pot on sauté mode. Add garlic and onion and sauté for 2-3 minutes.
4. Add remaining ingredients except for parmesan cheese and heavy cream and stir well. Seal pot with lid and cook on high for 12 minutes.
5. Once done, allow to release pressure naturally for 10 minutes then release remaining using quick release. Remove lid. Stir in cream and cheese and serve.

Nutrition: Calories: 381; Protein: 25.3 Grams; Fat: 12.9 Grams; Carbs: 9.7 Grams; Sodium: 480 mg; Cholesterol: 37 mg

105. Delicious Pasta Primavera

Preparation Time: 10 minutes
Cooking Time: 4 minutes
Servings: 4

Ingredients:

- 8 oz. whole wheat penne pasta
- 1 tbsp. fresh lemon juice
- 2 tbsp. fresh parsley, chopped
- 1/4 cup almonds slivered
- 1/4 cup parmesan cheese, grated
- 14 oz. can tomatoes, diced
- 1/2 cup prunes
- 1/2 cup zucchini, chopped
- 1/2 cup asparagus, cut into 1-inch pieces
- 1/2 cup carrots, chopped
- 1/2 cup broccoli, chopped
- 1 3/4 cups vegetable stock
- Pepper
- Salt

Directions:

3. Add stock, pars, tomatoes, prunes, zucchini, asparagus, carrots, and broccoli into the instant pot and stir well. Seal pot with lid and cook on high for 4 minutes.
4. Once done, release pressure using quick release. Remove lid. Add remaining ingredients and stir well and serve.

Nutrition: Calories: 381; Protein: 25.3 Grams; Fat: 12.9 Grams; Carbs: 9.7 Grams; Sodium: 480 mg; Cholesterol: 37 mg

106. Tuscan Chicken Linguine

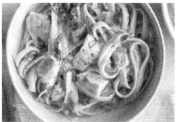

Preparation Time: 10 minutes
Cooking time: 25 minutes
Servings: 4

Ingredients

- 16 oz. linguine
- 2 tbsp. olive oil
- 4 chicken breasts
- 1 medium white onion, chopped
- 1 cup sundried tomatoes in oil, chopped
- 1 red bell pepper, deseeded and chopped
- 5 garlic cloves, minced
- ¾ cup chicken broth
- 1 ½ cups heavy cream
- ¾ cup grated Pecorino Romano cheese
- 1 cup baby kale, chopped Salt and black pepper to taste

Directions

1. In a pot of boiling water, cook the linguine pasta for 8-10 minutes until al dente. Drain and set aside.
2. Heat the olive oil in a large skillet, season the chicken with salt, black pepper, and cook in the oil until golden brown on the outside and cooked within, 7 to 8 minutes.
3. Transfer the chicken to a plate and cut into 4 slices each. Set aside. Add the onion, sundried tomatoes, bell pepper to the skillet and sauté until softened, 5 minutes. Mix in the garlic and cook until fragrant, 1 minute.
4. Deglaze the skillet with the chicken broth and mix in the heavy cream. Simmer for 2 minutes and stir in the Pecorino Romano cheese until melted, 2 minutes.
5. Once the cheese melts, stir in the kale to wilt and adjust the taste with salt and black pepper. Mix in the linguine and chicken until well coated in the sauce. Dish the food and serve warm.

Nutrition: Calories: 381; Protein: 25.3 Grams; Fat: 12.9 Grams; Carbs: 9.7 Grams; Sodium: 480 mg; Cholesterol: 37 mg

107. Classic Beef Lasagna

Preparation time: 20 minutes
Cooking time: 50 minutes
Servings: 4

Ingredients:

- 1 lb lasagna sheets
- 2 tbsp. olive oil
- 1 lb ground beef
- 1 medium white onion, chopped
- 1 tsp. Italian seasoning
- Salt and black pepper to taste
- 1 cup marinara sauce
- ½ cup grated Parmesan cheese

Directions:

1. Preheat oven to 350 F. Warm olive oil in a skillet and add the beef and onion. Cook until the beef is brown, 7-8 minutes.
2. Season with Italian seasoning, salt, and pepper. Cook for 1 minute and mix in the marinara sauce. Simmer for 3 minutes.
3. Spread a layer of the beef mixture in a lightly greased baking sheet and make a first single layer on the beef mixture. Top with a single layer of lasagna sheets.
4. Repeat the layering two more times using the remaining ingredients in the same quantities. Sprinkle with the Parmesan cheese.
5. Bake in the oven until the cheese melts and is bubbly with the sauce, 20 minutes. Remove the lasagna, allow cooling for 2 minutes and dish onto serving plates. Serve warm.

Nutrition: Calories: 381; Protein: 25.3 Grams; Fat: 12.9 Grams; Carbs: 9.7 Grams; Sodium: 480 mg; Cholesterol: 37 mg

108. Spicy Veggie Pasta Bake

Preparation time: 10 minutes
Cooking time: 35 minutes
Servings: 4
Ingredients:
- 16 oz. penne
- 1 tbsp. olive oil
- 1 cup mixed chopped bell peppers
- 1 yellow squash, chopped
- 1 red onion, halved and sliced
- 1 cup sliced white button mushrooms
- Salt and black pepper to taste
- ¼ tsp. red chili flakes
- 1 cup marinara sauce
- 1 cup grated mozzarella cheese
- 1 cup grated Parmesan cheese
- ¼ cup chopped fresh basil

Directions
1. In a pot of boiling water, cook the penne pasta for 8-10 minutes until al dente. Drain and set aside.
2. Heat the olive oil in a cast iron and sauté the bell peppers, squash, onion, and mushrooms. Cook until softened, 5 minutes.
3. Stir in garlic and cook until fragrant, 30 seconds. Season with salt, pepper, and red chili flakes. Mix in marinara sauce and cook for 5 minutes. Stir in the penne and spread the mozzarella and Parmesan cheeses on top. Bake in the oven until the cheeses melt and golden brown on top, 15 minutes. Allow cooling for 2 minutes and dish onto serving plates. Serve warm.

Nutrition: Calories: 381; Protein: 25.3 Grams; Fat: 12.9 Grams; Carbs: 9.7 Grams; Sodium: 480 mg; Cholesterol: 37 mg

109. Parmesan Spaghetti in Mushroom-Tomato Sauce

Preparation time: 10 minutes
Cooking time: 20 minutes
Servings: 4
Ingredients:
- 16 oz. spaghetti, cut in half

- 2 cups mushrooms, chopped
- 1 bell pepper, chopped
- ½ cup yellow onion, chopped
- 3 garlic cloves, minced
- ½ tsp. five-spice powder
- 4 tbsp. fresh parsley, chopped
- 1 tbsp. tomato paste
- 2 ripe tomatoes, chopped
- ½ cup Parmesan cheese, grated
- ¼ cup olive oil
- Salt and black pepper to taste

Directions:
1. Heat olive oil in a skillet over medium heat. Add in mushrooms, bell pepper, onion, and garlic and stir-fry for 4-5 minutes until tender.
2. Mix in salt, black pepper, 2 tbsp. of parsley, five-spice powder, tomato paste, and tomatoes; stir well and cook for 10-12 minutes.
3. In a pot with salted boiling water, add the pasta and cook until al dente, about 8-10 minutes, stirring occasionally.
4. Drain and stir in the vegetable mixture. Serve topped with Parmesan cheese and remaining fresh parsley.

Nutrition: Calories: 381; Protein: 25.3 Grams; Fat: 12.9 Grams; Carbs: 9.7 Grams; Sodium: 480 mg; Cholesterol: 37 mg

110. Mustard Chicken Farfalle

Preparation time: 10 minutes
Cooking time: 30 minutes
Servings: 4
Ingredients:
- 16 oz. farfalle
- 1 tbsp. olive oil
- 4 chicken breasts, cut into strips
- Salt and black pepper to taste
- 1 yellow onion, finely sliced
- 1 yellow bell pepper, sliced
- 1 garlic clove, minced
- 1 tbsp. wholegrain mustard
- 5 tbsp. heavy cream
- 1 cup chopped mustard greens
- 1 tbsp. chopped parsley

Directions:
1. In a pot of boiling water, cook the farfalle pasta for 8-10 minutes until al dente. Drain and set aside.
2. Heat the olive oil in a large skillet, season the chicken with salt, black pepper, and cook in the oil until golden brown, 10 minutes.
3. Set aside. Stir in the onion, bell pepper and cook until softened, 5 minutes. Mix in the garlic and cook until fragrant, 30 seconds.
4. Mix in the mustard and heavy cream; simmer for 2 minutes and mix in the chicken and mustard greens.
5. Allow wilting for 2 minutes and adjust the taste with salt and black pepper. Stir in the farfalle pasta, allow warming for 1 minute and dish the food onto serving plates. Garnish with the parsley and serve warm.

Nutrition: Calories: 381; Protein: 25.3 Grams; Fat: 12.9 Grams; Carbs: 9.7 Grams; Sodium: 480 mg; Cholesterol: 37 mg

111. Italian Mushroom Pizza

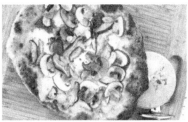

Preparation time: 10 minutes
Cooking time: 35 minutes
Servings: 4

Ingredients:

- For the Crust:
- 2 cups flour
- 1 cup lukewarm water
- 1 pinch of sugar
- 1 tsp. active dry yeast
- ¾ tsp. salt
- 2 tbsp. olive oil
- For the Topping
- 1 tsp. olive oil
- 2 medium Cremini mushrooms, sliced
- 1 garlic clove, minced
- ½ cup sugar-free tomato sauce
- 1 tsp. sugar 1 bay leaf
- 1 tsp. dried oregano
- 1tsp dried basil
- Salt and black pepper to taste
- ½ cup grated mozzarella cheese
- ½ cup grated Parmesan cheese
- 6 black olives, pitted and sliced

Directions:

1. Sift the flour and salt in a bowl and stir in yeast. Mix lukewarm water, olive oil, and sugar in another bowl.
2. Add the wet mixture to the dry mixture and whisk until you obtain a soft dough. Place the dough on a lightly floured work surface and knead it thoroughly for 4-5 minutes until elastic.
3. Transfer the dough to a greased bowl. Cover with cling film and leave to rise for 50-60 minutes in a warm place until doubled in size.
4. Roll out the dough to a thickness of around 12 inches. Preheat the oven to 400 F. Line a pizza pan with parchment paper.
5. Heat the olive oil in a medium skillet and sauté the mushrooms until softened, 5 minutes. Stir in the garlic and cook until fragrant, 30 seconds.
6. Mix in the tomato sauce, sugar, bay leaf, oregano, basil, salt, and black pepper. Cook for 2 minutes and turn the heat off.
7. Spread the sauce on the crust, top with the mozzarella and Parmesan cheeses, and then, the olives.
8. Bake in the oven until the cheeses melts, 15 minutes. Remove the pizza, slice, and serve warm.

Nutrition: Calories: 381; Protein: 25.3 Grams; Fat: 12.9 Grams; Carbs: 9.7 Grams; Sodium: 480 mg; Cholesterol: 37 mg

112. Chicken Bacon Ranch Pizza

Preparation time: 10 minutes
Cooking time: 35 minutes
Servings: 4

Ingredients:

- For the Crust:
- 2 cups flour
- 1 cup lukewarm water
- 1 pinch of sugar
- 1 tsp. active dry yeast
- ¾ tsp. salt
- 2 tbsp. olive oil
- For the ranch sauce
- 1 tbsp. butter
- 2 garlic cloves, minced
- 1 tbsp. cream cheese
- ¼ cup half and half
- 1 tbsp. dry Ranch seasoning mix
- For the Topping:
- 3 bacon slices, chopped
- 2 chicken breasts
- Salt and black pepper to taste
- 1 cup grated mozzarella cheese
- 6 fresh basil leaves

Directions:

1. Sift the flour and salt in a bowl and stir in yeast. Mix lukewarm water, olive oil, and sugar in another bowl.
2. Add the wet mixture to the dry mixture and whisk until you obtain a soft dough. Place the dough on a lightly floured work surface and knead it thoroughly for 4-5 minutes until elastic.
3. Transfer the dough to a greased bowl. Cover with cling film and leave to rise for 50-60 minutes in a warm place until doubled in size.
4. Roll out the dough to a thickness of around 12 inches. Preheat the oven to 400 F. Line a pizza pan with parchment paper.
5. In a bowl, mix the sauce's ingredients butter, garlic, cream cheese, half and half, and ranch mix. Set aside. Heat a grill pan over medium heat and cook the bacon until crispy and brown, 5 minutes.
6. Transfer to a plate and set aside. Season the chicken with salt, pepper and grill in the pan on both sides until golden brown, 10 minutes.
7. Remove to a plate, allow cooling and cut into thin slices. Spread the ranch sauce on the pizza crust, followed by the chicken and bacon, and then, mozzarella cheese and basil. Bake for 5 minutes or until the cheese melts. Slice and serve warm.

Nutrition: Calories: 381; Protein: 25.3 Grams; Fat: 12.9 Grams; Carbs: 9.7 Grams; Sodium: 480 mg; Cholesterol: 37 mg

113. Fall Baked Vegetable with Rigatoni

Preparation time: 10 minutes
Cooking time: 35 minutes
Servings: 6

Ingredients
- 1 lb pumpkin, chopped
- 1 zucchini, chopped
- 2 tbsp. grated Pecorino-Romano cheese
- 1 onion, chopped
- 1 lb rigatoni
- 2 tbsp. olive oil
- Salt and black pepper to taste
- ½ tsp. garlic powder
- ½ cup dry white wine

Directions
1. Preheat oven to 420 F. Combine zucchini, pumpkin, onion, and olive oil in a bowl. Arrange on a lined aluminum foil sheet and season with salt, pepper, and garlic powder.
2. Bake for 30 minutes until tender. In a pot of boiling water, cook rigatoni for 8-10 minutes until al dente. Drain and set aside. In a food processor, place ½ cup of the roasted veggies and wine and pulse until smooth.
3. Transfer to a skillet over medium heat. Stir in rigatoni and cook until heated through. Top with the remaining roasted vegetables and Pecorino cheese to serve.

Nutrition: Calories: 381; Protein: 25.3 Grams; Fat: 12.9 Grams; Carbs: 9.7 Grams; Sodium: 480 mg; Cholesterol: 37 mg

114. Walnut Pesto Pasta

Preparation time: 10 minutes
Cooking time: 10 minutes
Servings: 4
Ingredients
- 8 oz. whole-wheat pasta
- ¼ cup walnuts, chopped
- 3 garlic cloves, finely minced
- ½ cup fresh dill, chopped
- ¼ cup grated Parmesan cheese
- 3 tbsp. extra-virgin olive oil

Directions
1. Cook the whole-wheat pasta to pack instructions, drain and let it cool.
2. Place the olive oil, dill, garlic, Parmesan cheese, and walnuts in a food processor and blend for 15 seconds or until paste forms.
3. Pour over the cooled pasta and toss to combine. Serve immediately.

Nutrition: Calories: 381; Protein: 25.3 Grams; Fat: 12.9 Grams; Carbs: 9.7 Grams; Sodium: 480 mg; Cholesterol: 37 mg

115. Beef Carbonara

Preparation time: 10 minutes
Cooking time: 20 minutes
Servings: 4
Ingredients:
- 16 oz. linguine
- 4 bacon slices, chopped
- 1 ¼ cups heavy whipping cream
- ¼ cup mayonnaise
- Salt and black pepper to taste
- 4 egg yolks
- 1 cup grated Parmesan cheese

Directions:
1. In a pot of boiling water, cook the linguine pasta for 8-10 minutes until al dente. Drain and set aside.
2. Add the bacon to a skillet and cook over medium heat until crispy, 5 minutes. Set aside. Pour heavy cream into a pot and allow simmering for 5 minutes.
3. Whisk in mayonnaise and season with salt and pepper. Cook for 1 minute and spoon 2 tablespoons of the mixture into a medium bowl. Allow cooling and mix in the egg yolks. Pour the mixture into the pot and mix quickly.
4. Stir in Parmesan and fold in the pasta. Garnish with more Parmesan. Cook for 1 minute to warm the pasta.

Nutrition: Calories: 381; Protein: 25.3 Grams; Fat: 12.9 Grams; Carbs: 9.7 Grams; Sodium: 480 mg; Cholesterol: 37 mg

116. Coconut Flour Pizza

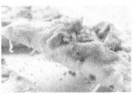

Preparation time: 10 minutes
Cooking Time: 35 minutes
Servings: 4
Ingredients
- 2 tablespoons psyllium husk powder
- ¾ cup coconut flour
- 1 teaspoon garlic powder
- ½ teaspoon salt
- ½ teaspoon baking soda
- 1 cup boiling water
- 1 teaspoon apple cider vinegar
- 3 eggs
- Toppings:
- 3 tablespoons tomato sauce
- 1½ oz. Mozzarella cheese
- 1 tablespoon basil, freshly chopped

Directions
1. Preheat the oven to 350 degrees f and grease a baking sheet. Mix coconut flour, salt, psyllium husk powder, and garlic powder until fully combined.
2. Add eggs, apple cider vinegar, and baking soda and knead with boiling water. Place the dough out on a baking sheet and top with the toppings.
3. Transfer in the oven and bake for about 20 minutes. Dish out and serve warm.

Nutrition: Calories: 381; Protein: 25.3 Grams; Fat: 12.9 Grams; Carbs: 9.7 Grams; Sodium: 480 mg; Cholesterol: 37 mg

117. Keto Pepperoni Pizza

Preparation time: 40 minutes
Cooking time: 10 minutes
Servings: 4
Ingredients
- Crust
- 6 oz. mozzarella cheese, shredded

- 4 eggs
- Topping
- 1 teaspoon dried oregano
- 1½ oz. pepperoni
- 3 tablespoons tomato paste
- 5 oz. mozzarella cheese, shredded
- Olives

Directions:
1. Preheat the oven to 400 degrees F and grease a baking sheet. Whisk together eggs and cheese in a bowl and spread on a baking sheet.
2. Transfer in the oven and bake for about 15 minutes until golden. Remove from the oven and allow it to cool.
3. Increase the oven temperature to 450 degrees F. spread the tomato paste on the crust and top with oregano, pepperoni, cheese, and olives on top.
4. Bake for another 10 minutes and serve hot.

Nutrition: Calories: 381; Protein: 25.3 Grams; Fat: 12.9 Grams; Carbs: 9.7 Grams; Sodium: 480 mg; Cholesterol: 37 mg

118. Fresh Bell Pepper Basil Pizza

Preparation time: 25 minutes
Cooking Time: 10 minutes
Servings: 3
Ingredients:
- Pizza Base
- ½ cup almond flour
- 2 tablespoons cream cheese
- 1 teaspoon Italian seasoning
- ½ teaspoon black pepper
- 6 ounces mozzarella cheese
- 2 tablespoons psyllium husk
- 2 tablespoons fresh Parmesan cheese
- 1 large egg
- ½ teaspoon salt
- Toppings
- 4 ounces cheddar cheese, shredded
- ¼ cup Marinara sauce
- 2/3 medium bell pepper
- 1 medium vine tomato
- 3 tablespoons basil, fresh chopped

Directions:
1. Preheat the oven to 400 degrees F and grease a baking dish. Microwave mozzarella cheese for about 30 seconds and top with the remaining pizza crust.
2. Add the remaining pizza ingredients to the cheese and mix together. Flatten the dough and transfer in the oven.
3. Bake for about 10 minutes and remove pizza from the oven. Top the pizza with the toppings and bake for another 10 minutes.
4. Remove pizza from the oven and allow to cool.

Nutrition: Calories: 381; Protein: 25.3 Grams; Fat: 12.9 Grams; Carbs: 9.7 Grams; Sodium: 480 mg; Cholesterol: 37 mg

119. Basil & Artichoke Pizza

Preparation time: 1 hour
Cooking time: 20 minutes
Servings: 4
Ingredients:
- 1 cup canned passata
- 2 cups flour
- 1 cup lukewarm water
- 1 pinch of sugar
- 1 tsp. active dry yeast
- ¾ tsp. salt 2 tbsp. olive oil
- 1 ½ cups frozen artichoke hearts
- ¼ cup grated Asiago cheese
- ½ onion, minced
- 3 garlic cloves, minced
- 1 tbsp. dried oregano
- 1 cup sun-dried tomatoes, chopped
- ½ tsp. red pepper flakes
- 5-6 basil leaves, torn

Directions:
1. Sift the flour and salt in a bowl and stir in yeast. Mix lukewarm water, olive oil, and sugar in another bowl.
2. Add the wet mixture to the dry mixture and whisk until you obtain a soft dough. Place the dough on a lightly floured work surface and knead it thoroughly for 4-5 minutes until elastic.
3. Transfer the dough to a greased bowl. Cover with cling film and leave to rise for 50-60 minutes in a warm place until doubled in size.
4. Roll out the dough to a thickness of around 12 inches. Preheat oven to 400 F. Warm oil in a saucepan over medium heat and sauté onion and garlic for 3-4 minutes.
5. Mix in tomatoes and oregano and bring to a boil. Decrease the heat and simmer for another 5 minutes.
6. Transfer the pizza crust to a baking sheet. Spread the sauce all over and top with artichoke hearts and sun-dried tomatoes.
7. Scatter the cheese and bake for 15 minutes until golden. Top with red pepper flakes and basil leaves and serve sliced.

Nutrition: Calories: 381; Protein: 25.3 Grams; Fat: 12.9 Grams; Carbs: 9.7 Grams; Sodium: 480 mg; Cholesterol: 37 mg

120. Spanish-Style Pizza de Jarmon

Preparation time: 10 minutes
Cooking time: 35 minutes
Servings: 4
Ingredients:
- For the crust
- 2 cups flour
- 1 cup lukewarm water
- 1 pinch of sugar
- 1 tsp. active dry yeast
- ¾ tsp. salt
- 2 tbsp. olive oil
- For the topping
- ½ cup tomato sauce

- ½ cup sliced mozzarella cheese
- 4 oz. jamon serrano, sliced
- 7 fresh basil leaves

Directions:
1. Sift the flour and salt in a bowl and stir in yeast. Mix lukewarm water, olive oil, and sugar in another bowl.
2. Add the wet mixture to the dry mixture and whisk until you obtain a soft dough. Place the dough on a lightly floured work surface and knead it thoroughly for 4-5 minutes until elastic.
3. Transfer the dough to a greased bowl. Cover with cling film and leave to rise for 50-60 minutes in a warm place until doubled in size.
4. Roll out the dough to a thickness of around 12 inches. Preheat the oven to 400 F. Line a pizza pan with parchment paper.
5. Spread the tomato sauce on the crust. Arrange the mozzarella slices on the sauce and then the jamon serrano. Bake for 15 minutes or until the cheese melts.
6. Remove from the oven and top with the basil. Slice and serve warm.

Nutrition: Calories: 381; Protein: 25.3 Grams; Fat: 12.9 Grams; Carbs: 9.7 Grams; Sodium: 480 mg; Cholesterol: 37 mg

121. Curry Chicken Pockets

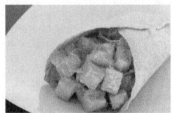

Preparation time: 10 minutes
Cooking time: 25 minutes
Servings: 4
Ingredients:
- 2 Cups Chicken, Cooked & Chopped
- ½ Cup Celery, Chopped
- 1/3 Cup Ricotta Cheese, Part Skim
- 1/ Cup Carrot, Shredded
- 1 Teaspoon Curry Powder
- 1 Tablespoon Apricot Preserved
- 10 Ounces Refrigerated Pizza Dough
- ¼ Teaspoon Sea Salt
- ¼ Teaspoon Ground Cinnamon

Directions:
1. Mix your carrot, ricotta, preserves, celery, chicken, cinnamon, salt and curry powder.
2. Spread the pizza dough and slice it into six equal squares.
3. Divide your mixture between each one, and then fold the corners of each towards the center and pinch them together. Put them on the baking sheet, baking at 375 for fifteen minutes. They should turn golden brown.
4. Allow them to cool before serving warm.

Nutrition: Calories: 415; Protein: 31.2 Grams; Fat: 32.7 Grams; Carbs: 14.7 Grams; Sodium: 277 mg; Cholesterol: 4.1 mg

122. Fajita Style Chili

Preparation time: 10 minutes
Cooking time: 5 hours
Servings: 4
Ingredients:
- 1 Teaspoon Fajita Seasoning
- 1 Tablespoon Chili Powder
- 2 lbs. Chicken Breasts, Boneless & Cubed
- ½ Teaspoon Cumin, Ground
- 2 Cloves Garlic, Minced
- Nonstick Cooking Spray as Needed
- 2 Cans (14.5 Ounces Each) Tomatoes, Diced
- ½ Green Bell Pepper, Julienned
- ½ Red Bell Pepper, Julienned
- ½ Yellow Bell Pepper, Julienned
- ½ Onion, Sliced
- 15 Ounces White Kidney Beans, Rinsed & Drained (Canned)
- 3 Tablespoons Sour Cream
- 3 Tablespoon Cheddar Cheese, Shredded & Reduced Fat
- 3 Tablespoons Guacamole

Directions:
1. Mix your chicken with fajita seasoning, garlic, cumin, and chili powder.
2. Grease a skillet and place it over medium heat. Add in your chicken, cooking until its golden brown.
3. Transfer it to a slow cooker, and then add in your tomatoes with their juices, vegetables, and beans. Cover, and cook on low for five hours.
4. Garnish with guacamole, cheese and sour cream before serving warm.

Nutrition: Calories: 495; Protein: 67.4 Grams; Fat: 11.5 Grams; Carbs: 10.2 Grams; Sodium: 212 mg; Cholesterol: 183 mg

123. Fun Fajita Wraps

Preparation time: 10 minutes
Cooking time: 10 minutes
Servings: 4
Ingredients:
- Nonstick Cooking Spray
- ¼ Teaspoon Garlic Powder
- ½ Teaspoon Chili Powder
- 12 Ounces Chicken Breasts, Skinless & Sliced into Strips
- 1 Green Sweet Pepper, Seeded & Sliced into Strips
- 2 Tortilla, 10 Inches & Whole Wheat
- 2 Tablespoons Ranch Salad Dressing, Reduced Calorie
- ½ Cup Salsa
- 1/3 Cup Cheddar Cheese, Shredded & Reduced Fat

Directions:
1. Mix your chicken strips with chili powder and garlic powder. Heat a skillet and grease with cooking spray. Place it over medium heat, and add in your sweet pepper and chicken. Cook for six minutes.
2. Toss your salad dressing in, and divide between tortillas.
3. Top with salsa and cheese, and roll your tortilla before slicing them in half. Serve warm.

Nutrition: Calories: 245, Protein: 38.5 Grams, Fat: 16.4 Grams, Carbs: 8.7 Grams, Sodium: 471 mg, Cholesterol: 143 mg

124. Classic Chicken Noodle Soup

Preparation time: 10 minutes
Cooking time: 20 minutes
Serves: 4
Ingredients:
- 1 Teaspoon Olive Oil
- 1 Cup Onion, Chopped
- 3 Cloves Garlic, Minced
- 1 Cup Celery, Chopped
- 1 Cup Carrots, Sliced & Peeled
- 4 Cups Chicken Broth
- 4 Ounces Linguini, Dried & Broken
- 1 Cup Chicken Breast, Cooked & Chopped
- 2 Tablespoons Parsley, Fresh

Directions:
1. Put a saucepan over medium heat, and heat up your oil. Stir in your onion and garlic, cooking until soften.
2. Add your celery and carrots. Cook for three minutes before adding your broth. Allow it to come to a boil before reducing it to simmer. Cook for five minutes before adding in your linguini.
3. Bring it to a boil and reduce the heat to simmer. Cook for ten more minutes.
4. Add in your parsley and chicken, and then cook until heated all the way through. Serve warm.

Nutrition: Calories: 381; Protein: 25.3 Grams; Fat: 12.9 Grams; Carbs: 9.7 Grams; Sodium: 480 mg; Cholesterol: 37 mg

125. Open Face Egg and Bacon Sandwich

Preparation time: 10 minutes
Cooking Time: 20 minutes
Servings: 1
Ingredients:
- ¼ oz. reduced fat cheddar, shredded
- ½ small jalapeno, thinly sliced
- ½ whole grain English muffin, split
- 1 large organic egg
- 1 thick slice of tomato
- 1-piece turkey bacon
- 2 thin slices red onion
- 4-5 sprigs fresh cilantro
- Cooking spray
- Pepper to taste

Directions:
1. On medium fire, place a skillet, cook bacon until crisp tender and set aside. In same skillet, drain oils, and place ½ of English muffin and heat for at least a minute per side.
2. Transfer muffin to a serving plate. Coat the same skillet with cooking spray and fry egg to desired doneness.
3. Once cooked, place egg on top of muffin. Add cilantro, tomato, onion, jalapeno and bacon on top of egg.
4. Serve and enjoy.

Nutrition: Calories: 381; Protein: 25.3 Grams; Fat: 12.9 Grams; Carbs: 9.7 Grams; Sodium: 480 mg; Cholesterol: 37 mg

126. Tuscan Stew

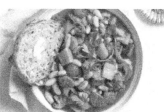

Preparation time: 10 minutes
Cooking time: 1 hour and 30 minutes
Servings: 6
Ingredients:
- Croutons:
- 1 Tablespoons Olive Oil
- 1 Slice Bread, Whole Grain & Cubed
- 2 Cloves Garlic, Quartered
- Soup:
- 1 Bay Leaf
- 2 Cups White Beans, Soaked Overnight & Drained
- 6 Cups Water
- ½ Teaspoon Sea Salt, Divided
- 1 Cup Yellow Onion, Chopped
- 2 Tablespoons Olive Oil
- 3 Carrots, Peeled & Chopped
- 6 Cloves Garlic, Chopped
- ¼ Teaspoon Ground Black Pepper
- 1 Tablespoons Rosemary, Fresh & Chopped
- 1 ½ Cups Vegetable Stock

Directions:
1. Add your oil to a skillet and heat it, and then cook your garlic for a minute. It should become fragrant. Allow it to sit for ten minutes before removing your garlic from the oil.
2. Return the pan with the oil to heat and then throw in your bread cubes. Cook for five minutes. They should be golden, and then set them to the side.
3. Mix your salt, water, bay leaf and white beans in the pot, boiling on high heat before reducing to a simmer.
4. Cover the beans and cook for one hour to one hour and ten minutes. They should be al dente.
5. Drain the beans, but reserve a half a cup of the cooking liquid. Discard the bay leaf, and transfer your beans to a bowl.
6. Mix the reserved liquid with ½ cup of beans, returning it to a boil. Mash with a fork to form a paste, and then place the pot on the stove. Heat the oil using the pot.
7. Add in your onions and carrots. Cook for seven minutes and add garlic, and then cook for a minute more. Add in your rosemary, salt, pepper, stock and bean mixture.
8. Allow it to come to a boil and then reduce the heat to let it simmer. Let it simmer for five minutes, and then top with croutons. Garnish with rosemary sprigs and enjoy.

Nutrition: Calories: 307; Protein: 16 Grams; Fat: 7 Grams; Carbs: 45 Grams; Sodium: 463 mg; Cholesterol: 68 mg

127. Tenderloin Fajitas

Preparation time: 10 minutes
Cooking time: 25 minutes
Servings: 8

Ingredients:

- ¼ Teaspoon Garlic Powder
- ¼ Teaspoon Ground Coriander
- 1 Tablespoon Chili Powder
- ½ Teaspoon Paprika
- ½ Teaspoon Oregano
- 1 lb. Pork Tenderloin, Sliced into Strips
- 8 Flour Tortillas, Whole Wheat & Warned
- 1 Small Onion, Sliced
- ½ Cup Cheddar Cheese, Shredded
- 4 Tomatoes, Diced
- 1 Cup Salsa
- 4 Cups Lettuce, Shredded

Directions:

1. Preheat a grill to 400, and then mix your coriander, garlic, oregano, paprika, and coriander in a bowl. Add in the pork slices, making sure they're well coated.
2. Arrange your pork and onions on a grilling grate, grilling for five minutes per side.
3. Stuff the tortillas with the mixture, topping with two tablespoons tomatoes, a tablespoon of cheese, ½ cup shredded lettuce and two tablespoons of salsa. Fold your tortillas and serve warm.

Nutrition: Calories: 250; Protein: 44 Grams; Fat: 9.8 Grams; Carbs: 21.1 Grams; Sodium: 671 mg; Cholesterol: 22 mg

128. Peanut Sauce Chicken Pasta

Preparation Time: 10 minutes
Cooking time: 20 minutes
Servings: 4
Ingredients:

- 2 Teaspoons Olive Oil
- 6 Ounces Spaghetti, Whole Wheat
- 10 Ounces Snap Peas, Fresh & Trimmed & Sliced into Strips
- 2 Cups Carrots, Julienned
- 2 Cups Chicken, Cooked & Shredded
- 1 Cup Thai Peanut Sauce
- 1 Cucumber, Halved Lengthwise & Sliced Diagonally
- Cilantro, Fresh & Chopped

Directions:

1. Start by cooking spaghetti as the package instructs, and then drain them and rinse the noodles using cold water.
2. Heat your greased skillet using oil, placing it over medium heat.
3. Once it's hot, add in your snap peas and carrot. Cook for eight minutes, and stir in your spaghetti, chicken and peanut sauce. Toss well, and garnish with cucumber and cilantro.

Nutrition: Calories: 403; Protein: 31 Grams; Fat: 15 Grams; Carbs: 43 Grams; Sodium: 432 mg; Cholesterol: 42 mg

129. Chicken Cherry Wraps

Preparation time: 10 minutes
Cooking time: 10 minutes
Serves: 4
Ingredients:

- ¼ Teaspoon Sea Salt, Fine
- ¼ Teaspoon Black Pepper
- 2 Teaspoons Olive oil
- ¾ lb. Chicken Breasts, Boneless & Cubed
- 1 Teaspoon Ginger, Ground
- 1 ½ Cups Carrots, Shredded
- 1 ¼ Cup Sweet Cherries, Fresh, Pitted & Chopped
- 4 Green Onions, Chopped
- 2 Tablespoons Rice Vinegar
- 1/3 Cup Almonds, Chopped Roughly
- 2 Tablespoons Rice Vinegar
- 2 Tablespoons Teriyaki Sauce, Low Sodium
- 1 Tablespoon Honey Raw
- 8 Large Lettuce Leaves

Directions:

1. Season your chicken using ginger, salt and pepper.
2. Get out a skillet, placing over medium heat and adding in your oil. Once your oil is hot cook your chicken for five minutes.
3. Throw in your cherries, green onions, carrots and almonds.
4. Add in your vinegar, teriyaki and honey before making sure it's mixed well, and your chicken is cooked all the way through.
5. Spread this on lettuce leaves to serve.

Nutrition: Calories: 257; Protein: 21 Grams; Fat: 10 Grams; Carbs: 21 Grams; Sodium: 381 mg; Cholesterol: 47 mg

130. Easy Barley Soup

Preparation time: 10 minutes
Cooking time: 20 minutes
Servings: 4
Ingredients:

- 1 Tablespoon Olive Oil
- 1 Onion, Chopped
- 5 Carrots, Chopped
- 2/3 Cup Barley, Quick Cooking
- 6 Cups Chicken Broth, Reduced Sodium
- ½ Teaspoon Black Pepper
- 2 Cups Baby Spinach, Fresh
- 2 Cups Turkey Breast, Cooked & Cubed

Directions:

1. Start by getting a saucepan and heat your oil over medium high heat.
2. Stir in your carrots and onion and sauté for five minutes before adding in your barley and broth. Bring it to a boil before reducing too low to simmer. Cook for fifteen minutes.
3. Stir in your pepper, spinach and turkey. Mix well before serving.

Nutrition: Calories: 208; Protein: 21 Grams; Fat: 4 Grams; Carbs: 23 Grams; Sodium: 662 mg; Cholesterol: 37 mg

131. Cauliflower Lunch Salad

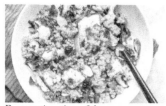

Preparation time: 2 hours
Cooking time: 10 minutes
Servings: 4
Ingredients:

- 1/3 cup low-sodium veggie stock
- 2 tablespoons olive oil
- 6 cups cauliflower florets, grated
- Black pepper to the taste
- ¼ cup red onion, chopped
- 1 red bell pepper, chopped
- Juice of ½ lemon
- ½ cup Kalamata olives halved
- 1 teaspoon mint, chopped
- 1 tablespoon cilantro, chopped

Directions:
1. Heat-up a pan with the oil over medium-high heat, add cauliflower, pepper and stock, stir, cook within 10 minutes, transfer to a bowl, and keep in the fridge for 2 hours.
2. Mix cauliflower with olives, onion, bell pepper, black pepper, mint, and cilantro, and lemon juice, toss to coat, and serve.

Nutrition: Calories: 102; Carbs: 3g; Fat: 10g; Protein: 0g; Sodium 97 mg

132. Cheesy Black Bean Wraps

Preparation time: 5 minutes
Cooking time: 10 minutes
Servings: 6
Ingredients:

- 2 Tablespoons Green Chili Peppers, Chopped
- 4 Green Onions, Diced
- 1 Tomato, Diced
- 1 Tablespoon Garlic, Chopped
- 6 Tortilla Wraps, Whole Grain & Fat Free
- ¾ Cup Cheddar Cheese, Shredded
- ¾ Cup Salsa
- 1 ½ Cups Corn Kernels
- 3 Tablespoons Cilantro, Fresh & Chopped
- 1 ½ Cup Black Beans, Canned & Drained

Directions:
1. Toss your chili peppers, corn, black beans, garlic, tomato, onions and cilantro in a bowl.
2. Heat the mixture in a microwave for a minute, and stir for a half a minute.
3. Spread the two tortillas between paper towels and microwave for twenty seconds. Warm the remaining tortillas the same way, and add a half a cup of bean mixture, two tablespoons of salsa and two tablespoons of cheese for each tortilla. Roll them up before serving.

Nutrition: Calories: 341; Protein: 19 Grams; Fat: 11 Grams; Carbs: 36.5 Grams; Sodium: 141 mg; Cholesterol: 0 mg

133. Arugula Risotto

Preparation time: 10 minutes
Cooking time: 15 minutes
Servings: 4
Ingredients:

- 1 Tablespoon Olive Oil
- ½ Cup Yellow Onion, Chopped
- 1 Cup Quinoa, Rinsed
- 1 Clove Garlic, Minced
- 2 ½ Cups Vegetable Stock, Low Sodium
- 2 Cups Arugula, Chopped & Stemmed
- 1 Carrot, Peeled & shredded
- ½ Cup Shiitake Mushrooms, Sliced
- ¼ Teaspoon Black Pepper
- ¼ Teaspoon Sea Salt, Fine
- ¼ Cup Parmesan Cheese, Grated

Directions:
1. Get a saucepan and place it over medium heat, heating up your oil. Cook for four minutes until your onions are softened, and then add in your garlic and quinoa. Cook for a minute.
2. Stir in your stock, and bring it to a boil. Reduce it to simmer, and cook for twelve minutes.
3. Add in your arugula, mushrooms and carrots, cooking for an additional two minutes.
4. Add in salt, pepper and cheese before serving.

Nutrition: Calories: 288; Protein: 6 Grams; Fat: 5 Grams; Carbs: 28 Grams; Sodium: 739 mg; Cholesterol: 0.5 mg

134. Vegetarian Stuffed Eggplant

Preparation Time: 10 minutes
Cooking time: 25 minutes
Servings: 2
Ingredients:

- 4 Ounces White Beans, Cooked
- 1 Tablespoons Olive Oil
- 1 cup Water
- 1 Eggplant
- ¼ Cup Onion, Chopped
- ½ Cup Bell Pepper, Chopped
- 1 Cup Canned Tomatoes, Unsalted
- ¼ Cup Tomato Liquid
- ¼ Cup Celery, Chopped
- 1 Cup Mushrooms, Fresh & Sliced
- ¾ Cup Breadcrumbs, Whole Wheat
- Black Pepper to Taste

Directions:
1. Preheat the oven to 350, and then grease a baking dish with cooking spray.
2. Trim the eggplant and cut it in half lengthwise. Scoop the pulp out using a spoon, leaving a shell that's a quarter of an inch thick.
3. Place the shells in the baking dish with their cut side up.

4. Add the water to the bottom of the dish, and dice the eggplant pulp into cubes, setting them to the side.
5. Add the oil into an iron skillet, heating it over medium heat.
6. Stir in peppers, chopped eggplants, and onions with your celery, mushrooms, tomatoes and tomato juice.
7. Cook for ten minutes on simmering heat, and then stir in your bread crumbs, beans and black pepper. Divide the mixture between eggshells.
8. Cover with foil, and bake for fifteen minutes. Serve warm.

Nutrition: Calories: 334; Protein: 26 Grams; Fat: 10 Grams; Carbs: 35 Grams; Sodium: 142 mg; Cholesterol: 162 mg

135. Vegetable Tacos

Preparation time: 10 minutes
Cooking time: 20 minutes
Servings: 4
Ingredients:
- 1 Tablespoon Olive Oil
- 1 Cup Red Onion, Chopped
- 1 Cup Yellow Summer Squash, Diced
- 1 Cup Green Zucchini, Diced
- 3 Cloves Garlic, Minced
- 4 Tomatoes, Seeded & Chopped
- 1 Jalapeno Chili, Seeded & Chopped
- 1 Cup Corn Kernels, Fresh
- 1 Cup Pinto Beans, Canned, Rinsed & Drained
- ½ Cup Cilantro, Fresh & Chopped
- 8 Corn Tortillas
- ½ Cup Smoke Flavored Salsa

Directions:
1. Get out a saucepan and add in your olive oil over medium heat, and stir in your onion. Cook until softened.
2. Add in your squash and zucchini, cooking for an additional five minutes.
3. Stir in your garlic, beans, tomatoes, jalapeño and corn. Cook for an additional five minutes before stirring in your cilantro and removing the pan from heat.
4. Warm each tortilla, in a nonstick skillet for twenty seconds per side.
5. Place the tortillas on a serving plate, spooning the vegetable mixture into each. Top with salsa, and roll to serve.

Nutrition: Calories: 310; Protein: 10 Grams; Fat: 6 Grams; Carbs: 54 Grams; Sodium: 97 mg; Cholesterol: 20 mg

136. Lemongrass and Chicken Soup

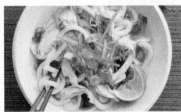

Preparation time: 10 minutes
Cooking time: 25 minutes

Servings: 4
Ingredients:
- 4 lime leaves, torn
- 4 cups veggie stock, low-sodium
- 1 lemongrass stalk, chopped
- 1 tablespoon ginger, grated
- 1-pound chicken breast, skinless, boneless, and cubed
- 8 ounces mushrooms, chopped
- 4 Thai chilies, chopped
- 13 ounces of coconut milk
- ¼ cup lime juice
- ¼ cup cilantro, chopped
- A pinch of black pepper

Directions:
1. Put the stock into a pot, bring to a simmer over medium heat, add lemongrass, ginger, and lime leaves, stir, cook for 10 minutes, strain into another pot, and heat up over medium heat again.
2. Add chicken, mushrooms, milk, cilantro, black pepper, chilies, and lime juice, stir, simmer for 15 minutes, ladle into bowls and serve.

Nutrition: Calories: 105; Carbs: 1g; Fat: 2g; Protein: 15g; Sodium 200 mg

137. Easy Lunch Salmon Steaks

Preparation time: 10 minutes
Cooking time: 20 minutes
Servings: 4
Ingredients:
- 1 big salmon fillet, cut into 4 steaks
- 3 garlic cloves, minced
- 1 yellow onion, chopped
- Black pepper to the taste
- 2 tablespoons olive oil
- ¼ cup parsley, chopped
- Juice of 1 lemon
- 1 tablespoon thyme, chopped
- 4 cups of water

Directions:
1. Heat a pan with the oil on medium-high heat, cook onion and garlic within 3 minutes.
2. Add black pepper, parsley, thyme, and water, and lemon juice, stir, bring to a gentle boil, add salmon steaks, cook them for 15 minutes, drain, divide between plates and serve with a side salad for lunch.

Nutrition: Calories: 110; Carbs: 3g; Fat: 4g; Protein: 15g; Sodium 330 mg

138. Light Balsamic Salad

Preparation time: 10 minutes
Cooking time: 0 minutes
Servings: 3
Ingredients:
- 1 orange, cut into segments
- 2 green onions, chopped
- 1 romaine lettuce head, torn

- 1 avocado, pitted, peeled, and cubed
- ¼ cup almonds, sliced
- For the salad dressing:
- 1 teaspoon mustard
- ¼ cup olive oil
- 2 tablespoons balsamic vinegar
- Juice of ½ orange
- Salt and black pepper

Directions:
1. In a salad bowl, mix oranges with avocado, lettuce, almonds, and green onions.
2. In another bowl, mix olive oil with vinegar, mustard, orange juice, salt, and pepper, whisk well, add this to your salad, toss and serve.

Nutrition: Calories: 35; Carbs: 5g; Fat: 2g; Protein: 0; Sodium 400 mg

139. Purple Potato Soup

Preparation time: 10 minutes
Cooking time: 1 hour and 15 minutes
Servings: 6
Ingredients:
- 6 purple potatoes, chopped
- 1 cauliflower head, florets separated
- Black pepper to the taste
- 4 garlic cloves, minced
- 1 yellow onion, chopped
- 3 tablespoons olive oil
- 1 tablespoon thyme, chopped
- 1 leek, chopped
- 2 shallots, chopped
- 4 cups chicken stock, low-sodium

Directions:
1. In a baking dish, mix potatoes with onion, cauliflower, garlic, pepper, thyme, and half of the oil, toss to coat, introduce in the oven and bake for 45 minutes at 400 degrees F.
2. Heat a pot with the rest of the oil over medium-high heat, add leeks and shallots, stir and cook for 10 minutes.
3. Add roasted veggies and stock, stir, bring to a boil, cook for 20 minutes, transfer soup to your food processor, blend well, divide into bowls, and serve.

Nutrition: Calories: 70; Carbs: 15g; Fat: 0g; Protein: 2g; Sodium 6 mg

140. Leeks Soup

Preparation time: 10 minutes
Cooking time: 1 hour and 15 minutes
Servings: 6
Ingredients:
- 2 gold potatoes, chopped
- 1 cup cauliflower florets
- Black pepper to the taste
- 5 leeks, chopped
- 4 garlic cloves, minced
- 1 yellow onion, chopped
- 3 tablespoons olive oil
- Handful parsley, chopped

- 4 cups low-sodium chicken stock

Directions:
1. Heat-up a pot with the oil over medium-high heat, add onion and garlic, stir and cook for 5 minutes.
2. Add potatoes, cauliflower, and black pepper, leeks, and stock, stir, bring to a simmer, cook over medium heat for 30 minutes, blend using an immersion blender, add parsley, stir, ladle into bowls and serve.

Nutrition: Calories: 125; Carbs: 29g; Fat: 1g; Protein: 4g; Sodium 52 mg

141. Rice with Chicken

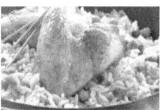

Preparation time: 10 minutes
Cooking time: 30 minutes
Servings: 4
Ingredients:
- ½ cup coconut aminos
- 1/3 cup rice wine vinegar
- 2 tablespoons olive oil
- 1 chicken breast, skinless, boneless, and cubed
- ½ cup red bell pepper, chopped
- A pinch of black pepper
- 2 garlic cloves, minced
- ½ teaspoon ginger, grated
- ½ cup carrots, grated
- 1 cup white rice
- 2 cups of water

Directions:
1. Heat-up a pan with the oil over medium-high heat, add the chicken, stir and brown for 4 minutes on each side.
2. Add aminos, vinegar, bell pepper, black pepper, garlic, ginger, carrots, rice and stock, stock, cover the pan and cook over medium heat for 20 minutes.
3. Divide everything into bowls and serve for lunch. Enjoy!

Nutrition: Calories: 70; Carbs: 13g; Fat: 2g; Protein: 2g; Sodium 5 mg

142. Tomato Soup

Preparation time: 10 minutes
Cooking time: 20 minutes
Servings: 4
Ingredients:
- 3 garlic cloves, minced
- 1 yellow onion, chopped
- 3 carrots, chopped
- 15 ounces tomato sauce, no-salt-added
- 1 tablespoon olive oil
- 15 ounces roasted tomatoes, no-salt-added
- 1 cup low-sodium veggie stock
- 1 tablespoon tomato paste, no-salt-added
- 1 tablespoon basil, dried

- ¼ teaspoon oregano, dried
- 3 ounces coconut cream
- A pinch of black pepper

Directions:
1. Heat-up a pot with the oil over medium heat, add garlic and onion, stir and cook for 5 minutes.
2. Add carrots, tomato sauce, tomatoes, stock, tomato paste, basil, oregano, and black pepper, stir, bring to a simmer, cook for 15 minutes, add cream, blend the soup using an immersion blender, divide into bowls and serve for lunch. Enjoy!

Nutrition: Calories: 90; Carbs: 20g; Fat: 0g; Protein: 2g; Sodium 480 mg

143. Cod Soup

Preparation time: 10 minutes
Cooking time: 25 minutes
Servings: 4

Ingredients:
- 1 yellow onion, chopped
- 12 cups low-sodium fish stock
- 1-pound carrots, sliced
- 1 tablespoon olive oil
- Black pepper to the taste
- 2 tablespoons ginger, minced
- 1 cup of water
- 1-pound cod, skinless, boneless, and cut into medium chunks

Directions:
1. Heat-up a pot with the oil over medium-high heat, add onion, stir and cook for 4 minutes. Add water, stock, ginger, and carrots, stir and cook for 10 minutes more.
2. Blend soup using an immersion blender, add the fish and pepper, stir, cook for 10 minutes more, ladle into bowls and serve. Enjoy!

Nutrition: Calories: 344; Carbs: 35g; Fat: 4g; Protein: 46g; Sodium 334 mg

144. Sweet Potato Soup

Preparation time: 10 minutes
Cooking time: 1 hour and 40 minutes
Servings: 6

Ingredients:
- 4 big sweet potatoes
- 28 ounces veggie stock
- A pinch of black pepper
- ¼ teaspoon nutmeg, ground
- 1/3 cup low-sodium heavy cream

Directions:
1. Put the sweet potatoes on a lined baking sheet, bake them at 350 degrees F for 1 hour and 30 minutes, cool them down, peel, roughly chop them, and put them in a pot.
2. Add stock, nutmeg, cream, and pepper pulse well using an immersion blender, heat the soup over medium heat, cook for 10 minutes, ladle into bowls and serve. Enjoy!

Nutrition: Calories: 110; Carbs: 23g; Fat: 1g; Protein: 2g; Sodium 140 mg

145. Sweet Potatoes and Zucchini Soup

Preparation time: 10 minutes
Cooking time: 20 minutes
Servings: 8

Ingredients:
- 4 cups veggie stock
- 2 tablespoons olive oil
- 2 sweet potatoes, peeled and cubed
- 8 zucchinis, chopped
- 2 yellow onions, chopped
- 1 cup of coconut milk
- A pinch of black pepper
- 1 tablespoon coconut aminos
- 4 tablespoons dill, chopped
- ½ teaspoon basil, chopped

Directions:
1. Heat-up a pot with the oil over medium heat, add onion, stir and cook for 5 minutes.
2. Add zucchinis, stock, basil, potato, and pepper, stir and cook for 15 minutes more.
3. Add milk, aminos, and dill, pulse using an immersion blender, ladle into bowls and serve for lunch.

Nutrition: Calories: 270; Carbs: 50g; Fat: 4g; Protein: 11g; Sodium 416 mg

146. Hearty Chicken Fried Rice

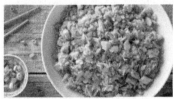

Preparation time: 10 minutes
Cooking time: 12 minutes
Servings: 4

Ingredients:
- 1 teaspoon olive oil
- 4 large egg whites
- 1 onion, chopped
- 2 garlic cloves, minced
- 12 ounces skinless chicken breasts, boneless, cut into ½ inch cubes
- ½ cup carrots, chopped
- ½ cup frozen green peas
- 2 cups long grain brown rice, cooked
- 3 tablespoons soy sauce, low sodium

Directions:
1. Coat skillet with oil, place it over medium-high heat.
2. Add egg whites and cook until scrambled.
3. Sauté onion, garlic and chicken breasts for 6 minutes.
4. Add carrots, peas and keep cooking for 3 minutes.
5. Stir in rice, season with soy sauce.
6. Add cooked egg whites, stir for 3 minutes.
7. Enjoy!

Nutrition: Calories: 353; Fat: 11g; Carbohydrates: 30g; Protein: 23g

147. Creamy Chicken Breast

Preparation time: 10 minutes
Cooking time: 20 minutes
Servings: 4
Ingredients:

- 1 tablespoon olive oil
- A pinch of black pepper
- 2 pounds chicken breasts, skinless, boneless, and cubed
- 4 garlic cloves, minced
- 2 and ½ cups low-sodium chicken stock
- 2 cups coconut cream
- ½ cup low-fat parmesan, grated
- 1 tablespoon basil, chopped

Directions:

1. Heat-up a pan with the oil over medium-high heat, add chicken cubes, and brown them for 3 minutes on each side.
2. Add garlic, black pepper, stock, and cream, toss, cover the pan and cook everything for 10 minutes more.
3. Add cheese and basil, toss, divide between plates and serve for lunch. Enjoy!

Nutrition: Calories 221; Fat 6g; Fiber 9g; Carbs 14g; Protein 7g; Sodium 197 mg

148. Indian Chicken Stew

Preparation time: 1 hour
Cooking time: 20 minutes
Servings: 4
Ingredients:

- 1-pound chicken breasts, skinless, boneless, and cubed
- 1 tablespoon garam masala
- 1 cup fat-free yogurt
- 1 tablespoon lemon juice
- A pinch of black pepper
- ¼ teaspoon ginger, ground
- 15 ounces tomato sauce, no-salt-added
- 5 garlic cloves, minced
- ½ teaspoon sweet paprika

Directions:

1. In a bowl, mix the chicken with garam masala, yogurt, lemon juice, black pepper, ginger, and fridge for 1 hour. Heat-up a pan over medium heat, add chicken mix, toss and cook for 5-6 minutes.
2. Add tomato sauce, garlic and paprika, toss, cook for 15 minutes, divide between plates and serve for lunch. Enjoy!

Nutrition: Calories 221; Fat 6g; Fiber 9g; Carbs 14g; Protein 16g; Sodium 4 mg

149. Chicken, Bamboo, and Chestnuts Mix

Preparation time: 10 minutes
Cooking time: 20 minutes
Servings: 4
Ingredients:

- 1-pound chicken thighs, boneless, skinless, and cut into medium chunks
- 1 cup low-sodium chicken stock
- 1 tablespoon olive oil
- 2 tablespoons coconut aminos
- 1-inch ginger, grated
- 1 carrot, sliced
- 2 garlic cloves, minced
- 8 ounces canned bamboo shoots, no-salt-added and drained
- 8 ounces water chestnuts

Directions:

1. Heat-up a pan with the oil over medium-high heat, add chicken, stir, and brown for 4 minutes on each side.
2. Add the stock, aminos, ginger, carrot, garlic, bamboo, and chestnuts, toss, cover the pan, and cook everything over medium heat for 12 minutes.
3. Divide everything between plates and serve. Enjoy!

Nutrition: Calories 281; Fat 7g; Fiber 9g; Carbs 14g; Protein 14g; Sodium 125mg

150. Salsa Chicken

Preparation time: 10 minutes
Cooking time: 25 minutes
Servings: 4
Ingredients:

- 1 cup mild salsa, no-salt-added
- ½ teaspoon cumin, ground
- Black pepper to the taste
- 1 tablespoon chipotle paste
- 1-pound chicken thighs, skinless and boneless
- 2 cups corn
- Juice of 1 lime
- ½ tablespoon olive oil
- 2 tablespoons cilantro, chopped
- 1 cup cherry tomatoes, halved
- 1 small avocado, pitted, peeled, and cubed

Directions:

1. In a pot, combine the salsa with the cumin, black pepper, chipotle paste, chicken thighs, and corn, toss, bring to a simmer and cook over medium heat for 25 minutes.
2. Add lime juice, oil, cherry tomatoes, and avocado, toss, divide into bowls and serve for lunch. Enjoy!

Nutrition: Calories 269; Fat 6g; Fiber 9g; Carbs 18g; Protein 7g; Sodium 500 mg

151. Hearty Roasted Cauliflower

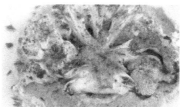

Preparation time: 5 minutes
Cooking time: 30 minutes
Servings: 8
Ingredients:

- 1 large cauliflower head
- 2 tablespoons melted coconut oil
- 2 tablespoons fresh thyme
- 1 teaspoon Celtic sea sunflower seeds
- 1 teaspoon fresh ground pepper
- 1 head roasted garlic
- 2 tablespoons fresh thyme for garnish

Directions:
1. Pre-heat your oven to 425 degrees F.
2. Rinse cauliflower and trim, core and sliced.
3. Lay cauliflower evenly on rimmed baking tray.
4. Drizzle coconut oil evenly over cauliflower, sprinkle thyme leaves.
5. Season with pinch of sunflower seeds and pepper.
6. Squeeze roasted garlic.
7. Roast cauliflower until slightly caramelized for about 30 minutes, making sure to turn once.
8. Garnish with fresh thyme leaves.
9. Enjoy!

Nutrition: Calories: 129; Fat: 11g; Carbohydrates: 6g; Protein: 7g

152. Cool Cabbage Fried Beef

Preparation time: 5 minutes
Cooking time: 15 minutes
Servings: 4

Ingredients:
- 1 pound beef, ground and lean
- ½ pound bacon
- 1 onion
- 1 garlic cloves, minced
- ½ head cabbage
- pepper to taste

Directions:
1. Take skillet and place it over medium heat.
2. Add chopped bacon, beef and onion until slightly browned.
3. Transfer to a bowl and keep it covered.
4. Add minced garlic and cabbage to the skillet and cook until slightly browned.
5. Return the ground beef mix to the skillet and simmer for 3-5 minutes over low heat.
6. Serve and enjoy!

Nutrition: Calories: 360; Fat: 22g; Net Carbohydrates: 5g; Protein: 34g

153. Fennel and Figs Lamb

Preparation time: 10 minutes
Cooking time: 40 minutes
Servings: 2

Ingredients:
- 6 ounces lamb racks
- 1 fennel bulbs, sliced
- pepper to taste
- 1 tablespoon olive oil
- 2 figs, cut in half
- 1/8 cup apple cider vinegar
- 1/2 tablespoon swerve

Directions:

1. Take a bowl and add fennel, figs, vinegar, swerve, oil and toss.
2. Transfer to baking dish.
3. Season with sunflower seeds and pepper.
4. Bake for 15 minutes at 400 degrees F.
5. Season lamb with sunflower seeds and pepper and transfer to a heated pan over medium-high heat.
6. Cook for a few minutes.
7. Add lamb to the baking dish with fennel and bake for 20 minutes.
8. Divide between plates and serve.
9. Enjoy!

Nutrition: Calories: 230; Fat: 3g; Carbohydrates: 5g; Protein: 10g

154. Black Berry Chicken Wings

Preparation time: 35 minutes
Cooking time: 50 minutes
Servings: 4

Ingredients:
- 3 pounds chicken wings, about 20 pieces
- ½ cup blackberry chipotle jam
- Pepper to taste
- ½ cup water

Directions:
1. Add water and jam to a bowl and mix well.
2. Place chicken wings in a zip bag and add two-thirds of marinade.
3. Season with pepper.
4. Let it marinate for 30 minutes.
5. Pre-heat your oven to 400 degrees F.
6. Prepare a baking sheet and wire rack, place chicken wings in wire rack and bake for 15 minutes.
7. Brush remaining marinade and bake for 30 minutes more.
8. Enjoy!

Nutrition: Calories: 502; Fat: 39g; Carbohydrates: 01.8g; Protein: 34g

155. Mushroom and Olive "Mediterranean" Steak

Preparation time: 10 minutes
Cooking time: 14 minutes
Servings: 2

Ingredients:
- 1/2 pound boneless beef sirloin steak, ¾ inch thick, cut into 4 pieces
- 1/2 large red onion, chopped
- 1/2 cup mushrooms
- 2 garlic cloves, thinly sliced
- 2 tablespoons olive oil
- 1/4 cup green olives, coarsely chopped
- 1/2 cup parsley leaves, finely cut

Directions:
1. Take a large sized skillet and place it over medium-high heat.
2. Add oil and let it heat up.
3. Add beef and cook until both sides are browned, remove beef and drain fat.
4. Add the rest of the oil to the skillet and heat.

5. Add onions, garlic and cook for 2-3 minutes.
6. Stir well.
7. Add mushrooms, olives and cook until the mushrooms are thoroughly done.
8. Return the beef to the skillet and reduce heat to medium.
9. Cook for 3-4 minutes (covered).
10. Stir in parsley.
11. Serve and enjoy!

Nutrition: Calories: 386; Fat: 30g; Carbohydrates: 11g; Protein: 21g

156. Generous Lemon Dredged Broccoli

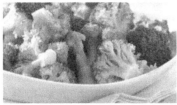

Preparation time: 10 minutes
Cooking time: 15 minutes
Servings: 4
Ingredients:
- 2 heads broccoli, separated into florets
- 2 teaspoons extra virgin olive oil
- 1 teaspoon sunflower seeds
- ½ teaspoon pepper
- 1 garlic clove, minced
- ½ teaspoon lemon juice

Directions:
1. Pre-heat your oven to a temperature of 400 degrees F.
2. Take a large sized bowl and add broccoli florets with some extra virgin olive oil, pepper, sea sunflower seeds and garlic.
3. Spread the broccoli out in a single even layer on a fine baking sheet.
4. Bake in your pre-heated oven for about 15-20 minutes until the florets are soft enough to be pierced with a fork.
5. Squeeze lemon juice over them generously before serving.
6. Enjoy!

Nutrition: Calories: 49; Fat: 2g; Carbohydrates: 4g; Protein: 3g

157. Tantalizing Almond butter Beans

Preparation time: 5 minutes
Cooking time: 12 minutes
Servings: 4
Ingredients:
- 2 garlic cloves, minced
- Red pepper flakes to taste
- Sunflower seeds to taste
- 2 tablespoons clarified butter
- 4 cups green beans, trimmed

Directions:
1. Bring a pot of water to boil, with added seeds for taste.
2. Once the water starts to boil, add beans and cook for 3 minutes.

3. Take a bowl of ice water and drain beans, plunge them into the ice water.
4. Once cooled, keep them on the side.
5. Take a medium skillet and place it over medium heat, add ghee and melt.
6. Add red pepper, sunflower seeds, garlic.
7. Cook for 1 minute.
8. Add beans and toss until coated well, cook for 3 minutes.
9. Serve and enjoy!

Nutrition: Calories: 93; Fat: 8g; Carbohydrates: 4g; Protein: 2g

158. Healthy Chicken Cream Salad

Preparation time: 5 minutes
Cooking time: 50 minutes
Servings: 3
Ingredients:
- 2 chicken breasts
- 1 ½ cups low fat cream
- 3 ounces celery
- 2 ounce green pepper, chopped
- ½ ounce green onion, chopped
- ½ cup low fat mayo
- 3 hard-boiled eggs, chopped

Directions:
1. Pre-heat your oven to 350 degrees F.
2. Take a baking sheet and place chicken, cover with cream.
3. Bake for 30-40 minutes.
4. Take a bowl and mix in the chopped celery, peppers, and onions.
5. Chop the baked chicken into bite-sized portions.
6. Peel and chop the hard boiled eggs.
7. Take a large salad bowl and mix in eggs, veggies and chicken.
8. Toss well and serve.
9. Enjoy!

Nutrition: Calories: 415; Fat: 24g; Carbohydrates: 4g; Protein: 40g

159. Generously Smothered Pork Chops

Preparation time: 10 minutes
Cooking time: 30 minutes
Servings: 4
Ingredients:
- 4 pork chops, bone-in
- 2 tablespoons of olive oil
- ¼ cup vegetable broth
- ½ pound Yukon gold potatoes, peeled and chopped
- 1 large onion, sliced
- 2 garlic cloves, minced
- 2 teaspoon rubbed sage
- 1 teaspoon thyme, ground
- Pepper as needed

Directions:
1. Pre-heat your oven to 350 degrees F.
2. Take a large sized skillet and place it over medium heat.
3. Add a tablespoon of oil and allow the oil to heat up.

4. Add pork chops and cook them for 4-5 minutes per side until browned.
5. Transfer chops to a baking dish.
6. Pour broth over the chops.
7. Add remaining oil to the pan and sauté potatoes, onion, and garlic for 3-4 minutes.
8. Take a large bowl and add potatoes, garlic, onion, thyme, sage, pepper.
9. Transfer this mixture to the baking dish (wish pork).
10. Bake for 20-30 minutes.
11. Serve and enjoy!

Nutrition: Calorie: 261; Fat: 10g; Carbohydrates: 1.3g; Protein: 2g

160. Crazy Lamb Salad

Preparation time: 10 minutes
Cooking time: 35 minutes
Servings: 4
Ingredients:

- 1 tablespoon olive oil
- 3 pound leg of lamb, bone removed, leg butterflied
- Salt and pepper to taste
- 1 teaspoon cumin
- Pinch of dried thyme
- 2 garlic cloves, peeled and minced
- For Salad
- 4 ounces feta cheese, crumbled
- ½ cup pecans
- 2 cups spinach
- 1 ½ tablespoons lemon juice
- ¼ cup olive oil
- 1 cup fresh mint, chopped

Directions:
1. Rub lamb with salt and pepper, 1 tablespoon oil, thyme, cumin, minced garlic.
2. Pre-heat your grill to medium-high and transfer lamb.
3. Cook for 40 minutes, making sure to flip it once.
4. Take a lined baking sheet and spread the pecans.
5. Toast in oven for 10 minutes at 350 degree F.
6. Transfer grilled lamb to cutting board and let it cool.
7. Slice.
8. Take a salad bowl and add spinach, 1 cup mint, feta cheese, ¼ cup olive oil, lemon juice, toasted pecans, salt, and pepper and toss well.
9. Add lamb slices on top.
10. Serve and enjoy!

Nutrition: Calories: 334; Fat: 33g; Carbohydrates: 5g; Protein: 7g

161. Chilled Chicken, Artichoke and Zucchini Platter

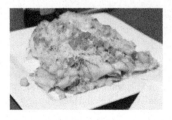

Preparation time: 10 minutes
Cooking time: 5 minutes
Servings: 4
Ingredients:

- 2 medium chicken breasts, cooked and cut into 1-inch cubes
- ¼ cup extra virgin olive oil
- 2 cups artichoke hearts, drained and roughly chopped
- 3 large zucchini, diced/cut into small rounds
- 1 can (15 ounce) chickpeas
- 1 cup Kalamata olives
- ½ teaspoon Fresh ground black pepper
- ½ teaspoon Italian seasoning
- ¼ cup parmesan, grated

Directions:
1. Take a large skillet and place it over medium heat, heat up olive oil.
2. Add zucchini and sauté for 5 minutes, season with salt and pepper.
3. Remove from heat and add all the listed ingredients to the skillet.
4. Stir until combined.
5. Transfer to glass container and store.
6. Serve and enjoy!

Nutrition: Calories: 457; Fat: 22g; Carbohydrates: 30g; Protein: 24g

162. Chicken and Carrot Stew

Preparation time: 15 minutes
Cooking time: 6 hours
Servings: 6
Ingredients:

- 4 chicken breasts, boneless and cubed
- 2 cups chicken broth
- 1 cup tomatoes, chopped
- 3 cups carrots, peeled and cubed
- 1 teaspoon thyme dried
- 1 cup onion, chopped
- 2 garlic clove, minced
- Pepper to taste

Directions:
1. Add all the ingredients to the Slow Cooker.
2. Stir and close the lid.
3. Cook for 6 hours.
4. Serve hot and enjoy!

Nutrition: Calories: 182; Fat: 4g; Carbohydrates: 10g; Protein: 39g

163. Tasty Spinach Pie

Preparation time: 10 minutes
Cooking time: 4 hours
Servings: 2
Ingredients:

- 10 ounces spinach
- 2 cups baby Bella mushrooms, chopped
- 1 red bell pepper, chopped
- 1 ½ cups low-fat cheese, shredded
- 8 whole eggs
- 1 cup coconut cream
- 2 tablespoons chives, chopped

- Pinch of pepper
- ½ cup almond flour
- ¼ teaspoon baking soda

Directions:
1. Take a bowl and add eggs, coconut cream, chives, pepper and whisk well.
2. Add almond flour, baking soda, cheese, mushrooms bell pepper, spinach and toss well.
3. Grease your cooker and transfer mix to the Slow Cooker.
4. Place lid and cook on LOW for 4 hours.
5. Slice and enjoy!

Nutrition: Calories: 201; Fat: 6g; Carbohydrates: 8g; Protein: 5g

164. Mesmerizing Carrot and Pineapple Mix

Preparation time: 10 minutes
Cooking time: 6 hours
Servings: 10

Ingredients:
- 1 cup raisins
- 6 cups water
- 23 ounces natural applesauce
- 2 tablespoons stevia
- 2 tablespoons cinnamon powder
- 14 ounces carrots, shredded
- 8 ounces canned pineapple, crushed
- 1 tablespoon pumpkin pie spice

Directions:
1. Add carrots, applesauce, raisins, stevia, cinnamon, pineapple, pumpkin pie spice to your Slow Cooker and gently stir.
2. Place lid and cook on LOW for 6 hours.
3. Serve and enjoy!

Nutrition: Calories: 179; Fat: 5g; Carbohydrates: 15g; Protein: 4g

165. Blackberry Chicken Wings

Preparation time: 35 minutes
Cooking time: 50 minutes
Servings: 4

Ingredients:
- 3 pounds chicken wings, about 20 pieces
- ½ cup blackberry chipotle jam
- Sunflower seeds and pepper to taste
- ½ cup water

Directions:
1. Add water and jam to a bowl and mix well.
2. Place chicken wings in a zip bag and add two-thirds of the marinade.
3. Season with sunflower seeds and pepper.
4. Let it marinate for 30 minutes.
5. Pre-heat your oven to 400 degrees F.
6. Prepare a baking sheet and wire rack, place chicken wings in wire rack and bake for 15 minutes.
7. Brush remaining marinade and bake for 30 minutes more.
8. Enjoy!

Nutrition: Calories: 502; Fat: 39g; Carbohydrates: 01.8g; Protein: 34g

166. Secret Asian Green Beans

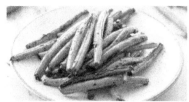

Preparation time: 10 minutes
Cooking time: 2 hours
Servings: 10

Ingredients:
- 16 cups green beans, halved
- 3 tablespoons olive oil
- ¼ cup tomato sauce, salt-free
- ½ cup coconut sugar
- ¾ teaspoon low sodium soy sauce
- Pinch of pepper

Directions:
1. Add green beans, coconut sugar, pepper tomato sauce, soy sauce, and oil to your Slow Cooker.
2. Stir well.
3. Place lid and cook on LOW for 3 hours.
4. Divide between serving platters and serve.
5. Enjoy!

Nutrition: Calories: 200; Fat: 4g; Carbohydrates: 12g; Protein: 3g

167. Excellent Acorn Mix

Preparation time: 10 minutes
Cooking time: 7 hours
Servings: 10

Ingredients:
- 2 acorn squash, peeled and cut into wedges
- 16 ounces cranberry sauce, unsweetened
- ¼ teaspoon cinnamon powder
- Pepper to taste

Directions:
1. Add acorn wedges to your Slow Cooker.
2. Add cranberry sauce, cinnamon, raisins and pepper.
3. Stir.
4. Place lid and cook on LOW for 7 hours.
5. Serve and enjoy!

Nutrition: Calories: 200; Fat: 3g; Carbohydrates: 15g; Protein: 2g

168. Crunchy Almond Chocolate Bars

Preparation time: 10 minutes
Cooking time: 2 hours and 30 minutes
Servings: 12

Ingredients:
- 1 egg white
- ¼ cup coconut oil, melted
- 1 cup coconut sugar
- ½ teaspoon vanilla extract
- 1 teaspoon baking powder

- 1 ½ cups almond meal
- ½ cup dark chocolate chips

Directions:
1. Take a bowl and add sugar, oil, vanilla extract, egg white, almond flour, baking powder and mix it well.
2. Fold in chocolate chips and stir.
3. Line Slow Cooker with parchment paper.
4. Grease.
5. Add the cookie mix and press on bottom.
6. Place lid and cook on LOW for 2 hours 30 minutes.
7. Take cookie sheet out and let it cool.
8. Cut in bars and enjoy!

Nutrition: Calories: 200; Fat: 2g; Carbohydrates: 13g; Protein: 6g

169. Lettuce and Chicken Platter

Preparation time: 10 minutes
Cooking time: 20 minutes
Servings: 6
Ingredients:
- 2 cups chicken, cooked and coarsely chopped
- ½ head ice berg lettuce, sliced and chopped
- 1 celery rib, chopped
- 1 medium apple, cut
- ½ red bell pepper, deseeded and chopped
- 6-7 green olives, pitted and halved
- 1 red onion, chopped
- For dressing
- 1 tablespoon raw honey
- 2 tablespoons lemon juice
- Salt and pepper to taste

Directions:
1. Cut the vegetables and transfer them to your Salad Bowl.
2. Add olives.
3. Chop the cooked chicken and transfer to your Salad bowl.
4. Prepare dressing by mixing the ingredients listed under Dressing.
5. Pour the dressing into the Salad bowl.
6. Toss and enjoy!

Nutrition: Calories: 296; Fat: 21g; Carbohydrates: 9g; Protein: 18g

170. Greek Lemon Chicken Bowl

Preparation time: 10 minutes
Cooking time: 15 minutes
Servings: 6
Ingredients:
- 2 cups chicken, cooked and chopped
- 2 cans chicken broth, fat free
- 2 medium carrots, chopped
- ¼ teaspoon pepper
- 2 tablespoons parsley, snipped
- ¼ cup lemon juice
- 1 can cream chicken soup, fat free, low sodium
- ½ cup onion, chopped
- 1 garlic clove, minced

Directions:
1. Take a pot and add all the ingredients except parsley into it.
2. Season with salt and pepper.
3. Bring the mix to a boil over medium-high heat.
4. Reduce the heat and simmer for 15 minutes.
5. Garnish with parsley.
6. Serve hot and enjoy!

Nutrition: Calories: 520; Fat: 33g; Carbohydrates: 31g; Protein: 30g

171. Garden Salad

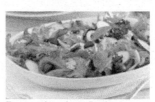

Preparation time: 5 minutes
Cooking time: 20 minutes
Servings: 6
Ingredients:
- 1 pound raw peanuts in shell
- 1 bay leaf
- 2 medium-sized chopped up tomatoes
- ½ cup diced up green pepper
- ½ cup diced up sweet onion
- ¼ cup finely diced hot pepper
- ¼ cup diced up celery
- 2 tablespoons olive oil
- ¾ teaspoon flavored vinegar
- ¼ teaspoon freshly ground black pepper

Directions:
1. Boil your peanuts for 1 minute and rinse them.
2. The skin will be soft, so discard the skin.
3. Add 2 cups of water to the Instant Pot.
4. Add bay leaf and peanuts.
5. Lock the lid and cook on HIGH pressure for 20 minutes.
6. Drain the water.
7. Take a large bowl and add the peanuts, diced up vegetables.
8. Whisk in olive oil, lemon juice, pepper in another bowl.
9. Pour the mixture over the salad and mix.
10. Enjoy!

Nutrition: Calories: 140; Fat: 4g; Carbohydrates: 24g; Protein: 5g

172. Spicy Cabbage Dish

Preparation time: 10 minutes
Cooking time: 4 hours
Servings: 4
Ingredients:
- 2 yellow onions, chopped
- 10 cups red cabbage, shredded
- 1 cup plums, pitted and chopped
- 1 teaspoon cinnamon powder
- 1 garlic clove, minced
- 1 teaspoon cumin seeds
- ¼ teaspoon cloves, ground
- 2 tablespoons red wine vinegar

- 1 teaspoon coriander seeds
- ½ cup water

Directions:
1. Add cabbage, onion, plums, garlic, cumin, cinnamon, cloves, vinegar, coriander and water to your Slow Cooker.
2. Stir well.
3. Place lid and cook on LOW for 4 hours.
4. Divide between serving platters.
5. Enjoy!

Nutrition: Calories: 197; Fat: 1g; Carbohydrates: 14g; Protein: 3g

173. Extreme Balsamic Chicken

Preparation time: 10 minutes
Cooking time: 35 minutes
Servings: 4

Ingredients:
- 3 boneless chicken breasts, skinless
- Sunflower seeds to taste
- ¼ cup almond flour
- 2/3 cups low-fat chicken broth
- 1 ½ teaspoons arrowroot
- ½ cup low sugar raspberry preserve
- 1 ½ tablespoons balsamic vinegar

Directions:
1. Cut chicken breast into bite-sized pieces and season them with seeds.
2. Dredge the chicken pieces in flour and shake off any excess.
3. Take a non-stick skillet and place it over medium heat.
4. Add chicken to the skillet and cook for 15 minutes, making sure to turn them half-way through.
5. Remove chicken and transfer to platter.
6. Add arrowroot, broth, raspberry preserve to the skillet and stir.
7. Stir in balsamic vinegar and reduce heat to low, stir-cook for a few minutes.
8. Transfer the chicken back to the sauce and cook for 15 minutes more.
9. Serve and enjoy!

Nutrition: Calories: 546; Fat: 35g; Carbohydrates: 11g; Protein: 44g

174. Enjoyable Spinach and Bean Medley

Preparation time: 10 minutes
Cooking time: 4 hours
Servings: 4

Ingredients:
- 5 carrots, sliced
- 1 ½ cups great northern beans, dried
- 2 garlic cloves, minced
- 1 yellow onion, chopped
- Pepper to taste
- ½ teaspoon oregano, dried
- 5 ounces baby spinach
- 4 ½ cups low sodium veggie stock
- 2 teaspoons lemon peel, grated

- 3 tablespoon lemon juice

Directions:
1. Add beans, onion, carrots, garlic, oregano and stock to your Slow Cooker.
2. Stir well.
3. Place lid and cook on HIGH for 4 hours.
4. Add spinach, lemon juice and lemon peel.
5. Stir and let it sit for 5 minutes.
6. Divide between serving platters and enjoy!

Nutrition: Calories: 219; Fat: 8g; Carbohydrates: 14g; Protein: 8g

175. Tantalizing Cauliflower and Dill Mash

Preparation time: 10 minutes
Cooking time: 6 hours
Servings: 6

Ingredients:
- 1 cauliflower head, florets separated
- 1/3 cup dill, chopped
- 6 garlic cloves
- 2 tablespoons olive oil
- Pinch of black pepper

Directions:
1. Add cauliflower to Slow Cooker
2. Add dill, garlic and water to cover them.
3. Place lid and cook on HIGH for 5 hours.
4. Drain the flowers.
5. Season with pepper and add oil, mash using potato masher.
6. Whisk and serve.
7. Enjoy!

Nutrition: Calories: 207; Fat: 4g; Carbohydrates: 14g; Protein: 3g

176. Traditional Black Bean Chili

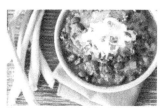

Preparation time: 10 minutes
Cooking time: 4 hours
Servings: 4

Ingredients:
- 1 ½ cups red bell pepper, chopped
- 1 cup yellow onion, chopped
- 1 ½ cups mushrooms, sliced
- 1 tablespoon olive oil
- 1 tablespoon chili powder
- 2 garlic cloves, minced
- 1 teaspoon chipotle chili pepper, chopped
- ½ teaspoon cumin, ground
- 16 ounces canned black beans, drained and rinsed
- 2 tablespoons cilantro, chopped
- 1 cup tomatoes, chopped

Directions:
1. Add red bell peppers, onion, dill, mushrooms, chili powder, garlic, chili pepper, cumin, black beans, and tomatoes to your Slow Cooker.
2. Stir well.
3. Place lid and cook on HIGH for 4 hours.
4. Sprinkle cilantro on top.
5. Serve and enjoy!

Nutrition: Calories: 211; Fat: 3g; Carbohydrates: 22g; Protein: 5g

177. Very Wild Mushroom Pilaf

Preparation time: 10 minutes
Cooking time: 3 hours
Servings: 4
Ingredients:
- 1 cup wild rice
- 2 garlic cloves, minced
- 6 green onions, chopped
- 2 tablespoons olive oil
- ½ pound baby Bella mushrooms
- 2 cups water

Directions:
1. Add rice, garlic, onion, oil, mushrooms and water to your Slow Cooker.
2. Stir well until mixed.
3. Place lid and cook on LOW for 3 hours.
4. Stir pilaf and divide between serving platters.
5. Enjoy!

Nutrition: Calories: 210; Fat: 7g; Carbohydrates: 16g; Protein: 4g

178. Green Palak Paneer

Preparation time: 5 minutes
Cooking time: 10 minutes
Servings: 4
Ingredients:
- 1 pound spinach
- 2 cups cubed Paneer (vegan)
- 2 tablespoons coconut oil
- 1 teaspoon cumin
- 1 chopped up onion
- 1-2 teaspoons hot green chili minced up
- 1 teaspoon minced garlic
- 15 cashews
- 4 tablespoons almond milk
- 1 teaspoon Garam masala
- Flavored vinegar as needed

Directions:
1. Add cashews and milk to a blender and blend well.
2. Set your pot to Sauté mode and add coconut oil; allow the oil to heat up.
3. Add cumin seeds, garlic, green chilies, ginger and sauté for 1 minute.
4. Add onion and sauté for 2 minutes.
5. Add chopped spinach, flavored vinegar and a cup of water.
6. Lock up the lid and cook on HIGH pressure for 10 minutes.

7. Quick-release the pressure.
8. Add ½ cup of water and blend to a paste.
9. Add cashew paste, Paneer and Garam Masala and stir thoroughly.
10. Serve over hot rice!

Nutrition: Calories: 367; Fat: 26g; Carbohydrates: 21g; Protein: 16g

179. Sporty Baby Carrots

Preparation time: 5 minutes
Cooking time: 5 minutes
Servings: 4
Ingredients:
- 1 pound baby carrots
- 1 cup water
- 1 tablespoon clarified ghee
- 1 tablespoon chopped up fresh mint leaves
- Sea flavored vinegar as needed

Directions:
1. Place a steamer rack on top of your pot and add the carrots.
2. Add water.
3. Lock the lid and cook at HIGH pressure for 2 minutes.
4. Do a quick release.
5. Pass the carrots through a strainer and drain them.
6. Wipe the insert clean.
7. Return the insert to the pot and set the pot to Sauté mode.
8. Add clarified butter and allow it to melt.
9. Add mint and sauté for 30 seconds.
10. Add carrots to the insert and sauté well.
11. Remove them and sprinkle with bit of flavored vinegar on top.
12. Enjoy!

Nutrition: Calories: 131; Fat: 10g; Carbohydrates: 11g; Protein: 1g

180. Saucy Garlic Greens

Preparation time: 5 minutes
Cooking time: 20 minutes
Servings: 4
Ingredients:
- 1 bunch of leafy greens
- Sauce
- ½ cup cashews soaked in water for 10 minutes
- ¼ cup water
- 1 tablespoon lemon juice
- 1 teaspoon coconut aminos
- 1 clove peeled whole clove
- 1/8 teaspoon of flavored vinegar

Directions:
1. Make the sauce by draining and discarding the soaking water from your cashews and add the cashews to a blender.
2. Add fresh water, lemon juice, flavored vinegar, coconut aminos, and garlic.
3. Blitz until you have a smooth cream and transfer to bowl.
4. Add ½ cup of water to the pot.
5. Place the steamer basket to the pot and add the greens in the basket.
6. Lock the lid and steam for 1 minute.

7. Quick-release the pressure.
8. Transfer the steamed greens to strainer and extract excess water.
9. Place the greens into a mixing bowl.
10. Add lemon garlic sauce and toss.
11. Enjoy!

Nutrition: Calories: 77; Fat: 5g; Carbohydrates: 0g; Protein: 2g

181. Parmesan Baked Chicken

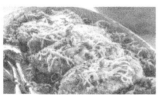

Preparation time: 5 minutes
Cooking time: 20 minutes
Servings: 2
Ingredients:
- 2 tablespoons ghee
- 2 boneless chicken breasts, skinless
- Pink sunflower seeds
- Freshly ground black pepper
- ½ cup mayonnaise, low fat
- ¼ cup parmesan cheese, grated
- 1 tablespoon dried Italian seasoning, low fat, low sodium
- ¼ cup crushed pork rinds

Directions:
1. Preheat your oven to 425 degrees F.
2. Take a large baking dish and coat with ghee.
3. Pat chicken breasts dry and wrap with a towel.
4. Season with sunflower seeds and pepper.
5. Place in baking dish.
6. Take a small bowl and add mayonnaise, parmesan cheese, Italian seasoning.
7. Slather mayo mix evenly over chicken breast.
8. Sprinkle crushed pork rinds on top.
9. Bake for 20 minutes until topping is browned.
10. Serve and enjoy!

Nutrition: Calories: 850; Fat: 67g; Carbohydrates: 2g; Protein: 60g

182. Buffalo Chicken Lettuce Wraps

Preparation time: 35 minutes
Cooking time: 10 minutes
Servings: 2
Ingredients:
- 3 chicken breasts, boneless and cubed
- 20 slices of almond butter lettuce leaves
- ¾ cup cherry tomatoes halved
- 1 avocado, chopped
- ¼ cup green onions, diced
- ½ cup ranch dressing
- ¾ cup hot sauce

Directions:
1. Take a mixing bowl and add chicken cubes and hot sauce, mix.
2. Place in the fridge and let it marinate for 30 minutes.

3. Preheat your oven to 400 degrees F.
4. Place coated chicken on a cookie pan and bake for 9 minutes.
5. Assemble lettuce serving cups with equal amounts of lettuce, green onions, tomatoes, ranch dressing, and cubed chicken.
6. Serve and enjoy!

Nutrition: Calories: 106; Fat: 6g; Net Carbohydrates: 2g; Protein: 5g

183. Crazy Japanese Potato and Beef Croquettes

Preparation time: 10 minutes
Cooking time: 20 minutes
Servings: 10
Ingredients:
- 3 medium russet potatoes, peeled and chopped
- 1 tablespoon almond butter
- 1 tablespoon vegetable oil
- 3 onions, diced
- ¾ pound ground beef
- 4 teaspoons light coconut aminos
- All-purpose flour for coating
- 2 eggs, beaten
- Panko bread crumbs for coating
- ½ cup oil, frying

Directions:
1. Take a saucepan and place it over medium-high heat; add potatoes and sunflower seeds water, boil for 16 minutes.
2. Remove water and put potatoes in another bowl, add almond butter and mash the potatoes.
3. Take a frying pan and place it over medium heat, add 1 tablespoon oil and let it heat up.
4. Add onions and stir fry until tender.
5. Add coconut aminos to beef to onions.
6. Keep frying until beef is browned.
7. Mix the beef with the potatoes evenly.
8. Take another frying pan and place it over medium heat; add half a cup of oil.
9. Form croquettes using the mashed potato mixture and coat them with flour, then eggs and finally breadcrumbs.
10. Fry patties until golden on all sides.
11. Enjoy!

Nutrition: Calories: 239; Fat: 4g; Carbohydrates: 20g; Protein: 10g

184. Spicy Chili Crackers

Preparation time: 15 minutes
Cooking time: 60 minutes
Servings: 30 crackers
Ingredients:
- ¾ cup almond flour
- ¼ cup coconut four
- ¼ cup coconut flour
- ½ teaspoon paprika
- ½ teaspoon cumin
- 1 ½ teaspoons chili pepper spice
- 1 teaspoon onion powder
- ½ teaspoon sunflower seeds

- 1 whole egg
- ¼ cup unsalted almond butter

Directions:
1. Preheat your oven to 350 degrees F.
2. Line a baking sheet with parchment paper and keep it on the side.
3. Add ingredients to your food processor and pulse until you have a nice dough.
4. Divide dough into two equal parts.
5. Place one ball on a sheet of parchment paper and cover with another sheet; roll it out.
6. Cut into crackers and repeat with the other ball.
7. Transfer the prepped dough to a baking tray and bake for 8-10 minutes.
8. Remove from oven and serve.
9. Enjoy!

Nutrition: Total Carbs: 2.8g, Fiber: 1, Protein: 1.6g, Fat: 4.1g

185. Golden Eggplant Fries

Preparation time: 10 minutes
Cooking time: 15 minutes
Servings: 8
Ingredients:
- 2 eggs
- 2 cups almond flour
- 2 tablespoons coconut oil, spray
- 2 eggplant, peeled and cut thinly
- Sunflower seeds and pepper

Directions:
1. Preheat your oven to 400 degrees F.
2. Take a bowl and mix with sunflower seeds and black pepper.
3. Take another bowl and beat eggs until frothy.
4. Dip the eggplant pieces into the eggs.
5. Then coat them with the flour mixture.
6. Add another layer of flour and egg.
7. Then, take a baking sheet and grease with coconut oil on top.
8. Bake for about 15 minutes.
9. Serve and enjoy!

Nutrition: Calories: 212, Fat: 15.8g, Carbohydrates: 12.1g, Protein: 8.6g

186. Chicken and Carrot Stew

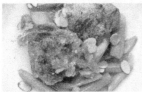

Preparation time: 15 minutes
Cooking time: 6 minutes
Servings: 4
Ingredients:
- 4 boneless chicken breast, cubed
- 3 cups of carrots, peeled and cubed
- 1 cup onion, chopped
- 1 cup tomatoes, chopped
- 1 teaspoon of dried thyme

- 2 cups of chicken broth
- 2 garlic cloves, minced
- Sunflower seeds and pepper as needed

Directions:
1. Add all of the listed ingredients to a Slow Cooker.
2. Stir and close the lid.
3. Cook for 6 hours.
4. Serve hot and enjoy!

Nutrition: Calories: 182, Fat: 3g, Carbohydrates: 10g, Protein: 39g

187. The Delish Turkey Wrap

Preparation time: 10 minutes
Cooking time: 10 minutes
Servings: 6
Ingredients:
- 1 ¼ pounds ground turkey, lean
- 4 green onions, minced
- 1 tablespoon olive oil
- 1 garlic clove, minced
- 2 teaspoons chili paste
- 8-ounce water chestnut, diced
- 3 tablespoons hoisin sauce
- 2 tablespoon coconut aminos
- 1 tablespoon rice vinegar
- 12 almond butter lettuce leaves
- 1/8 teaspoon sunflower seeds

Directions:
1. Take a pan and place it over medium heat, add turkey and garlic to the pan.
2. Heat for 6 minutes until cooked.
3. Take a bowl and transfer turkey to the bowl.
4. Add onions and water chestnuts.
5. Stir in hoisin sauce, coconut aminos, and vinegar and chili paste.
6. Toss well and transfer mix to lettuce leaves.
7. Serve and enjoy!

Nutrition: Calories: 162; Fat: 4g; Net Carbohydrates: 7g; Protein: 23g

188. Almond butternut Chicken

Preparation time: 15 minutes
Cooking time: 30 minutes
Servings: 4
Ingredients:
- ½ pound Nitrate free bacon
- 6 chicken thighs, boneless and skinless
- 2-3 cups almond butternut squash, cubed
- Extra virgin olive oil
- Fresh chopped sage
- Sunflower seeds and pepper as needed

Directions:
1. Prepare your oven by preheating it to 425 degrees F.
2. Take a large skillet and place it over medium-high heat, add bacon and fry until crispy.
3. Take a slice of bacon and place it on the side, crumble the bacon.
4. Add cubed almond butternut squash in the bacon grease and sauté, season with sunflower seeds and pepper.

5. Once the squash is tender, remove skillet and transfer to a plate.
6. Add coconut oil to the skillet and add chicken thighs, cook for 10 minutes.
7. Season with sunflower seeds and pepper.
8. Remove skillet from stove and transfer to oven.
9. Bake for 12-15 minutes, top with the crumbled bacon and sage.
10. Enjoy!

Nutrition: Calories: 323; Fat: 19g; Carbohydrates: 8g; Protein: 12g

189. Zucchini Zoodles with Chicken and Basil

Preparation time: 10 minutes
Cooking time: 10 minutes
Servings: 3
Ingredients:
- 2 chicken fillets, cubed
- 2 tablespoons ghee
- 1 pound tomatoes, diced
- ½ cup basil, chopped
- ¼ cup almond milk
- 1 garlic clove, peeled, minced
- 1 zucchini, shredded

Directions:
1. Sauté cubed chicken in ghee until no longer pink.
2. Add tomatoes and season with sunflower seeds.
3. Simmer and reduce liquid.
4. Prepare your zucchini Zoodles by shredding zucchini in a food processor.
5. Add basil, garlic, coconut almond milk to the chicken and cook for a few minutes.
6. Add half of the zucchini Zoodles to a bowl and top with creamy tomato basil chicken.
7. Enjoy!

Nutrition: Calories: 540; Fat: 27g; Carbohydrates: 13g; Protein: 59g

190. Duck with Cucumber and Carrots

Preparation time: 10 minutes
Cooking time: 40 minutes
Servings: 8
Ingredients:
- 1 duck, cut up into medium pieces
- 1 chopped cucumber, chopped
- 1 tablespoon low sodium vegetable stock
- 2 carrots, chopped
- 2 cups of water
- Black pepper as needed
- 1-inch ginger piece, grated

Directions:
1. Add duck pieces to your Instant Pot.
2. Add cucumber, stock, carrots, water, ginger, pepper and stir.
3. Lock up the lid and cook on LOW pressure for 40 minutes.
4. Release the pressure naturally.
5. Serve and enjoy!

Nutrition: Calories: 206; Fats: 7g; Carbs: 28g; Protein: 16g

191. Epic Mango Chicken

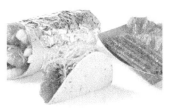

Preparation time: 25 minutes
Cooking time: 10 minutes
Servings: 4
Ingredients:
- 2 medium mangoes, peeled and sliced
- 10-ounce coconut almond milk
- 4 teaspoons vegetable oil
- 4 teaspoons spicy curry paste
- 14-ounce chicken breast halves, skinless and boneless, cut in cubes
- 4 medium shallots
- 1 large English cucumber, sliced and seeded

Directions:
1. Slice half of the mangoes and add the halves to a bowl.
2. Add mangoes and coconut almond milk to a blender and blend until you have a smooth puree.
3. Keep the mixture on the side.
4. Take a large-sized pot and place it over medium heat, add oil and allow the oil to heat up.
5. Add curry paste and cook for 1 minute until you have a nice fragrance, add shallots and chicken to the pot and cook for 5 minutes.
6. Pour mango puree in to the mix and allow it to heat up.
7. Serve the cooked chicken with mango puree and cucumbers.
8. Enjoy!

Nutrition: Calories: 398; Fat: 20g; Carbohydrates: 32g; Protein: 26g

192. Chicken and Cabbage Platter

Preparation time: 9 minutes
Cooking time: 14 minutes
Servings: 2
Ingredients:
- ½ cup sliced onion
- 1 tablespoon sesame garlic-flavored oil
- 2 cups shredded Bok-Choy
- 1/2 cups fresh bean sprouts
- 1 1/2 stalks celery, chopped
- 1 ½ teaspoons minced garlic
- 1/2 teaspoon stevia
- 1/2 cup chicken broth
- 1 tablespoon coconut aminos
- 1/2 tablespoon freshly minced ginger
- 1/2 teaspoon arrowroot
- 2 boneless chicken breasts, cooked and sliced thinly

Directions:

1. Shred the cabbage with a knife.
2. Slice onion and add to your platter alongside the rotisserie chicken.
3. Add a dollop of mayonnaise on top and drizzle olive oil over the cabbage.
4. Season with sunflower seeds and pepper according to your taste.
5. Enjoy!

Nutrition: Calories: 368; Fat: 18g; Net Carbohydrates: 8g; Protein: 42g; Fiber: 3g; Carbohydrates: 11g

193. Hearty Chicken Liver Stew

Preparation time: 10 minutes
Cooking time: 20 minutes
Servings: 2
Ingredients:
- 10 ounces chicken livers
- 1-ounce onion, chopped
- 2 ounces sour cream
- 1 tablespoon olive oil
- Sunflower seeds to taste

Directions:
1. Take a pan and place it over medium heat.
2. Add oil and let it heat up.
3. Add onions and fry until just browned.
4. Add livers and season with sunflower seeds.
5. Cook until livers are half cooked.
6. Transfer the mix to a stew pot.
7. Add sour cream and cook for 20 minutes.
8. Serve and enjoy!

Nutrition: Calories: 146; Fat: 9g; Carbohydrates: 2g; Protein: 15g

194. Chicken Quesadilla

Preparation time: 10 minutes
Cooking time: 35 minutes
Servings: 2
Ingredients:
- ¼ cup ranch dressing
- ½ cup cheddar cheese, shredded
- 20 slices bacon, center-cut
- 2 cups grilled chicken, sliced

Directions:
1. Re-heat your oven to 400 degrees F.
2. Line baking sheet using parchment paper.
3. Weave bacon into two rectangles and bake for 30 minutes.
4. Lay grilled chicken over bacon square, drizzling ranch dressing on top.
5. Sprinkle cheddar cheese and top with another bacon square.
6. Bake for 5 minutes more.
7. Slice and serve.
8. Enjoy!

Nutrition: Calories: 619, Fat: 35g, Carbohydrates: 2g, Protein: 79g

195. Mustard Chicken

Preparation time: 10 minutes
Cooking time: 40 minutes
Servings: 2
Ingredients:
- 2 chicken breasts
- 1/4 cup chicken broth
- 2 tablespoons mustard
- 1 1/2 tablespoons olive oil
- 1/2 teaspoon paprika
- 1/2 teaspoon chili powder
- 1/2 teaspoon garlic powder

Directions:
1. Take a small bowl and mix mustard, olive oil, paprika, chicken broth, garlic powder, chicken broth, and chili.
2. Add chicken breast and marinate for 30 minutes.
3. Take a lined baking sheet and arrange the chicken.
4. Bake for 35 minutes at 375 degrees F.
5. Serve and enjoy!

Nutrition: Calories: 531; Fat: 23g; Carbohydrates: 10g; Protein: 64g

196. Fascinating Spinach and Beef Meatballs

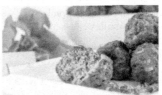

Preparation time: 10 minutes
Cooking time: 20 minutes
Servings: 4
Ingredients:
- ½ cup onion
- 4 garlic cloves
- 1 whole egg
- ¼ teaspoon oregano
- Pepper as needed
- 1 pound lean ground beef
- 10 ounces spinach

Directions:
1. Preheat your oven to 375 degrees F.
2. Take a bowl and mix in the rest of the ingredients, and using your hands, roll into meatballs.
3. Transfer to a sheet tray and bake for 20 minutes.
4. Enjoy!

Nutrition: Calorie: 200, Fat: 8g, Carbohydrates: 5g, Protein: 29g

197. Juicy and Peppery Tenderloin

Preparation time: 10 minutes
Cooking time: 20 minutes
Servings: 4
Ingredients:
- 2 teaspoons sage, chopped
- Sunflower seeds and pepper

- 2 1/2 pounds beef tenderloin
- 2 teaspoons thyme, chopped
- 2 garlic cloves, sliced
- 2 teaspoons rosemary, chopped
- 4 teaspoons olive oil

Directions:
1. Preheat your oven to 425 degrees F.
2. Take a small knife and cut incisions in the tenderloin; insert one slice of garlic into the incision.
3. Rub meat with oil.
4. Take a bowl and add sunflower seeds, sage, thyme, rosemary, pepper and mix well.
5. Rub the spice mix over tenderloin.
6. Put rubbed tenderloin into the roasting pan and bake for 10 minutes.
7. Lower temperature to 350 degrees F and cook for 20 minutes more until an internal thermometer reads 145 degrees F.
8. Transfer tenderloin to a cutting board and let sit for 15 minutes; slice into 20 pieces and enjoy!

Nutrition: Calorie: 183, Fat: 9g, Carbohydrates: 1g, Protein: 24g

198. Healthy Avocado Beef Patties

Preparation time: 15 minutes
Cooking time: 10 minutes
Servings: 2
Ingredients:
- 1 pound 85% lean ground beef
- 1 small avocado, pitted and peeled
- Fresh ground black pepper as needed

Directions:
1. Pre-heat and prepare your broiler to high.
2. Divide beef into two equal-sized patties.
3. Season the patties with pepper accordingly.
4. Broil the patties for 5 minutes per side.
5. Transfer the patties to a platter.
6. Slice avocado into strips and place them on top of the patties.
7. Serve and enjoy!

Nutrition: Calories: 568, Fat: 43g, Net Carbohydrates: 9g, Protein: 38g

199. Ravaging Beef Pot Roast

Preparation time: 10 minutes
Cooking time: 75 minutes
Servings: 4

Ingredients:
- 3 ½ pounds beef roast
- 4 ounces mushrooms, sliced
- 12 ounces beef stock
- 1-ounce onion soup mix
- ½ cup Italian dressing, low sodium, and low fat

Directions:
1. Take a bowl and add the stock, onion soup mix and Italian dressing.
2. Stir.
3. Put beef roast in pan.
4. Add mushrooms, stock mix to the pan and cover with foil.
5. Preheat your oven to 300 degrees F.
6. Bake for 1 hour and 15 minutes.
7. Let the roast cool.
8. Slice and serve.
9. Enjoy with the gravy on top!

Nutrition: Calories: 700, Fat: 56g, Carbohydrates: 10g, Protein: 70g

200. Lovely Faux Mac and Cheese

Preparation time: 15 minutes
Cooking time: 45 minutes
Servings: 4
Ingredients:
- 5 cups cauliflower florets
- Sunflower seeds and pepper to taste
- 1 cup coconut almond milk
- ½ cup vegetable broth
- 2 tablespoons coconut flour, sifted
- 1 organic egg, beaten
- 1 cup cashew cheese

Directions:
1. Preheat your oven to 350 degrees F.
2. Season florets with sunflower seeds and steam until firm.
3. Place florets in a greased ovenproof dish.
4. Heat coconut almond milk over medium heat in a skillet, make sure to season the oil with sunflower seeds and pepper.
5. Stir in broth and add coconut flour to the mix, stir.
6. Cook until the sauce begins to bubble.
7. Remove heat and add beaten egg.
8. Pour the thick sauce over the cauliflower and mix in cheese.
9. Bake for 30-45 minutes.
10. Serve and enjoy!

Nutrition: Calories: 229; Fat: 14g; Carbohydrates: 9g; Protein: 15g

DINNER

201. The Almond Breaded Chicken Goodness

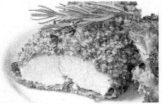

Preparation Time: 15 minutes
Cooking Time: 15 minutes
Servings: 3
Ingredients:
4.   2 large chicken breasts, boneless and skinless
5.   1/3 cup lemon juice
6.   1 ½ cups seasoned almond meal
7.   2 tablespoons coconut oil
8.   Lemon pepper, to taste
9.   Parsley for decoration
Directions:
- Slice chicken breast in half. Pound out each half until ¼ inch thick.
- Take a pan and place it over medium heat, add oil and heat it up. Dip each chicken breast slice into lemon juice and let it sit for 2 minutes.
- Turnover and the let the other side sit for 2 minutes as well. Transfer to almond meal and coat both sides.
- Add coated chicken to the oil and fry for 4 minutes per side, making sure to sprinkle lemon pepper liberally.
- Transfer to a paper lined sheet and repeat until all chicken are fried. Garnish with parsley and enjoy!

Nutrition: Calories: 128; Protein: 21 Grams; Fat: 4 Grams; Carbs: 3 Grams; Sodium: 81 mg; Cholesterol: 55 mg

202. Almond butter Pork Chops

Preparation Time: 5 minutes
Cooking Time: 25 minutes
Servings: 3
Ingredients:
3.   1 tablespoon almond butter, divided
4.   2 boneless pork chops
5.   Pepper to taste
6.   1 tablespoon dried Italian seasoning, low fat and low sodium
7.   1 tablespoon olive oil
Directions:
- Pre-heat your oven to 350 degrees F. Pat pork chops dry with a paper towel and place them in a baking dish.
- Season with pepper, and Italian seasoning. Drizzle olive oil over pork chops. Top each chop with ½ tablespoon almond butter.
- Bake for 25 minutes. Transfer pork chops on two plates and top with almond butter juice. Serve and enjoy!

Nutrition: Calories: 128; Protein: 21 Grams; Fat: 4 Grams; Carbs: 3 Grams; Sodium: 81 mg; Cholesterol: 55 mg

203. Healthy Mediterranean Lamb Chops

Preparation Time: 10 minutes
Cooking Time: 10 minute
Servings: 2
Ingredients:
2.   4 lamb shoulder chops,
3.   8 ounces each
4.   2 tablespoons Dijon mustard
5.   2 tablespoons Balsamic vinegar
6.   ½ cup olive oil
7.   2 tablespoons shredded fresh basil
Directions:
- Pat your lamb chop dry using a kitchen towel and arrange them on a shallow glass baking dish. Take a bowl and a whisk in Dijon mustard, balsamic vinegar, pepper and mix them well.
- Whisk in the oil very slowly into the marinade until the mixture is smooth Stir in basil. Pour the marinade over the lamb chops and stir to coat both sides well.
- Cover the chops and allow them to marinate for 1-4 hours (chilled). Take the chops out and leave them for 30 minutes to allow the temperature to reach a normal level.
- Pre-heat your grill to medium heat and add oil to the grate. Grill the lamb chops for 5-10 minutes per side until both sides are browned. Once the center reads 145 degrees F, the chops are ready, serve and enjoy!

Nutrition: Calories: 128; Protein: 21 Grams; Fat: 4 Grams; Carbs: 3 Grams; Sodium: 81 mg; Cholesterol: 55 mg

204. Brown Butter Duck Breast

Preparation Time: 5 minutes
Cooking Time: 25 minutes
Servings: 3
Ingredients:
2.   1 whole 6 ounce duck breast, skin on
3.   Pepper to taste
4.   1 head radicchio
5.   4 ounces, core removed
6.   ¼ cup unsalted butter
7.   6 fresh sage leaves, sliced
Directions:
- Pre-heat your oven to 400 degree F. Pat duck breast dry with paper towel. Season with pepper.
- Place duck breast in skillet and place it over medium heat, sear for 3-4 minutes each side. Turn breast over and transfer skillet to oven.
- Roast for 10 minutes (uncovered). Cut radicchio in half. Remove and discard the woody white core and thinly slice the leaves. Keep them on the side.
- Remove skillet from oven. Transfer duck breast, fat side up to cutting board and let it rest. Re-heat your skillet over medium heat.
- Add unsalted butter, sage and cook for 3-4 minutes. Cut duck into 6 equal slices. Divide radicchio between 2 plates, top with slices of duck breast and drizzle browned butter and sage. Enjoy!

Nutrition: Calories: 128; Protein: 21 Grams; Fat: 4 Grams; Carbs: 3 Grams; Sodium: 81 mg; Cholesterol: 55 mg

205. Chipotle Lettuce Chicken

Preparation Time: 10 minutes
Cooking Time: 25 minutes
Servings: 6

Ingredients:

2. 1 pound chicken breast, cut into strips
3. Splash of olive oil
4. 1 red onion, finely sliced
5. 14 ounces tomatoes
6. 1 teaspoon chipotle, chopped
7. ½ teaspoon cumin
8. Lettuce as needed
9. Fresh coriander leaves
10. Jalapeno chilies, sliced
11. Fresh tomato slices for garnish
12. Lime wedges

Directions:

- Take a non-stick frying pan and place it over medium heat. Add oil and heat it up.
- Add chicken and cook until brown. Keep the chicken on the side.
- Add tomatoes, sugar, chipotle, cumin to the same pan and simmer for 25 minutes until you have a nice sauce. Add chicken into the sauce and cook for 5 minutes.
- Transfer the mix to another place. Use lettuce wraps to take a portion of the mixture and serve with a squeeze of lemon. Enjoy!

Nutrition: Calories: 128; Protein: 21 Grams; Fat: 4 Grams; Carbs: 3 Grams; Sodium: 81 mg; Cholesterol: 55 mg

206. Zucchini Beef Sauté with Coriander Greens

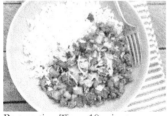

Preparation Time: 10 minutes
Cooking Time: 10 minutes
Servings: 4

Ingredients:

- 10 ounces beef, sliced into
- 1-2 inch strips
- 1 zucchini, cut into 2-inch strips
- ¼ cup parsley, chopped
- 3 garlic cloves, minced
- 2 tablespoons tamari sauce
- 4 tablespoons avocado oil

Directions:

1. Add 2 tablespoons avocado oil in a frying pan over high heat.
2. Place strips of beef and brown for a few minutes on high heat.

3. Once the meat is brown, add zucchini strips and sauté until tender.
4. Once tender, add tamari sauce, garlic, parsley and let them sit for a few minutes more.
5. Serve immediately and enjoy!

Nutrition: Calories: 128; Protein: 21 Grams; Fat: 4 Grams; Carbs: 3 Grams; Sodium: 81 mg; Cholesterol: 55 mg

207. Walnuts and Asparagus Delight

Preparation Time: 5 minutes
Cooking Time: 5 minutes
Servings: 4

Ingredients:

- 1 ½ tablespoons olive oil
- ¾ pound asparagus, trimmed
- ¼ cup walnuts, chopped
- Sunflower seeds and pepper to taste

Directions:

1. Place a skillet over medium heat add olive oil and let it heat up.
2. Add asparagus, sauté for 5 minutes until browned.
3. Season with sunflower seeds and pepper.
4. Remove heat.
5. Add walnuts and toss.
6. Serve warm!

Nutrition: Calories: 128; Protein: 21 Grams; Fat: 4 Grams; Carbs: 3 Grams; Sodium: 81 mg; Cholesterol: 55 mg

208. Beef Soup

Preparation Time: 10 minutes
Cooking Time: 40 minutes
Servings: 4

Ingredients:

- 1 pound ground beef, lean
- 1 cup mixed vegetables, frozen
- 1 yellow onion, chopped
- 6 cups vegetable broth
- 1 cup low-fat cream
- Pepper to taste

Directions:

1. Take a stockpot and add all the ingredients the except heavy cream, salt, and black pepper.
2. Bring to a boil.
3. Reduce heat to simmer.
4. Cook for 40 minutes.
5. Once cooked, warm the heavy cream.
6. Then add once the soup is cooked.
7. Blend the soup till smooth by using an immersion blender.
8. Season with salt and black pepper.
9. Serve and enjoy!

Nutrition: Calories: 128; Protein: 21 Grams; Fat: 4 Grams; Carbs: 3 Grams; Sodium: 81 mg; Cholesterol: 55 mg

209. Clean Chicken and Mushroom Stew

Preparation Time: 10 minutes
Cooking Time: 35 minutes
Servings: 4
Ingredients:
- 4 chicken breast halves, cut into bite sized pieces
- 1 pound mushrooms, sliced (5-6 cups)
- 1 bunch spring onion, chopped
- 4 tablespoons olive oil
- 1 teaspoon thyme
- Sunflower seeds and pepper as needed

Directions:
1. Take a large deep frying pan and place it over medium-high heat.
2. Add oil and let it heat up.
3. Add chicken and cook for 4-5 minutes per side until slightly browned.
4. Add spring onions and mushrooms, season with sunflower seeds and pepper according to your taste. Stir.
5. Cover with lid and bring the mix to a boil. Reduce heat and simmer for 25 minutes. Serve!

Nutrition: Calories: 128; Protein: 21 Grams; Fat: 4 Grams; Carbs: 3 Grams; Sodium: 81 mg; Cholesterol: 55 mg

210. Zucchini Zoodles with Chicken and Basil

Preparation Time: 10 minutes
Cooking Time: 10 minutes
Servings: 4
Ingredients:
- 2 chicken fillets, cubed
- 2 tablespoons ghee
- 1 pound tomatoes, diced
- ½ cup basil, chopped
- ¼ cup coconut almond milk
- 1 garlic clove, peeled, minced
- 1 zucchini, shredded

Directions:
1. Sauté cubed chicken in ghee until no longer pink.
2. Add tomatoes and season with sunflower seeds.
3. Simmer and reduce the liquid.
4. Prepare your zucchini Zoodles by shredding zucchini in a food processor.
5. Add basil, garlic, coconut almond milk to chicken and cook for a few minutes.
6. Add half of the zucchini Zoodles to a bowl and top with creamy tomato basil chicken. Enjoy!

Nutrition: Calories: 128; Protein: 21 Grams; Fat: 4 Grams; Carbs: 3 Grams; Sodium: 81 mg; Cholesterol: 55 mg

211. Pan-Seared Lamb Chops

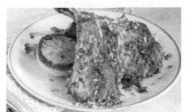

Preparation Time: 10 minutes
Cooking Time: 4-6 minutes
Servings: 4
Ingredients:
- 4 garlic cloves, peeled
- Salt, to taste
- 1 teaspoon black mustard seeds, crushed finely
- 2 teaspoons ground cumin
- 1 teaspoon ground ginger
- 1 teaspoon ground coriander
- ½ teaspoon ground cinnamon
- Freshly ground black pepper, to taste
- 1 tablespoon coconut oil
- 8 medium lamb chops, trimmed

Directions:
1. Place garlic cloves onto a cutting board and sprinkle with a few salt.
2. With a knife, crush the garlic till a paste forms.
3. In a bowl, mix together garlic paste and spices.
4. With a clear, crisp knife, make 3-4 cuts on both side in the chops.
5. Rub the chops with garlic mixture generously.
6. In a large skillet, melt butter on medium heat.
7. Add chops and cook for approximately 2-3 minutes per side or till desired doneness.

Nutrition: Calories: 128; Protein: 21 Grams; Fat: 4 Grams; Carbs: 3 Grams; Sodium: 81 mg; Cholesterol: 55 mg

212. Lamb & Pineapple Kebabs

Preparation Time: 15 minutes
Cooking Time: 10 minutes
Servings: 4-6
Ingredients:
- 1 large pineapple, cubed into
- 1½-inch size, divided
- 1 (½-inch) piece fresh ginger, chopped
- 2 garlic cloves, chopped
- Salt, to taste
- 16-24-ounce lamb shoulder steak, trimmed and cubed into 1½-inch size
- Fresh mint leaves coming from a bunch
- Ground cinnamon, to taste

Directions:
1. In a blender, add about 1½ servings of pineapple, ginger, garlic and salt and pulse till smooth.
2. Transfer the amalgamation right into a large bowl.
3. Add chops and coat with mixture generously.
4. Refrigerate to marinate for about 1-2 hours.
5. Preheat the grill to medium heat. Grease the grill grate.

6. Thread lam, remaining pineapple and mint leaves onto pre-soaked wooden skewers.
7. Grill the kebabs approximately 10 min, turning occasionally.

Nutrition: Calories: 128; Protein: 21 Grams; Fat: 4 Grams; Carbs: 3 Grams; Sodium: 81 mg; Cholesterol: 55 mg

213. Spiced Pork One

Preparation Time: 15 minutes
Cooking Time: 60 minutes 52 minutes
Servings: 4
Ingredients:
- 1 (2-inch) piece fresh ginger, chopped
- 5-10 garlic cloves, chopped
- 1 teaspoon ground cumin
- ½ teaspoon ground turmeric 1 tablespoon hot paprika
- 1 tablespoon red pepper flakes
- Salt, to taste
- 2 tablespoons cider vinegar
- 2 pounds pork shoulder, trimmed and cubed into 1½-inch size
- 2 cups domestic hot water, divided
- 1 (1-inch wide) ball tamarind pulp
- ¼ cup olive oil
- 1 teaspoon black mustard seeds, crushed
- 4 green cardamoms
- 5 whole cloves
- 1 (3-inch) cinnamon stick
- 1 cup onion, chopped finely
- 1 large red bell pepper, seeded and chopped

Directions:
1. In a food processor, add ginger, garlic, cumin, turmeric, paprika, red pepper flakes, salt and cider vinegar and pulse till smooth.
2. Transfer the amalgamation in to a large bowl.
3. Add pork and coat with mixture generously.
4. Keep aside, covered for around an hour at room temperature.
5. In a bowl, add 1 cup of warm water and tamarind and make aside till water becomes cool.
6. With the hands, crush the tamarind to extract the pulp.
7. Add remaining cup of hot water and mix till well combined.
8. Through a fine sieve, strain the tamarind juice inside a bowl.
9. In a sizable skillet, heat oil on medium-high heat.
10. Add mustard seeds, green cardamoms, cloves and cinnamon stick and sauté for about 4 minutes.
11. Add onion and sauté for approximately 5 minutes.
12. Add pork and stir fry for approximately 6 minutes.
13. Stir in tamarind juice and convey with a boil.
14. Reduce the heat to medium-low and simmer 1½ hours.
   15. Stir in bell pepper and cook for about 7 minutes.

Nutrition: Calories: 128; Protein: 21 Grams; Fat: 4 Grams; Carbs: 3 Grams; Sodium: 81 mg; Cholesterol: 55 mg

214. Pork chops in Creamy Sauce

Preparation Time: 15 minutes

Cooking Time: 14 minutes
Servings: 4
Ingredients:
- 2 garlic cloves, chopped
- 1 small jalapeño pepper, chopped
- ¼ cup fresh cilantro leaves
- 1½ teaspoons ground turmeric, divided
- 1 tablespoon fish sauce
- 2 tablespoons fresh lime juice
- 1 (13½-ounce) can coconut milk
- 4 (½-inch thick) pork chops
- Salt, to taste
- 1 tablespoon coconut oil
- 1 shallot, chopped finely

Directions:
1. In a blender, add garlic, jalapeño pepper, cilantro, 1 teaspoon of ground turmeric, fish sauce, lime juice and coconut milk and pulse till smooth.
2. Sprinkle the pork with salt and remaining turmeric evenly.
3. In a skillet, melt butter on medium-high heat.
4. Add shallots and sauté approximately 1 minute.
5. Add chops and cook for approximately 2 minutes per side.
6. Transfer the chops inside a bowl.
7. Add coconut mixture and convey to your boil.
8. Reduce heat to medium and simmer, stirring occasionally for approximately 5 minutes.
9. Stir in pork chops and cook for about 3-4 minutes.
10. Serve hot.

Nutrition: Calories: 128; Protein: 21 Grams; Fat: 4 Grams; Carbs: 3 Grams; Sodium: 81 mg; Cholesterol: 55 mg

215. Decent Beef and Onion Stew

Preparation Time: 10 minutes
Cooking Time 1-2 hours
Servings: 4
Ingredients:
- 2 pounds lean beef, cubed
- 3 pounds shallots, peeled
- 5 garlic cloves, peeled, whole
- 3 tablespoons tomato paste
- 1 bay leaves
- ¼ cup olive oil
- 3 tablespoons lemon juice

Directions:
1. Take a stew pot and place it over medium heat.
2. Add olive oil and let it heat up.
3. Add meat and brown.
4. Add remaining ingredients and cover with water.
5. Bring the whole mix to a boil.
6. Reduce heat to low and cover the pot.
7. Simmer for 1-2 hours until beef is cooked thoroughly.
8. Serve hot!

Nutrition: Calories: 128; Protein: 21 Grams; Fat: 4 Grams; Carbs: 3 Grams; Sodium: 81 mg; Cholesterol: 55 mg

216. Ground Beef with Cabbage

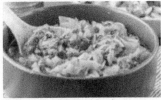

Preparation Time: 10 minutes
Cooking Time: 45 minutes
Servings: 4
Ingredients:

- 1 tbsp. olive oil
- 1 onion, sliced thinly
- 2 teaspoons fresh ginger, minced
- 4 garlic cloves, minced
- 1 pound lean ground beef
- 1½ tablespoons fish sauce
- 2 tablespoons fresh lime juice
- 1 small head purple cabbage, shredded
- 2 tablespoons peanut butter
- ½ cup fresh cilantro, chopped

Directions:

1. In a large skillet, heat oil on medium heat.
2. Add onion, ginger and garlic and sauté for about 4-5 minutes.
3. Add beef and cook for approximately 7-8 minutes, getting into pieces using the spoon.
4. Drain off the extra liquid in the skillet.
5. Stir in fish sauce and lime juice and cook for approximately 1 minute.
6. Add cabbage and cook approximately 4-5 minutes or till desired doneness.
7. Stir in peanut butter and cilantro and cook for about 1 minute.
8. Serve hot.

Nutrition: Calories: 128; Protein: 21 Grams; Fat: 4 Grams; Carbs: 3 Grams; Sodium: 81 mg; Cholesterol: 55 mg

217. Beef & Veggies Chili

Preparation Time: 15 minutes
Cooking Time: 1 hour
Servings: 6-8
Ingredients:

- 2 pounds lean ground beef
- ½ head cauliflower, chopped into large pieces
- 1 onion, chopped
- 6 garlic cloves, minced
- 2 cups pumpkin puree
- 1 teaspoon dried oregano, crushed
- 1 teaspoon dried thyme, crushed
- 1 teaspoon ground cumin
- 1 teaspoon ground turmeric
- 1-2 teaspoons chili powder
- 1 teaspoon paprika
- 1 teaspoon cayenne pepper
- ¼ teaspoon red pepper flakes, crushed
- Salt and freshly ground black pepper, to taste
- 1 (26-ounce) can tomatoes, drained
- ½ cup water
- 1 cup beef broth

Directions:

1. Heat a substantial pan on medium-high heat.
2. Add beef and stir fry for around 5 minutes.
3. Add cauliflower, onion and garlic and stir fry for approximately 5 minutes.
4. Add spices and herbs and stir to mix well.
5. Stir in remaining ingredients and provide to a boil.
6. Reduce heat to low and simmer, covered approximately 30-45 minutes.
7. Serve hot.

Nutrition: Calories: 128; Protein: 21 Grams; Fat: 4 Grams; Carbs: 3 Grams; Sodium: 81 mg; Cholesterol: 55 mg

218. Beef Meatballs in Tomato Gravy

Preparation Time: 20 minutes
Cooking Time: 37 minutes
Servings: 4
Ingredients:

- For Meatballs:
- 1 pound lean ground beef
- 1 organic egg, bea10
- 1 tablespoon fresh ginger, minced
- 1 garlic oil, minced
- 2 tablespoons fresh cilantro, chopped finely
- 2 tablespoons tomato paste
- 1/3 cup almond meal
- 1 tablespoon ground cumin
- Pinch of ground cinnamon
- Salt and freshly ground black pepper, to taste
- ¼ cup coconut oil
- For Tomato Gravy:
- 2 tablespoons coconut oil
- ½ of small onion, chopped
- 2 garlic cloves, chopped
- 1 teaspoon fresh lemon zest, grated finely
- 2 cups tomatoes, chopped finely
- Pinch of ground cinnamon
- 1 teaspoon red pepper flakes, crushed
- ¾ cup chicken broth
- Salt and freshly ground black pepper, to taste
- ¼ cup fresh parsley, chopped

Directions:

1. For meatballs in a sizable bowl, add all ingredients except oil and mix till well combined.
2. Make about 1-inch sized balls from mixture.
3. In a substantial skillet, melt coconut oil on medium heat.
4. Add meatballs and cook for approximately 3-5 minutes or till golden brown all sides.
5. Transfer the meatballs in to a bowl.
6. For gravy in a big pan, melt coconut oil on medium heat.
7. Add onion and garlic and sauté approximately 4 minutes.
8. Add lemon zest and sauté approximately 1 minute.
9. Add tomatoes, cinnamon, red pepper flakes and broth and simmer approximately 7 minutes.

10. Stir in salt, black pepper and meatballs and reduce the warmth to medium-low.
11. Simmer for approximately twenty minutes.
12. Serve hot with all the garnishing of parsley.

Nutrition: Calories: 128; Protein: 21 Grams; Fat: 4 Grams; Carbs: 3 Grams; Sodium: 81 mg; Cholesterol: 55 mg

219. Spicy Lamb Curry

Preparation Time: 15 minutes
Cooking Time: 2 hours 45 minutes
Servings: 6-8
Ingredients:
- For Spice Mixture:
- 4 teaspoons ground coriander
- 4 teaspoons ground coriander
- 4 teaspoons ground cumin
- ¾ teaspoon ground ginger
- 2 teaspoons ground cinnamon
- ½ teaspoon ground cloves
- ½ teaspoon ground cardamom
- 2 tablespoons sweet paprika
- ½ tablespoon cayenne pepper
- 2 teaspoons chili powder
- 2 teaspoons salt
- For Curry:
- 1 tablespoon coconut oil
- 2 pounds boneless lamb, trimmed and cubed into 1-inch size
- Salt and freshly ground black pepper, to taste
- 2 cups onions, chopped
- 1¼ cups water
- 1 cup coconut milk

Directions:
1. For spice mixture in a bowl, mix together all spices. Keep aside.
2. Season the lamb with salt and black pepper.
3. . In a large Dutch oven, heat oil on medium-high heat.
4. Add lamb and stir fry for around 5 minutes.
5. Add onion and cook approximately 4-5 minutes.
6. Stir in spice mixture and cook approximately 1 minute.
7. Add water and coconut milk and provide to some boil on high heat.
8. Reduce the heat to low and simmer, covered for approximately 1-120 minutes or till desired doneness of lamb.
9. Uncover and simmer for approximately 3-4 minutes.
10. Serve hot.

Nutrition: Calories: 128; Protein: 21 Grams; Fat: 4 Grams; Carbs: 3 Grams; Sodium: 81 mg; Cholesterol: 55 mg

220. Ground Lamb with Harissa

Preparation Time: 15 minutes
Cooking Time: 1 hour 11 minutes
Servings: 4
Ingredients:
- 1 tablespoon extra-virgin olive oil
- 2 red peppers, seeded and chopped finely
- 1 yellow onion, chopped finely
- 2 garlic cloves, chopped finely
- 1 teaspoon ground cumin
- ½ teaspoon ground turmeric
- ¼ teaspoon ground cinnamon
- ¼ teaspoon ground ginger
- 1½ pound lean ground lamb
- Salt, to taste
- 1 (14½-ounce) can diced tomatoes
- 2 tablespoons harissa
- 1 cup water
- Chopped fresh cilantro, for garnishing

Directions:
1. In a sizable pan, heat oil on medium-high heat.
2. Add bell pepper, onion and garlic and sauté for around 5 minutes.
3. Add spices and sauté for around 1 minute.
4. Add lamb and salt and cook approximately 5 minutes, getting into pieces.
5. Stir in tomatoes, harissa and water and provide with a boil.
6. Reduce the warmth to low and simmer, covered for about 1 hour.
7. Serve hot while using garnishing of harissa.

Nutrition: Calories: 128; Protein: 21 Grams; Fat: 4 Grams; Carbs: 3 Grams; Sodium: 81 mg; Cholesterol: 55 mg

221. Roasted Lamb Chops

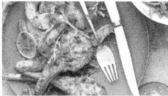

Preparation Time: 15 minutes
Cooking Time: 30 minutes
Servings: 4
Ingredients:
- For Lamb Marinade:
- 4 garlic cloves, chopped
- 1 (2-inch) piece fresh ginger, chopped
- 2 green chilies, seeded and chopped
- 1 teaspoon fresh lime zest
- 2 teaspoons garam masala
- 1 teaspoon ground coriander
- 1 teaspoon ground cumin
- ½ teaspoon ground cinnamon
- 1 teaspoon coconut oil, melted
- 2 tablespoons fresh lime juice
- 6-7 tablespoons plain Greek yogurt
- 1 (8-bone) rack of lamb, trimmed
- 2 onions, sliced
- For Relish:
- ½ of garlic herb, chopped
- 1 (1-inch) piece fresh ginger, chopped
- ¼ cup fresh cilantro, chopped
- ¼ cup fresh mint, chopped
- 1 green chili, seeded and chopped
- 1 teaspoon fresh lime zest

- 1 teaspoon organic honey
- 2 tablespoons fresh apple juice
- 2 tablespoons fresh lime juice

Directions:
1. For chops in a very mixer, add all ingredients except yogurt, chops and onions and pulse till smooth.
2. Transfer the mixture in a large bowl with yogurt and stir to combine well.
3. Add chops and coat with mixture generously.
4. Refrigerate to marinate for approximately twenty four hours.
5. Preheat the oven to 375 degrees F. Linea roasting pan with a foil paper.
6. Place the onion wedges in the bottom of prepared roasting pan.
7. Arrange rack of lamb over onion wedges.
8. Roast approximately half an hour.
9. Meanwhile for relish in the blender, add all ingredients and pulse till smooth.
10. Serve chops and onions alongside relish.

Nutrition: Calories: 128; Protein: 21 Grams; Fat: 4 Grams; Carbs: 3 Grams; Sodium: 81 mg; Cholesterol: 55 mg

222. Baked Meatballs & Scallions

Preparation Time: 20 minutes
Cooking Time: 35 minutes
Servings: 4-6
Ingredients:
- For Meatballs:
- 1 lemongrass stalk, outer skin peeled and chopped
- 1 (1½-inch) piece fresh ginger, sliced
- 3 garlic cloves, chopped
- 1 cup fresh cilantro leaves, chopped roughly
- ½ cup fresh basil leaves, chopped roughly
- 2 tablespoons plus 1 teaspoon fish sauce
- 2 tablespoons water
- 2 tablespoons fresh lime juice
- ½ pound lean ground pork
- 1 pound lean ground lamb
- 1 carrot, peeled and grated
- 1 organic egg, bea10 For Scallions:
- 16 stalks scallions, trimmed
- 2 tablespoons coconut oil, melted
- Salt, to taste
- ½ cup water

Directions:
1. Preheat the oven to 375 degrees F. Grease a baking dish.
2. In a blender, add lemongrass, ginger, garlic, fresh herbs, fish sauce, water and lime juice and pulse till chopped finely.
3. Transfer the amalgamation in a bowl with remaining ingredients and mix till well combined.
4. Make about 1-inch balls from mixture.
5. Arrange the balls into prepared baking dish in a single layer.
6. In another rimmed baking dish, arrange scallion stalks in a very single layer.
7. Drizzle with coconut oil and sprinkle with salt.
8. Pour water in the baking dish 1nd with a foil paper cover it tightly.

9. Bake the scallion for around a half-hour.
10. Bake the meatballs for approximately 30-35 minutes. Pork with Bell Pepper.
11. This stir fry not simply tastes wonderful but additionally is packed with nutritious benefits.

Nutrition: Calories: 128; Protein: 21 Grams; Fat: 4 Grams; Carbs: 3 Grams; Sodium: 81 mg; Cholesterol: 55 mg

223. Pork Chili

Preparation Time: 45 minutes
Cooking Time: 60 minutes
Servings: 4
Ingredients:
- 2 tablespoons extra-virgin organic olive oil
- 2 pound ground pork
- 1 medium red bell pepper, seeded and chopped
- 1 medium onion, chopped
- 5 garlic cloves, chopped finely
- 1 (2-inch) part of hot pepper, minced
- 1 tablespoon ground cumin
- 1 teaspoon ground turmeric
- 3 tablespoon chili powder
- ½ teaspoon chipotle chili powder
- Salt and freshly ground black pepper, to taste
- 1 cup chicken broth
- 1 (28-ounce) can fire-roasted crushed tomatoes
- 2 medium bokchoy heads, sliced
- 1 avocado, peeled, pitted and chopped

Directions:
1. In a sizable pan, heat oil on medium heat.
2. Add pork and stir fry for about 5 minutes.
3. Add bell pepper, onion, garlic, hot pepper and spices and stir fry for approximately 5 minutes.
4. Add broth and tomatoes and convey with a boil.
5. Stir in bokchoy and cook, covered for approximately twenty minutes.
6. Uncover and cook approximately 20-half an hour.
7. Serve hot while using topping of avocado.

Nutrition: Calories: 128; Protein: 21 Grams; Fat: 4 Grams; Carbs: 3 Grams; Sodium: 81 mg; Cholesterol: 55 mg

224. Baked Pork & Mushroom Meatballs

Preparation Time: 15 minutes
Cooking Time: 15 minutes
Servings: 6
Ingredients:
- 1 pound lean ground pork
- 1 organic egg white, bea10
- 4 fresh shiitake mushrooms, stemmed and minced
- 1 tablespoon fresh parsley, minced
- 1 tablespoon fresh basil leaves, minced
- 1 tablespoon fresh mint leaves, minced
- 2 teaspoons fresh lemon zest, grated finely
- 1½ teaspoons fresh ginger, grated finely
- Salt and freshly ground black pepper, to taste

Directions:

1. Preheat the oven to 425 degrees F. Arrange the rack inside center of oven.
2. Line a baking sheet with a parchment paper.
3. . In a sizable bowl, add all ingredients and mix till well combined.
4. Make small equal-sized balls from mixture.
5. Arrange the balls onto prepared baking sheet in a single layer.
6. Bake for approximately 12-quarter-hour or till done completely.

Nutrition: Calories: 128; Protein: 21 Grams; Fat: 4 Grams; Carbs: 3 Grams; Sodium: 81 mg; Cholesterol: 55 mg

225. Citrus Beef with Bok Choy

Preparation Time: 15 minutes
Cooking Time: 11 minutes
Servings: 4
Ingredients:
- For Marinade:
- 2 minced garlic cloves
- 1 (1-inch) piece fresh ginger, grated
- 1/3 cup fresh orange juice
- ½ cup coconut aminos
- 2 teaspoons fish sauce
- 2 teaspoons Sriracha
- 1¼ pound sirloin steak, trimmed and sliced thinly
- For Veggies:
- 2 tablespoons coconut oil, divided
- 3-4 wide strips of fresh orange zest
- 1 jalapeño pepper, sliced thinly
- ½ pound string beans, stemmed and halved crosswise
- 1 tablespoon arrowroot powder
- ½ pound bokchoy, chopped
- 2 teaspoons sesame seeds

Directions:
1. For marinade in a big bowl, mix together garlic, ginger, orange juice, coconut aminos, fish sauce and Sriracha.
2. Add beef and coat with marinade generously.
3. Refrigerate to marinate for around couple of hours.
4. In a substantial skillet, heat oil on medium-high heat.
5. Add orange zest and sauté approximately 2 minutes.
6. Remove beef from bowl, reserving the marinade.
7. In the skillet, add beef and increase the heat to high.
8. Stir fry for about 2-3 minutes or till browned.
9. With a slotted spoon, transfer the beef and orange strips right into a bowl.
10. With a paper towel, wipe out the skillet.
11. In a similar skillet, heat remaining oil on medium-high heat.
12. Add jalapeño pepper and string beans and stir fry for about 3-4 minutes.
13. Meanwhile add arrowroot powder in reserved marinade and stir to mix.
14. . In the skillet, add marinade mixture, beef and bokchoy and cook for about 1-2 minutes.
15. Serve hot with garnishing of sesame seeds.

Nutrition: Calories: 128; Protein: 21 Grams; Fat: 4 Grams; Carbs: 3 Grams; Sodium: 81 mg; Cholesterol: 55 mg

226. Ground Beef with Greens & Tomatoes

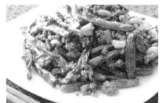

Preparation Time: 15 minutes
Cooking Time: 15 minutes
Servings: 4
Ingredients:
- 1 tbsp. organic olive oil
- ½ of white onion, chopped
- 2 garlic cloves, chopped finely
- 1 jalapeño pepper, chopped finely
- 1 pound lean ground beef
- 1 teaspoon ground coriander
- 1 teaspoon ground cumin
- ½ teaspoon ground turmeric
- ½ teaspoon ground ginger
- ½ teaspoon ground cinnamon
- ½ teaspoon ground fennel seeds
- Salt and freshly ground black pepper, to taste
- 8 fresh cherry tomatoes, quartered
- 8 collard greens leaves, stemmed and chopped
- 1 teaspoon fresh lemon juice

Directions:
1. In a big skillet, heat oil on medium heat.
2. Add onion and sauté for approximately 4 minutes.
3. Add garlic and jalapeño pepper and sauté for approximately 1 minute.
4. Add beef and spices and cook approximately 6 minutes breaking into pieces while using spoon.
5. Stir in tomatoes and greens and cook, stirring gently for about 4 minutes.
6. Stir in lemon juice and take away from heat.

Nutrition: Calories: 128; Protein: 21 Grams; Fat: 4 Grams; Carbs: 3 Grams; Sodium: 81 mg; Cholesterol: 55 mg

227. Curried Beef Meatballs

Preparation Time: 20 minutes
Cooking Time: 22 minutes
Servings: 6
Ingredients:
- For Meatballs:
- 1 pound lean ground beef
- 2 organic eggs, bea10
- 3 tablespoons red onion, minced
- ¼ cup fresh basil leaves, chopped
- 1 (1-inch) fresh ginger piece, chopped finely
- 4 garlic cloves, chopped finely
- 3 Thai bird's eye chilies, minced
- 1 teaspoon coconut sugar
- 1 tablespoon red curry paste
- Salt, to taste
- 1 tablespoon fish sauce

- 2 tablespoons coconut oil
- For Curry:
- 1 red onion, chopped
- Salt, to taste
- 4 garlic cloves, minced
- 1 (1-inch) fresh ginger piece, minced
- 2 Thai bird's eye chilies, minced
- 2 tablespoons red curry paste
- 1 (14-ounce) coconut milk
- Salt and freshly ground black pepper, to taste
- Lime wedges, for serving

Directions:
1. For meatballs in a large bowl, add all ingredients except oil and mix till well combined.
2. Make small balls from mixture.
3. In a large skillet, melt coconut oil on medium heat.
4. Add meatballs and cook for about 3-5 minutes or till golden brown all sides.
5. Transfer the meatballs right into a bowl.
6. In the same skillet, add onion as well as a pinch of salt and sauté for around 5 minutes.
7. Add garlic, ginger and chilies and sauté for about 1 minute.
8. Add curry paste and sauté for around 1 minute.
9. Add coconut milk and meatballs and convey to some gentle simmer.
10. Reduce the warmth to low and simmer, covered for around 10 minutes.
11. Serve using the topping of lime wedges.

Nutrition: Calories: 128; Protein: 21 Grams; Fat: 4 Grams; Carbs: 3 Grams; Sodium: 81 mg; Cholesterol: 55 mg

228. Grilled Skirt Steak Coconut

Preparation Time: 45 minutes
Cooking Time: 8-9 minutes
Servings: 4
Ingredients:
- 2 teaspoons fresh ginger herb, grated finely
- 2 teaspoons fresh lime zest, grated finely
- ¼ cup coconut sugar
- 2 teaspoons fish sauce
- 2 tablespoons fresh lime juice
- ½ cup coconut milk
- 1 pound beef skirt steak, trimmed and cut into 4-inch slices lengthwise
- Salt, to taste

Directions:
1. In a sizable sealable bag, mix together all ingredients except steak and salt.
2. Add steak and coat with marinade generously.
3. Seal the bag and refrigerate to marinate for about 4-12 hours.
4. Preheat the grill to high heat. Grease the grill grate.
5. Remove steak from refrigerator and discard the marinade.
6. With a paper towel, dry the steak and sprinkle with salt evenly.
7. Cook the steak for approximately 3½ minutes.
8. Flip the medial side and cook for around 2½-5 minutes or till desired doneness.

9. Remove from grill pan and keep side for approximately 5 minutes before slicing. 10. With a clear, crisp knife cut into desired slices and serve.

Nutrition: Calories: 128; Protein: 21 Grams; Fat: 4 Grams; Carbs: 3 Grams; Sodium: 81 mg; Cholesterol: 55 mg

229. Lamb with Prunes

Preparation Time: 15 minutes
Cooking Time: 40 minutes
Servings: 6
Ingredients:
- 3 tablespoons coconut oil
- 2 onions, chopped finely
- 1 (1-inch) piece fresh ginger, minced
- 3 garlic cloves, minced
- ½ teaspoon ground turmeric
- 2 ½ pound lamb shoulder, trimmed and cubed into 3-inch size
- Salt and freshly ground black pepper, to taste
- ½ teaspoon saffron threads, crumbled
- 1 cinnamon stick
- 3 cups water
- 1 cup runes, pitted and halved

Directions:
1. In a big pan, melt coconut oil on medium heat.
2. Add onions, ginger, garlic cloves and turmeric and sauté for about 3-5 minutes.
3. Sprinkle the lamb with salt and black pepper evenly.
4. In the pan, add lamb and saffron threads and cook for approximately 4-5 minutes.
5. Add cinnamon stick and water and produce to some boil on high heat.
6. Reduce the temperature to low and simmer, covered for around 1½-120 minutes or till desired doneness of lamb.
7. Stir in prunes and simmer for approximately 20-a half-hour.
8. . Remove cinnamon stick and serve hot.

Nutrition: Calories: 128; Protein: 21 Grams; Fat: 4 Grams; Carbs: 3 Grams; Sodium: 81 mg; Cholesterol: 55 mg

230. Ground Lamb with Peas

Preparation Time: 15 minutes
Cooking Time: 55 minutes
Servings: 4
Ingredients:
- 1 tablespoon coconut oil
- 3 dried red chilies
- 1 (2-inch) cinnamon stick
- 3 green cardamom pods
- ½ teaspoon cumin seeds
- 1 medium red onion, chopped
- 1 (¾-inch) piece fresh ginger, minced
- 4 garlic cloves, minced
- 1½ teaspoons ground coriander
- ½ teaspoon garam masala
- ½ teaspoon ground cumin
- ½ teaspoon ground turmeric
- ¼ teaspoon ground nutmeg

- 2 bay leaves
- 1 pound lean ground lamb
- ½ cup Roma tomatoes, chopped
- 1-1½ cups water
- 1 cup fresh green peas, shelled
- 2 tablespoons plain Greek yogurt, whipped
- ¼ cup fresh cilantro, chopped
- Salt and freshly ground black pepper, to taste

Directions:
1. In a Dutch oven, melt coconut oil medium-high heat.
2. Add red chilies, cinnamon stick, cardamom pods and cumin seeds and sauté for around thirty seconds.
3. Add onion and sauté for about 3-4 minutes.
4. Add ginger, garlic cloves and spices and sauté for around thirty seconds.
5. Add lamb and cook approximately 5 minutes.
6. Add tomatoes and cook approximately 10 min.
7. Stir in water and green peas and cook, covered approximately 25-thirty minutes.
8. Stir in yogurt, cilantro, salt and black pepper and cook for around 4-5 minutes.
9. Serve hot.

Nutrition: Calories: 128; Protein: 21 Grams; Fat: 4 Grams; Carbs: 3 Grams; Sodium: 81 mg; Cholesterol: 55 mg

231. Basil Halibut

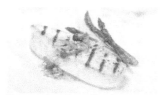

Preparation time: 10 minutes
Cooking time: 20 minutes
Servings: 4

Ingredients:
- 4 Halibut Fillets, 4 Ounces Each
- 2 Teaspoons Olive Oil
- 1 Tablespoon Garlic, Minced
- 2 Tomatoes, Diced
- 2 Tablespoons Basil, Fresh & Chopped
- 1 Teaspoon Oregano, Fresh & Chopped

Directions:
1. Heat the oven to 350, and then get out a 9 by 13-inch pan. Spray it down with cooking spray.
2. Toss the basil, olive oil garlic, oregano and tomato together in a bowl. Pour this over your fish in the pan.
3. Bake the twelve minutes. Your fish should be flakey.

Nutrition: Calories: 128; Protein: 21 Grams; Fat: 4 Grams; Carbs: 3 Grams; Sodium: 81 mg; Cholesterol: 55 mg

232. Beef with Mushroom & Broccoli

Preparation Time: 45 minutes
Cooking Time: 12 minutes
Servings: 4

Ingredients:
- For Beef Marinade:

- 1 garlic clove, minced
- 1 (2-inch) piece fresh ginger, minced
- Salt and freshly ground black pepper, to taste
- 3 tablespoons white wine vinegar
- ¾ cup beef broth
- 1 pound flank steak, trimmed and sliced into thin strips
- For Vegetables:
- 2 tablespoons coconut oil, divided
- 2 minced garlic cloves
- 3 cups broccoli Rabe, chopped
- 4-ounce shiitake mushrooms, halved
- 8-ounce Cremini mushrooms, sliced

Directions:
1. For marinade in a substantial bowl, mix together all ingredients except beef.
2. Add beef and coat with marinade generously.
3. Refrigerate to marinate for around quarter-hour.
4. In a substantial skillet, heat oil on medium-high heat.
5. Remove beef from bowl, reserving the marinade.
6. Add beef and garlic and cook for about 3-4 minutes or till browned.
7. With a slotted spoon, transfer the beef in a bowl.
8. In exactly the same skillet, add reserved marinade, broccoli and mushrooms and cook for approximately 3-4 minutes.
9. Stir in beef and cook for about 3-4 minutes.

Nutrition: Calories: 128; Protein: 21 Grams; Fat: 4 Grams; Carbs: 3 Grams; Sodium: 81 mg; Cholesterol: 55 mg

233. Beef with Zucchini Noodles

Preparation Time: 15 minutes
Cooking Time: 9 minutes
Servings: 4

Ingredients:
- 1 teaspoon fresh ginger, grated
- 2 medium garlic cloves, minced
- ¼ cup coconut aminos
- 2 tablespoons fresh lime juice
- 1½ pound NY strip steak, trimmed and sliced thinly
- 2 medium zucchinis, spiralized with Blade C
- Salt, to taste
- 3 tablespoons essential olive oil
- 2 medium scallions, sliced
- 1 teaspoon red pepper flakes, crushed
- 2 tablespoons fresh cilantro, chopped

Directions:
1. In a big bowl, mix together ginger, garlic, coconut aminos and lime juice.
2. Add beef and coat with marinade generously.
3. Refrigerate to marinate approximately 10 minutes.
4. Place zucchini noodles over a large paper towel and sprinkle with salt.
5. Keep aside for around 10 minutes.
6. In a big skillet, heat oil on medium-high heat.
7. Add scallion and red pepper flakes and sauté for about 1 minute.
8. Add beef with marinade and stir fry for around 3-4 minutes or till browned.
9. Add zucchini and cook for approximately 3-4 minutes.

10. Serve hot with all the topping of cilantro.
Nutrition: Calories: 128; Protein: 21 Grams; Fat: 4 Grams; Carbs: 3 Grams; Sodium: 81 mg; Cholesterol: 55 mg

234. Spiced Ground Beef

Preparation Time: 10 minutes
Cooking Time: 22 minutes
Servings: 5
Ingredients:
- 2 tablespoons coconut oil
- 2 whole cloves
- 2 whole cardamoms
- 1 (2-inch) piece cinnamon stick
- 2 bay leaves
- 1 teaspoon cumin seeds
- 2 onions, chopped
- Salt, to taste
- ½ tablespoon garlic paste
- ½ tablespoon fresh ginger paste
- 1 pound lean ground beef
- 1½ teaspoons fennel seeds powder
- 1 teaspoon ground cumin
- 1½ teaspoons red chili powder
- 1/8 teaspoon ground turmeric
- Freshly ground black pepper, to taste
- 1 cup coconut milk
- ¼ cup water
- ¼ cup fresh cilantro, chopped

Directions:
1. In a sizable pan, heat oil on medium heat.
2. Add cloves, cardamoms, cinnamon stick, bay leaves and cumin seeds and sauté for about 20-a few seconds.
3. Add onion and 2 pinches of salt and sauté for about 3-4 minutes.
4. Add garlic-ginger paste and sauté for about 2 minutes.
5. Add beef and cook for about 4-5 minutes, entering pieces using the spoon.
6. Cover and cook approximately 5 minutes.
7. Stir in spices and cook, stirring for approximately 2-2½ minutes.
8. Stir in coconut milk and water and cook for about 7-8 minutes.
9. Season with salt and take away from heat.
10. Serve hot using the garnishing of cilantro.

Nutrition: Calories: 128; Protein: 21 Grams; Fat: 4 Grams; Carbs: 3 Grams; Sodium: 81 mg; Cholesterol: 55 mg

235. Ground Beef with Veggies

Preparation Time: 45 minutes
Cooking Time: 20 minutes
Servings: 4-5
Ingredients
- 1-2 tablespoons coconut oil
- 1 red onion, sliced
- 2 red jalapeño peppers, seeded and sliced
- 2 minced garlic cloves

- 1 pound lean ground beef
- 1 small head broccoli, chopped
- ½ of head cauliflower, chopped
- 3 carrots, peeled and sliced
- 3 celery ribs, sliced
- Chopped fresh thyme, to taste
- Dried sage, to taste
- Ground turmeric, to taste
- Salt and freshly ground black pepper, to taste

Directions:
1. In a large skillet, melt coconut oil on medium heat.
2. Add onion, jalapeño peppers and garlic and sauté for about 5 minutes.
3. Add beef and cook for around 4-5 minutes, entering pieces using the spoon.
4. Add remaining ingredients and cook, stirring occasionally for about 8-10 min.
5. Serve hot.

Nutrition: Calories: 128; Protein: 21 Grams; Fat: 4 Grams; Carbs: 3 Grams; Sodium: 81 mg; Cholesterol: 55 mg

236. Shrimp & Corn Chowder

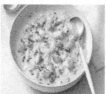

Preparation time: 20 minutes
Cooking time: 30 minutes
Servings: 6
Ingredients:
- 2 Carrots, Peeled & Sliced
- 1 Yellow Onion, Sliced
- 3 Tablespoons Olive Oil
- 2 Celery Stalks, Diced
- 4 Baby Red Potatoes, Diced
- 4 Cloves Garlic, Peeled & Minced
- ¼ Cup All Purpose Flour
- 3 Cups Vegetable Stock, Unsalted
- ½ Cup Milk
- ¾ Teaspoon Sea Salt, Fine
- ¼ Teaspoon Black Pepper
- ¼ Teaspoon Cayenne Pepper
- 4 Cups Corn Kernels Fresh
- 1 lb. Shrimp, Peeled & Deveined
- 2 Scallions Sliced Thin

Directions:
1. Get out a stockpot and heat your oil using medium heat. Once your oil is hot adding in your carrots, celery, potatoes and onion. Cook for seven minutes. The vegetable should soften. Stir and then add in your garlic. Cook for a minute more.
2. Make a flour roux, and increase the heat to medium high. Whisk and bring it to a simmer. Make sure to whisk any lumps out. Whisk in your milk, salt, pepper and cayenne. Allow it to simmer until it thickens. This should take about eight minutes.
3. Add in your shrimp and corn, and cook for another five minutes.

4. Divide between bowls to serve warm.

Nutrition: Calories: 340; Protein: 23 Grams; Fat: 9 Grams; Carbs: 45 Grams; Sodium: 473 mg; Cholesterol: 115 mg

237. Leek & Cauliflower Soup

Preparation time: 20 minutes
Cooking time: 20 minutes
Servings: 6
Ingredients:
- 1 Tablespoon Olive Oil
- 1 Leek, Trimmed & Sliced Thin
- 1 Yellow Onion, Peeled & Diced
- 1 Head Cauliflower, Chopped into Florets
- 3 Cloves Garlic, Minced
- 2 Tablespoons Thyme, Fresh & Chopped
- 1 Teaspoon Smoked Paprika
- 1 ¼ Teaspoons Sea Salt, Fine
- 1/4Teaspoon Ground Cayenne Pepper
- 1 Tablespoon Heavy Cream
- 3 Cups Vegetable Stock, Unsalted
- ½ Lemon, Juiced & Zested

Directions:
1. Heat your oil in a stockpot over medium heat, and add in your leek, onion, and cauliflower. Cook for five minutes or until the onion begins to soften. Add in your garlic, thyme, smoked paprika, salt, pepper and cayenne. Pour in your vegetable stock and bring it to a simmer, cooking for fifteen minutes. Your cauliflower should be very tender.
2. Remove from heat and stir in your lemon juice, lemon zest and cream. Use an immersion blender to puree, and serve warm.

Nutrition: Calories: 92; Protein: 5 Grams; Fat: 4 Grams; Carbs: 13 Grams; Sodium: 556 mg; Cholesterol: 3 mg

238. Easy Beef Brisket

Preparation time: 2 hours
Cooking time: 1 hour and 10 minutes
Servings: 4
Ingredients:
- 1 Teaspoon Thyme
- 4 Cloves Garlic, Peeled & Smashed
- 1 ½ Cups Onion, chopped
- 2 ½ lbs. Beef Brisket, Chopped
- 1 Tablespoons Olive Oil
- ¼ Teaspoon Black Pepper
- 14.5 Ounces Tomatoes & Liquid, Canned
- ¼ Cup Red Wine Vinegar
- 1 Cup Beef Stock, Low Sodium

Directions:
1. Turn the oven to 350, and then grease a Dutch oven using a tablespoon of oil. Place it over medium heat.
2. Add in your pepper and brisket. Cook until it browns, and then place your brisket on a plate.
3. Put your onions in the pot, and cook until golden brown. Stir in your garlic and thyme, cooking for another full minute before adding in the stock, vinegar and tomatoes.
4. Cook until it comes to a boil and add in your brisket again.

5. Reduce to a simmer, and cook for three hours in the oven until tender.

Nutrition: Calories: 299; Protein: 10.2 Grams; Fat: 9 Grams; Carbs: 21.4 Grams; Sodium: 372 mg; Cholesterol: 101 mg

239. Coconut Shrimp

Preparation time: 10 minutes
Cooking time: 15 minutes
Servings: 4
Ingredients:
- ¼ Cup Coconut, Sweetened
- ½ Teaspoon Sea Salt, Fine
- ¼ Cup Panko Breadcrumbs
- ½ Cup Coconut Milk
- 12 Large Shrimp, Peeled & Deveined

Directions:
1. Preheat your oven to 375, and then get out a baking pan. Spray it with cooking spray before setting it aside.
2. Grind your panko with coconut and salt in a food processor.
3. Add this mixture to a bowl and pour the coconut milk in another bowl.
4. Dip the shrimp in the coconut mixture and then dredge it through the panko mixture. Put the coated shrimp on the baking pan, and then bake for fifteen minutes. Serve warm.

Nutrition: Calories: 249; Protein: 35 Grams; Fat: 1.7 Grams; Carbs: 1.8 Grams; Sodium: 79 mg; Cholesterol: 78 mg

240. Asian Salmon

Preparation time: 10 minutes
Cooking time: 20 minutes
Servings: 2
Ingredients:
- 1 Cup Fresh Fruit, Diced
- ¼ Teaspoon Black Pepper
- 2 Salmon Fillets, 4 Ounces Each
- ¼ Teaspoon Sesame Oil
- 1 Teaspoon Soy Sauce, Low Sodium
- 2 Cloves Garlic, Minced
- ½ Cup Pineapple Juice, Sugar Free

Directions:
1. Start by getting out a bowl and mix your garlic, soy sauce, ginger and pineapple juice together. Place your fish in the dough and make sure it's covered. It marinates for an hour.
2. Flip the fillets after thirty minutes, and then heat the oven to 375.
3. Get out aluminum squares and grease them with cooking spray. Put the salmon fillet on each square, and drizzle with pepper, diced fruit and sesame oil. Fold the aluminum sheet to seal the fish, and then place them on the baking sheet.
4. Bake for ten minutes per side before serving.

Nutrition: Calories: 247; Protein: 27 Grams; Fat: 7 Grams; Carbs: 19 Grams; Sodium: 350 mg; Cholesterol: 120 mg

241. Fennel Sauce Tenderloin

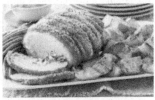

Preparation Time: 10 minutes
Cooking Time: 25 minutes
Servings: 4

Ingredients:

- 1 Fennel Bulb, Cored & Sliced
- 1 Sweet Onion, Sliced
- ½ Cup Dry White Wine
- 1 Teaspoon Fennel Seeds
- 4 Pork Tenderloin Fillets
- 2 Tablespoons Olive Oil
- 12 Ounces Chicken Broth, Low Sodium
- Fennel Fronds for Garnish
- Orange Slices for Garnish

Directions:

1. Thin your pork tenderloin by spreading them between parchment sheets and pounding with a mallet.
2. Heat a skillet, and add in your oil. Place it over medium heat, and cook your fennel seeds for three minutes.
3. Add the pork to the pan, cooking for an additional three minutes per side.
4. Transfer your pork to a platter before setting it to the side, and add in your fennel and onion.
5. Cook for five minutes, and then place the vegetables to the side.
6. Pour in your broth and wine, and bring it to a boil over high heat. Cook until the liquid has reduced by half.
7. Return your pork to the skillet, and cook for another five minutes.
8. Stir in your onion mixture, covering again. Cook for two more minutes, and serve warm.

Nutrition: Calories: 276; Protein: 23.4 Grams; Fat: 24 Grams; Carbs: 14 Grams; Sodium: 647 mg; Cholesterol: 49 mg

242. Beefy Fennel Stew

Preparation time: 20 minutes
Cooking time: 1 hour and 20 minutes
Servings: 4

Ingredients:

- 1 lb. Lean Beef, Boneless & Cubed
- 2 Tablespoons Olive Oil
- ½ Fennel Bulb, Sliced
- 3 Tablespoons All Purpose Flour
- 3 Shallots, Large & Chopped
- ¾ Teaspoon Black Pepper, Divided
- 2 Thyme Sprigs, Fresh
- 1 Bay Leaf
- ½ Cup Red Wine
- 3 Cups Vegetable Stock
- 4 Carrots, Peeled & Sliced into 1 Inch Pieces
- 4 White Potatoes, Large & Cubed
- 18 Small Boiling Onions, Halved

- 1/3 Cup Flat Leaf Parsley, Fresh & Chopped
- 3 Portobello Mushrooms, Chopped

Directions:

1. Get out a shallow container and add in your flour. Dredge the beef cubes through it, shaking off the excess flour.
2. Get out a saucepan and add in your oil, heating it over medium heat.
3. Add your beef, and cook for five minutes.
4. Add in your fennel and shallots, cooking for seven minutes. Stir in your pepper, bay leaf and thyme. Cook for a minute more.
5. Add your beef to the pan with your stock and wine.
6. Boil it and reduce it to a simmer. Cover, cooking for forty-five minutes.
7. Add in your onions, potatoes, carrots and mushrooms. Cook for another half hour, which should leave your vegetables tender.
8. Remove the thyme sprigs and bay leaf before serving warm. Garnish with parsley.

Nutrition: Calories: 244; Protein: 21 Grams; Fat: 8 Grams; Carbs: 22.1 Grams; Sodium: 587 mg; Cholesterol: 125 mg

243. Currant Pork Chops

Preparation time: 10 minutes
Cooking time: 20 minutes
Servings: 6

Ingredients:

- 2 Tablespoons Dijon Mustard
- 6 Pork Loin Chops, Center Cut
- 2 Teaspoons Olive Oil
- 1/3 Cup Wine Vinegar
- ¼ Cup Black Currant Jam
- 6 Orange Slices
- 1/8 Teaspoon Black Pepper

Directions:

1. Start by mixing your mustard and jam together in a bowl.
2. Get out a nonstick skillet, and grease it with olive oil before placing it over medium heat. Cook your chops for five minutes per side, and then top with a tablespoon of the jam mixture. Cover, and allow it to cook for two minutes. Transfer them to a serving plate.
3. Pour your wine vinegar in the same skillet, and scape the bits up to deglaze the pan, mixing well. Drizzle this over your pork chops.
4. Garnish with pepper and orange slices before serving warm.

Nutrition: Calories: 265; Protein: 25 Grams; Fat: 6 Grams; Carbs: 11 Grams; Sodium: 120 mg; Cholesterol: 22 mg

244. Spicy Tomato Shrimp

Preparation time: 10 minutes
Cooking time: 25 minutes
Servings: 6

Ingredients:

- ¾ lb. Shrimp, Uncooked, Peeled & Deveined
- 2 Tablespoons Tomato Paste
- ½ Teaspoon Garlic, Minced
- ½ Teaspoon Olive Oil

- 1 ½ Teaspoons Water
- ½ Teaspoon Oregano, Chopped
- ½ Teaspoon Chipotle Chili Powder

Directions:
1. Rinse and dry the shrimp before setting them to the side.
2. Get out a bowl and mix your tomato paste, water, chili powder, oil, oregano and garlic. Spread this over your shrimp, and make sure they're coated on both sides.
3. Marinate for about twenty minutes or until you're ready to grill. Preheat a gas grill to medium heat, and then grease the grate with oil. Place it six inches from the heat source. Skewer the shrimp, and for four minutes per side. Serve warm.

Nutrition: Calories: 185; Protein: 16.9 Grams; Fat: 1 Gram; Carbs: 12.4 Grams; Sodium: 394 mg; Cholesterol: 15 mg

245. Beef Stir Fry

Preparation time: 20 minutes
Cooking time: 20 minutes
Servings: 4

Ingredients:
- 1 Head Broccoli Chopped into Florets
- 1 Red Bell Pepper, Sliced Thin
- 1 ½ Cups Brown Rice
- 2 Scallions, Sliced Thin
- 2 Tablespoons Sesame Seeds
- ¼ Teaspoon Black Pepper
- 1 lb. Flank Steak, Sliced Thin
- 2 Tablespoons Canola Oil
- ¾ Cup Stir Fry Sauce

Directions:
1. Start by heating your oil in a large wok over medium-high heat. Add in your steak, seasoning with pepper. Cook for four minutes or until crisp. Remove it from the skillet.
2. Place your broccoli in the skillet and cook for four minutes. Toss occasionally. It should be tender but crisp.
3. Put your steak back in the skillet, and pour in your sauce. Allow it to simmer for three minutes.
4. Serve over rice with sesame seeds and scallions.

Nutrition: Calories: 408; Protein: 31 Grams; Fat: 18 Grams; Carbs: 36 Grams; Sodium: 461 mg; Cholesterol: 57 mg

246. Grilled Chicken with Lemon and Fennel

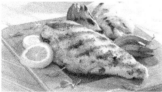

Preparation time: 5 minutes
Cooking time: 25 minutes
Servings: 4

Ingredients:
- 2 cups chicken fillets , cut and skewed
- 1 large fennel bulb
- 2 garlic cloves
- 1 jar green olives

- 1 lemon

Directions:
1. Pre-heat your grill to medium-high.
2. Crush garlic cloves.
3. Take a bowl and add olive oil and season with sunflower seeds and pepper.
4. Coat chicken skewers with the marinade.
5. Transfer them under the grill and grill for 20 minutes, making sure to turn them halfway through until golden.
6. Zest half of the lemon and cut the other half into quarters.
7. Cut the fennel bulb into similarly sized segments.
8. Brush olive oil all over the garlic clove segments and cook for 3-5 minutes.
9. Chop them and add them to the bowl with the marinade.
10. Add lemon zest and olives.
11. Once the meat is ready, serve with the vegetable mix.
12. Enjoy!

Nutrition: Calories: 649; Fat: 16g; Carbohydrates: 33g; Protein: 18g

247. Caramelized Pork Chops and Onion

Preparation time: 5 minutes
Cooking time: 40 minutes
Servings: 4

Ingredients:
- 4-pound chuck roast
- 4 ounces green Chili, chopped
- 2 tablespoons of chili powder
- ½ teaspoon of dried oregano
- ½ teaspoon of cumin, ground
- 2 garlic cloves, minced

Directions:
1. Rub the chops with a seasoning of 1 teaspoon of pepper and 2 teaspoons of sunflower seeds.
2. Take a skillet and place it over medium heat, add oil and allow the oil to heat up
3. Brown the seasoned chop both sides.
4. Add water and onion to the skillet and cover, lower the heat to low and simmer for 20 minutes.
5. Turn the chops over and season with more sunflower seeds and pepper.
6. Cover and cook until the water fully evaporates and the beer shows a slightly brown texture.
7. Remove the chops and serve with a topping of the caramelized onion.
8. Serve and enjoy!

Nutrition: Calorie: 47; Fat: 4g; Carbohydrates: 4g; Protein: 0.5g

248. Hearty Pork Belly Casserole

Preparation time: 5 minutes
Cooking time: 25 minutes
Servings: 4

Ingredients:
- 8 pork belly slices, cut into small pieces
- 3 large onions, chopped
- 4 tablespoons lemon

- Juice of 1 lemon
- Seasoning as you needed

Directions:
1. Take a large pressure cooker and place it over medium heat.
2. Add onions and sweat them for 5 minutes.
3. Add pork belly slices and cook until the meat browns and onions become golden.
4. Cover with water and add honey, lemon zest, sunflower seeds, pepper, and close the pressure seal.
5. Pressure cook for 40 minutes.
6. Serve and enjoy with a garnish of fresh chopped parsley if you prefer.

Nutrition: Calories: 753; Fat: 41g; Carbohydrates: 68g; Protein: 30g

249. Apple Pie Crackers

Preparation time: 10 minutes
Cooking time: 120 minutes
Servings: 100 crackers
Ingredients:
- 2 tablespoons + 2 teaspoons avocado oil
- 1 medium Granny Smith apple, roughly chopped
- ¼ cup Erythritol
- 1/4 cup sunflower seeds, ground
- 1 ¾ cups roughly ground flax seeds
- 1/8 teaspoon Ground cloves
- 1/8 teaspoon ground cardamom
- 3 tablespoons nutmeg
- ¼ teaspoon ground ginger

Directions:
1. Pre-heat your oven to 225 degrees F.
2. Line two baking sheets with parchment paper and keep them on the side.
3. Add oil, apple, Erythritol to a bowl and mix.
4. Transfer to food processor and add remaining ingredients, process until combined.
5. Transfer batter to baking sheets, spread evenly and cut into crackers.
6. Bake for 1 hour, flip and bake for another hour.
7. Let them cool and serve.
8. Enjoy!

Nutrition: Total Carbs: 0.9g (%); Fiber: 0.5g; Protein: 0.4g (%); Fat: 2.1g (%)

250. Paprika Lamb Chops

Preparation time: 10 minutes
Cooking time: 15 minutes
Servings: 4
Ingredients:
- 1 lamb rack, cut into chops
- pepper to taste
- 1 tablespoon paprika
- 1/2 cup cumin powder
- 1/2 teaspoon chili powder

Directions:
1. Take a bowl and add paprika, cumin, chili, pepper, and stir.
2. Add lamb chops and rub the mixture.

3. Heat grill over medium-temperature and add lamb chops, cook for 5 minutes.
4. Flip and cook for 5 minutes more, flip again.
5. Cook for 2 minutes, flip and cook for 2 minutes more.
6. Serve and enjoy!

Nutrition: Calories: 200; Fat: 5g; Carbohydrates: 4g; Protein: 8g

251. Sweet and Sour Cabbage and Apples

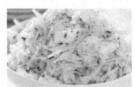

Preparation time: 15 minutes
Cooking time: 8 hours
Servings: 4
Ingredients:
- ¼ cup honey
- ¼ cup apple cider vinegar
- 2 tablespoons Orange Chili-Garlic Sauce
- 1 teaspoon sea salt
- 3 sweet tart apples, peeled, cored and sliced
- 2 heads green cabbage, cored and shredded
- 1 sweet red onion, thinly sliced

Directions:
1. Take a small bowl and whisk in honey, orange-chili garlic sauce, vinegar.
2. Stir well.
3. Add honey mix, apples, onion and cabbage to your Slow Cooker and stir.
4. Close lid and cook on LOW for 8 hours.
5. Serve and enjoy!

Nutrition: Calories: 164; Fat: 1g; Carbohydrates: 41g; Protein: 4g

252. Delicious Aloo Palak

Preparation time: 10 minutes
Cooking time: 6-8 hours
Servings: 6
Ingredients:
- 2 pounds red potatoes, chopped
- 1 small onion, diced
- 1 red bell pepper, seeded and diced
- ¼ cup fresh cilantro, chopped
- 1/3 cup low-sodium veggie broth
- 1 teaspoon salt
- ½ teaspoon Garam masala
- ½ teaspoon ground cumin
- ¼ teaspoon ground turmeric
- ¼ teaspoon ground coriander
- ¼ teaspoon freshly ground black pepper
- 2 pounds fresh spinach, chopped

Directions:
1. Add potatoes, bell pepper, onion, cilantro, broth and seasoning to your Slow Cooker.
2. Mix well.
3. Add spinach on top.

4. Place lid and cook on LOW for 6-8 hours.
5. Stir and serve.
6. Enjoy!
Nutrition: Calories: 205; Fat: 1g; Carbohydrates: 44g; Protein: 9g

253. Orange and Chili Garlic Sauce

Preparation time: 15 minutes
Cooking time: 8 hours
Servings: 5
Ingredients:
- ½ cup apple cider vinegar
- 4 pounds red jalapeno peppers, stems, seeds and ribs removed, chopped
- 10 garlic cloves, chopped
- ½ cup tomato paste
- Juice of 1 orange zest
- ½ cup honey
- 2 tablespoons soy sauce
- 2 teaspoons salt

Directions:
- Add vinegar, garlic, peppers, tomato paste, orange juice, honey, zest, soy sauce and salt to your Slow Cooker.
- Stir and close lid.
- Cook on LOW for 8 hours.
- Use as needed!

Nutrition: Calories: 33; Fat: 1g; Carbohydrates: 8g; Protein: 1g

254. Tantalizing Mushroom Gravy

Preparation time: 5 minutes
Cooking time: 5-8 hours
Servings: 2
Ingredients:
- 1 cup button mushrooms, sliced
- ¾ cup low-fat buttermilk
- 1/3 cup water
- 1 medium onion, finely diced
- 2 garlic cloves, minced
- 2 tablespoons extra virgin olive oil
- 2 tablespoons all-purpose flour
- 1 tablespoon fresh rosemary, minced
- Freshly ground black pepper

Directions:
1. Add the listed ingredients to your Slow Cooker.
2. Place lid and cook on LOW for 5-8 hours.
3. Serve warm and use as needed!

Nutrition: Calories: 54; Fat: 4g; Carbohydrates: 4g; Protein: 2g

255. Everyday Vegetable Stock

Preparation time: 5 minutes
Cooking time: 8-12 hours

Servings: 10
Ingredients:
- 2 celery stalks (with leaves), quartered
- 4 ounces mushrooms, with stems
- 2 carrots, unpeeled and quartered
- 1 onion, unpeeled, quartered from pole to pole
- 1 garlic head, unpeeled, halved across middle
- 2 fresh thyme sprigs
- 10 peppercorns
- ½ teaspoon salt
- Enough water to fill 3 quarters of Slow Cooker

Directions:
1. Add celery, mushrooms, onion, carrots, garlic, thyme, salt, peppercorn and water to your Slow Cooker.
2. Stir and cover.
3. Cook on LOW for 8-12 hours.
4. Strain the stock through a fine mesh cloth/metal mesh and discard solids.
5. Use as needed.

Nutrition: Calories: 38; Fat: 5g; Carbohydrates: 1g; Protein: 0g

256. The Vegan Lovers Refried Beans

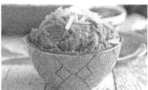

Preparation time: 5 minutes
Cooking time: 10 hours
Servings: 12
Ingredients:
- 4 cups vegetable broth
- 4 cups water
- 3 cups dried pinto beans
- 1 onion, chopped
- 2 jalapeno peppers, minced
- 4 garlic cloves, minced
- 1 tablespoon chili powder
- 2 teaspoon ground cumin
- 1 teaspoon sweet paprika
- 1 teaspoon salt
- ½ teaspoon fresh ground black pepper

Directions:
1. Add the listed ingredients to your Slow Cooker.
2. Cover and cook on HIGH for 10 hours.
3. If there's any extra liquid, ladle the liquid up and reserve it in a bowl.
4. Use an immersion blender to blend the mixture (in the Slow Cooker) until smooth.
5. Add the reserved liquid.
6. Serve hot and enjoy!

Nutrition: Calories: 91, Fat: 0g; Carbohydrates: 16g; Protein: 5g

257. Cool Apple and Carrot Harmony

Preparation time: 10 minutes
Cooking time: 10 minutes
Servings: 6
Ingredients:
- 1 cup apple juice
- 1 pound baby carrots
- 1 tablespoon cornstarch
- 1 tablespoon mint, chopped

Directions:
1. Add apple juice, carrots, cornstarch and mint to your Instant Pot.
2. Stir and lock the lid.
3. Cook on HIGH pressure for 10 minutes.
4. Perform a quick release.
5. Divide the mix amongst plates and serve.
6. Enjoy!

Nutrition: Calories: 161; Fat: 2g; Carbohydrates: 9g; Protein: 8g

258. Mac and Chokes

Preparation time: 5 minutes
Cooking time: 20 minutes
Servings: 6
Ingredients:
- 1 tablespoon of olive oil
- 1 large sized diced onion
- 10 minced garlic cloves
- 1 can artichoke hearts
- 1 pound uncooked macaroni shells
- 12 ounce baby spinach
- 4 cups vegetable broth
- 1 teaspoon red pepper flakes
- 4 ounces vegan cheese
- ¼ cup cashew cream

Directions:
1. Set the pot to Sauté mode and add oil, allow the oil to heat up and add onions.
2. Cook for 2 minutes.
3. Add garlic and stir well.
4. Add artichoke hearts and sauté for 1 minute more.
5. Add uncooked pasta and 3 cups of broth alongside 2 cups of water.
6. Mix well.
7. Lock the lid and cook on HIGH pressure for 4 minutes.
8. Quick release the pressure.
9. Open the pot and stir.
10. Add extra water, fold in spinach and cook on Sauté mode for a few minutes.
11. Add cashew cream and grated vegan cheese.
12. Add pepper flakes and mix well.
13. Enjoy!

Nutrition: Calories: 649; Fat: 29g; Carbohydrates: 64g; Protein: 34g

259. Black Eyed Peas and Spinach Platter

Preparation time: 10 minutes
Cooking time: 8 hours
Servings: 4
Ingredients:
- 1 cup black eyed peas, soaked overnight and drained
- 2 cups low-sodium vegetable broth
- 1 can (15 ounces) tomatoes, diced with juice
- 8 ounces ham, chopped
- 1 onion, chopped
- 2 garlic cloves, minced
- 1 teaspoon dried oregano
- 1 teaspoon salt
- ½ teaspoon freshly ground black pepper
- ½ teaspoon ground mustard
- 1 bay leaf

Directions:
1. Add the listed ingredients to your Slow Cooker and stir.
2. Place lid and cook on LOW for 8 hours.
3. Discard the bay leaf.
4. Serve and enjoy!

Nutrition: Calories: 209; Fat: 6g; Carbohydrates: 22g; Protein: 17g

260. Humble Mushroom Rice

Preparation time: 10 minutes
Cooking time: 3 hours
Servings: 3
Ingredients:
- ½ cup rice
- 2 green onions chopped
- 1 garlic clove, minced
- ¼ pound baby Portobello mushrooms, sliced
- 1 cup vegetable stock

Directions:
1. Add rice, onions, garlic, mushrooms, and stock to your Slow Cooker.
2. Stir well and place lid.
3. Cook on LOW for 3 hours...
4. Stir and divide amongst serving platters.
5. Enjoy!

Nutrition: Calories: 200; Fat: 6g; Carbohydrates: 28g; Protein: 5g

261. Chipotle Lettuce Chicken

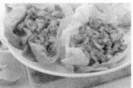

Preparation time: 10 minutes
Cooking time: 25 minutes
Servings: 6
Ingredients:
- 1 pound chicken breast, cut into strips
- Splash of olive oil

- 1 red onion, finely sliced
- 14 ounces tomatoes
- 1 teaspoon chipotle, chopped
- ½ teaspoon cumin
- Lettuce as needed
- Fresh coriander leaves
- Jalapeno chilies, sliced
- Fresh tomato slices for garnish
- Lime wedges

Directions:
1. Take a non-stick frying pan and place it over medium heat.
2. Add oil and heat it up.
3. Add chicken and cook until brown.
4. Keep the chicken on the side.
5. Add tomatoes, sugar, chipotle, cumin to the same pan and simmer for 25 minutes until you have a nice sauce.
6. Add chicken into the sauce and cook for 5 minutes.
7. Transfer the mix to another place.
8. Use lettuce wraps to take a portion of the mixture and serve with a squeeze of lemon.
9. Enjoy!

Nutrition: Calories: 332; Fat: 15g; Carbohydrates: 13g; Protein: 34g

262. Balsamic Chicken and Vegetables

Preparation time: 15 minutes
Cooking time: 25 minutes
Servings: 2
Ingredients:
- 4 chicken thigh, boneless and skinless
- 5 stalks of asparagus, halved
- 1 pepper, cut in chunks
- 1/2 red onion, diced
- ½ cup carrots, sliced
- 1 garlic cloves, minced
- 2-ounces mushrooms, diced
- ¼ cup balsamic vinegar
- 1 tablespoon olive oil
- ½ teaspoon stevia
- ½ tablespoon oregano
- Sunflower seeds and pepper as needed

Directions:
1. Pre-heat your oven to 425 degrees F.
2. Take a bowl and add all of the vegetables and mix.
3. Add spices and oil and mix.
4. Dip the chicken pieces into spice mix and coat them well.
5. Place the veggies and chicken onto a pan in a single layer.
6. Cook for 25 minutes.
7. Serve and enjoy!

Nutrition: Calories: 401; Fat: 17g; Net Carbohydrates: 11g; Protein: 48g

263. Cream Dredged Corn Platter

Preparation time: 10 minutes
Cooking time: 4 hours

Servings: 3
Ingredients:
- 3 cups corn
- 2 ounces cream cheese, cubed
- 2 tablespoons milk
- 2 tablespoons whipping cream
- 2 tablespoons butter, melted
- Salt and pepper as needed
- 1 tablespoon green onion, chopped

Directions:
1. Add corn, cream cheese, milk, whipping cream, butter, salt and pepper to your Slow Cooker.
2. Give it a nice toss to mix everything well.
3. Place lid and cook on LOW for 4 hours.
4. Divide the mix amongst serving platters.
5. Serve and enjoy!

Nutrition: Calories: 261; Fat: 11g; Carbohydrates: 17g; Protein: 6g

264. Exuberant Sweet Potatoes

Preparation time: 5 minutes
Cooking time: 7-8 hours
Servings: 4
Ingredients:
- 6 sweet potatoes, washed and dried

Directions:
1. Loosely ball up 7-8 pieces of aluminum foil in the bottom of your Slow Cooker, covering about half of the surface area.
2. Prick each potato 6-8 times using a fork.
3. Wrap each potato with foil and seal them.
4. Place wrapped potatoes in the cooker on top of the foil bed.
5. Place lid and cook on LOW for 7-8 hours.
6. Use tongs to remove the potatoes and unwrap them.
7. Serve and enjoy!

Nutrition: Calories: 129; Fat: 0g; Carbohydrates: 30g; Protein: 2g

265. Ethiopian Cabbage Delight

Preparation time: 15 minutes
Cooking time: 6-8 hours
Servings: 6
Ingredients:
- ½ cup water
- 1 head green cabbage, cored and chopped
- 1 pound sweet potatoes, peeled and chopped
- 3 carrots, peeled and chopped
- 1 onion, sliced
- 1 teaspoon extra virgin olive oil
- ½ teaspoon ground turmeric
- ½ teaspoon ground cumin
- ¼ teaspoon ground ginger

Directions:
1. Add water to your Slow Cooker.

2. Take a medium bowl and add cabbage, carrots, sweet potatoes, onion and mix.
3. Add olive oil, turmeric, ginger, cumin and toss until the veggies are fully coated.
4. Transfer veggie mix to your Slow Cooker.
5. Cover and cook on LOW for 6-8 hours.
6. Serve and enjoy!

Nutrition: Calories: 155; Fat: 2g; Carbohydrates: 35g; Protein: 4g

266. Amazing Sesame Breadsticks

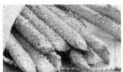

Preparation time: 10 minutes
Cooking time: 20 minutes
Servings: 5
Ingredients:
- 1 egg white
- 2 tablespoons almond flour
- 1 teaspoon Himalayan pink sunflower seeds
- 1 tablespoon extra-virgin olive oil
- ½ teaspoon sesame seeds

Directions:
1. Pre-heat your oven to 320 degrees F.
2. Line a baking sheet with parchment paper and keep it on the side.
3. Take a bowl and whisk in egg whites, add flour and half of sunflower seeds and olive oil.
4. Knead until you have a smooth dough.
5. Divide into 4 pieces and roll into breadsticks.
6. Place on prepared sheet and brush with olive oil, sprinkle sesame seeds and remaining sunflower seeds.
7. Bake for 20 minutes.
8. Serve and enjoy!

Nutrition: Total Carbs: 1.1g; Fiber: 1g; Protein: 1.6g; Fat: 5g

267. Brown Butter Duck Breast

Preparation time: 5 minutes
Cooking time: 25 minutes
Servings: 3
Ingredients:
- 1 whole 6 ounce duck breast, skin on
- Pepper to taste
- 1 head radicchio, 4 ounces, core removed
- ¼ cup unsalted butter
- 6 fresh sage leaves, sliced

Directions:
1. Pre-heat your oven to 400 degree F.
2. Pat duck breast dry with paper towel.
3. Season with pepper.
4. Place duck breast in skillet and place it over medium heat, sear for 3-4 minutes each side.
5. Turn breast over and transfer skillet to oven.
6. Roast for 10 minutes (uncovered).

7. Cut radicchio in half.
8. Remove and discard the woody white core and thinly slice the leaves.
9. Keep them on the side.
10. Remove skillet from oven.
11. Transfer duck breast, fat side up to cutting board and let it rest.
12. Re-heat your skillet over medium heat.
13. Add unsalted butter, sage and cook for 3-4 minutes.
14. Cut duck into 6 equal slices.
15. Divide radicchio between 2 plates, top with slices of duck breast and drizzle browned butter and sage.
16. Enjoy!

Nutrition: Calories: 393; Fat: 33g; Carbohydrates: 2g; Protein: 22g

268. Generous Garlic Bread Stick

Preparation time: 15 minutes
Cooking time: 15 minutes
Servings: 8
Ingredients:
- ¼ cup almond butter, softened
- 1 teaspoon garlic powder
- 2 cups almond flour
- ½ tablespoon baking powder
- 1 tablespoon Psyllium husk powder
- ¼ teaspoon sunflower seeds
- 3 tablespoons almond butter, melted
- 1 egg
- ¼ cup boiling water

Directions:
1. Pre-heat your oven to 400 degrees F.
2. Line baking sheet with parchment paper and keep it on the side.
3. Beat almond butter with garlic powder and keep it on the side.
4. Add almond flour, baking powder, husk, sunflower seeds in a bowl and mix in almond butter and egg, mix well.
5. Pour boiling water in the mix and stir until you have a nice dough.
6. Divide the dough into 8 balls and roll into breadsticks.
7. Place on baking sheet and bake for 15 minutes.
8. Brush each stick with garlic almond butter and bake for 5 minutes more.
9. Serve and enjoy!

Nutrition: Total Carbs: 7g; Fiber: 2g; Protein: 7g; Fat: 24g

269. Cauliflower Bread Stick

Preparation time: 10 minutes
Cooking time: 48 minutes
Servings: 5
Ingredients:
- 1 cup cashew cheese/ kite ricotta cheese
- 1 tablespoon organic almond butter
- 1 whole egg
- ½ teaspoon Italian seasoning
- ¼ teaspoon red pepper flakes
- 1/8 teaspoon kosher sunflower seeds

- 2 cups cauliflower rice, cooked for 3 minutes in microwave
- 3 teaspoons garlic, minced
- Parmesan cheese, grated

Directions:
1. Pre-heat your oven to 350 degrees F.
2. Add almond butter in a small pan and melt over low heat
3. Add red pepper flakes, garlic to the almond butter and cook for 2-3 minutes.
4. Add garlic and almond butter mix to the bowl with cooked cauliflower and add the Italian seasoning.
5. Season with sunflower seeds and mix, refrigerate for 10 minutes.
6. Add cheese and eggs to the bowl and mix.
7. Place a layer of parchment paper at the bottom of a 9 x 9 baking dish and grease with cooking spray, add egg and mozzarella cheese mix to the cauliflower mix.
8. Add mix to the pan and smooth to a thin layer with the palms of your hand.
9. Bake for 30 minutes, take out from oven and top with few shakes of parmesan and mozzarella.
10. Cook for 8 minutes more.
11. Enjoy!

Nutrition: Total Carbs: 11.5g; Fiber: 2g; Protein: 10.7g; Fat: 20g

270. Bacon and Chicken Garlic Wrap

Preparation time: 15 minutes
Cooking time: 10 minutes
Servings: 4

Ingredients:
- 1 chicken fillet, cut into small cubes
- 8-9 thin slices bacon, cut to fit cubes
- 6 garlic cloves, minced

Directions:
1. Pre-heat your oven to 400 degrees F.
2. Line a baking tray with aluminum foil.
3. Add minced garlic to a bowl and rub each chicken piece with it.
4. Wrap a bacon piece around each garlic chicken bite.
5. Secure with toothpick.
6. Transfer bites to baking sheet, keeping a little bit of space between them.
7. Bake for about 15-20 minutes until crispy.
8. Serve and enjoy!

Nutrition: Calories: 260; Fat: 19g; Carbohydrates: 5g; Protein: 22g

271. The Almond Breaded Chicken Goodness

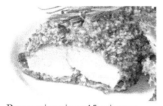

Preparation time: 15 minutes
Cooking time: 15 minutes
Servings: 3

Ingredients:
- 2 large chicken breasts, boneless and skinless
- 1/3 cup lemon juice
- 1 ½ cups seasoned almond meal
- 2 tablespoons coconut oil
- Lemon pepper, to taste
- Parsley for decoration

Directions:
1. Slice chicken breast in half.
2. Pound out each half until ¼ inch thick.
3. Take a pan and place it over medium heat, add oil and heat it up.
4. Dip each chicken breast slice into lemon juice and let it sit for 2 minutes.
5. Turnover and the let the other side sit for 2 minutes as well.
6. Transfer to almond meal and coat both sides.
7. Add coated chicken to the oil and fry for 4 minutes per side, making sure to sprinkle lemon pepper liberally.
8. Transfer to a paper lined sheet and repeat until all chicken are fried.
9. Garnish with parsley and enjoy!

Nutrition: Calories: 325; Fat: 24g; Carbohydrates: 3g; Protein: 16g

272. South-Western Pork Chops

Preparation time: 10 minutes
Cooking time: 15 minutes
Servings: 4

Ingredients:
- Cooking spray as needed
- 4-ounce pork loin chop, boneless and fat rimmed
- 1/3 cup salsa
- 2 tablespoons fresh lime juice
- ¼ cup fresh cilantro, chopped

Directions:
1. Take a large sized non-stick skillet and spray it with cooking spray.
2. Heat until hot over high heat.
3. Press the chops with your palm to flatten them slightly.
4. Add them to the skillet and cook on 1 minute for each side until they are nicely browned.
5. Lower the heat to medium-low.
6. Combine the salsa and lime juice.
7. Pour the mix over the chops.
8. Simmer uncovered for about 8 minutes until the chops are perfectly done.
9. If needed, sprinkle some cilantro on top.
10. Serve!

Nutrition: Calorie: 184; Fat: 4g; Carbohydrates: 4g; Protein: 0.5g

273. Almond butter Pork Chops

Preparation time: 5 minutes
Cooking time: 25 minutes
Servings: 2

Ingredients:
- 1 tablespoon almond butter, divided

- 2 boneless pork chops
- Pepper to taste
- 1 tablespoon dried Italian seasoning, low fat and low sodium
- 1 tablespoon olive oil

Directions:
1. Pre-heat your oven to 350 degrees F.
2. Pat pork chops dry with a paper towel and place them in a baking dish.
3. Season with pepper, and Italian seasoning.
4. Drizzle olive oil over pork chops.
5. Top each chop with ½ tablespoon almond butter.
6. Bake for 25 minutes.
7. Transfer pork chops on two plates and top with almond butter juice.
8. Serve and enjoy!

Nutrition: Calories: 333; Fat: 23g; Carbohydrates: 1g; Protein: 31g

274. Chicken Salsa

Preparation time: 4 minutes
Cooking time: 14 minutes
Servings: 1
Ingredients:
- 2 chicken breasts
- 1 cup salsa
- 1 taco seasoning mix
- 1 cup plain Greek Yogurt
- ½ cup of kite ricotta/cashew cheese, cubed

Directions:
1. Take a skillet and place over medium heat.
2. Add chicken breast, ½ cup of salsa and taco seasoning.
3. Mix well and cook for 12-15 minutes until the chicken is done.
4. Take the chicken out and cube them.
5. Place the cubes on toothpick and top with cheddar.
6. Place yogurt and remaining salsa in cups and use as dips.
7. Enjoy!

Nutrition: Calories: 359; Fat: 14g; Net Carbohydrates: 14g; Protein: 43g

275. Healthy Mediterranean Lamb Chops

Preparation time: 10 minutes
Cooking time: 10 minutes
Servings: 4
Ingredients:
- 4 lamb shoulder chops, 8 ounces each
- 2 tablespoons Dijon mustard
- 2 tablespoons Balsamic vinegar
- ½ cup olive oil
- 2 tablespoons shredded fresh basil

Directions:
1. Pat your lamb chop dry using a kitchen towel and arrange them on a shallow glass baking dish.
2. Take a bowl and a whisk in Dijon mustard, balsamic vinegar, pepper and mix them well.
3. Whisk in the oil very slowly into the marinade until the mixture is smooth

4. Stir in basil.
5. Pour the marinade over the lamb chops and stir to coat both sides well.
6. Cover the chops and allow them to marinate for 1-4 hours (chilled).
7. Take the chops out and leave them for 30 minutes to allow the temperature to reach a normal level.
8. Pre-heat your grill to medium heat and add oil to the grate.
9. Grill the lamb chops for 5-10 minutes per side until both sides are browned.
10. Once the center reads 145 degrees F, the chops are ready, serve and enjoy!

Nutrition: Calories: 521; Fat: 45g; Carbohydrates: 3.5g; Protein: 22g

276. Amazing Grilled Chicken and Blueberry Salad

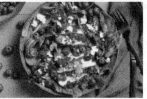

Preparation time: 10 minutes
Cooking time: 25 minutes
Servings: 5
Ingredients:
- 5 cups mixed greens
- 1 cup blueberries
- ¼ cup slivered almonds
- 2 cups chicken breasts, cooked and cubed
- For dressing
- ¼ cup olive oil
- ¼ cup apple cider vinegar
- ¼ cup blueberries
- 2 tablespoons honey
- Sunflower seeds and pepper to taste

Directions:
1. Take a bowl and add greens, berries, almonds, chicken cubes and mix well.
2. Take a bowl and mix the dressing ingredients, pour the mix into a blender and blitz until smooth.
3. Add dressing on top of the chicken cubes and toss well.
4. Season more and enjoy!

Nutrition: Calories: 266; Fat: 17g; Carbohydrates: 18g; Protein: 10g

277. Clean Chicken and Mushroom Stew

Preparation time: 10 minutes
Cooking time: 35 minutes
Servings: 4
Ingredients:
- 4 chicken breast halves, cut into bite sized pieces
- 1 pound mushrooms, sliced (5-6 cups)
- 1 bunch spring onion, chopped
- 4 tablespoons olive oil
- 1 teaspoon thyme

- Sunflower seeds and pepper as needed

Directions:
1. Take a large deep frying pan and place it over medium-high heat.
2. Add oil and let it heat up.
3. Add chicken and cook for 4-5 minutes per side until slightly browned.
4. Add spring onions and mushrooms, season with sunflower seeds and pepper according to your taste.
5. Stir.
6. Cover with lid and bring the mix to a boil.
7. Reduce heat and simmer for 25 minutes.
8. Serve!

Nutrition: Calories: 247; Fat: 12g; Carbohydrates: 10g; Protein: 23g

278. Elegant Pumpkin Chili Dish

Preparation time: 10 minutes
Cooking time: 15 minutes
Servings: 4
Ingredients:
- 3 cups yellow onion, chopped
- 8 garlic cloves, chopped
- 1 pound turkey, ground
- 2 cans (15 ounces each) fire roasted tomatoes
- 2 cups pumpkin puree
- 1 cup chicken broth
- 4 teaspoons chili spice
- 1 teaspoon ground cinnamon
- 1 teaspoon sea sunflower seeds

Directions:
1. Take a large sized pot and place it over medium-high heat.
2. Add coconut oil and let the oil heat up.
3. Add onion and garlic, sauté for 5 minutes.
4. Add ground turkey and break it while cooking, cook for 5 minutes.
5. Add remaining ingredients and bring the mix to simmer.
6. Simmer for 15 minutes over low heat (lid off).
7. Pour chicken broth.
8. Serve with desired salad.
9. Enjoy!

Nutrition: Calories: 312; Fat: 16g; Carbohydrates: 14g; Protein: 27g

279. Zucchini Zoodles with Chicken and Basil

Preparation time: 10 minutes
Cooking time: 10 minutes
Servings: 2
Ingredients:
- 2 chicken fillets, cubed
- 2 tablespoons ghee
- 1 pound tomatoes, diced
- ½ cup basil, chopped
- ¼ cup coconut almond milk
- 1 garlic clove, peeled, minced
- 1 zucchini, shredded

Directions:
1. Sauté cubed chicken in ghee until no longer pink.
2. Add tomatoes and season with sunflower seeds.
3. Simmer and reduce the liquid.
4. Prepare your zucchini Zoodles by shredding zucchini in a food processor.
5. Add basil, garlic, coconut almond milk to chicken and cook for a few minutes.
6. Add half of the zucchini Zoodles to a bowl and top with creamy tomato basil chicken.
7. Enjoy!

Nutrition: Calories: 540; Fat: 27g; Carbohydrates: 13g; Protein: 59g

280. Tasty Roasted Broccoli

Preparation time: 5 minutes
Cooking time: 20 minutes
Servings: 4
Ingredients:
- 4 cups broccoli florets
- 1 tablespoon olive oil
- Sunflower seeds and pepper to taste

Directions:
1. Pre-heat your oven to 400 degrees F.
2. Add broccoli in a zip bag alongside oil and shake until coated.
3. Add seasoning and shake again.
4. Spread broccoli out on baking sheet, bake for 20 minutes.
5. Let it cool and serve.
6. Enjoy!

Nutrition: Calories: 62; Fat: 4g; Carbohydrates: 4g; Protein: 4g

281. Zucchini Beef Sauté with Coriander Greens

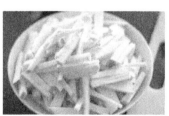

Preparation time: 10 minutes
Cooking time: 10 minutes
Servings: 4
Ingredients:
- 10 ounces beef, sliced into 1-2 inch strips
- 1 zucchini, cut into 2-inch strips
- ¼ cup parsley, chopped
- 3 garlic cloves, minced
- 2 tablespoons tamari sauce
- 4 tablespoons avocado oil

Directions:
1. Add 2 tablespoons avocado oil in a frying pan over high heat.
2. Place strips of beef and brown for a few minutes on high heat.
3. Once the meat is brown, add zucchini strips and sauté until tender.

4. Once tender, add tamari sauce, garlic, parsley and let them sit for a few minutes more.
5. Serve immediately and enjoy!

Nutrition: Calories: 500; Fat: 40g; Carbohydrates: 5g; Protein: 31g

282. Hearty Lemon and Pepper Chicken

Preparation time: 5 minutes
Cooking time: 15 minutes
Servings: 4

Ingredients:
- 2 teaspoons olive oil
- 1 ¼ pounds skinless chicken cutlets
- 2 whole eggs
- ¼ cup panko crumbs
- 1 tablespoon lemon pepper
- Sunflower seeds and pepper to taste
- 3 cups green beans
- ¼ cup parmesan cheese
- ¼ teaspoon garlic powder

Directions:
1. Pre-heat your oven to 425 degrees F.
2. Take a bowl and stir in seasoning, parmesan, lemon pepper, garlic powder, panko.
3. Whisk eggs in another bowl.
4. Coat cutlets in eggs and press into panko mix.
5. Transfer coated chicken to a parchment lined baking sheet.
6. Toss the beans in oil, pepper, add sunflower seeds, and lay them on the side of the baking sheet.
7. Bake for 15 minutes.
8. Enjoy!

Nutrition: Calorie: 299; Fat: 10g; Carbohydrates: 10g; Protein: 43g

283. Walnuts and Asparagus Delight

Preparation time: 5 minutes
Cooking time: 5 minutes
Servings: 4

Ingredients:
- 1 ½ tablespoons olive oil
- ¾ pound asparagus, trimmed
- ¼ cup walnuts, chopped
- Sunflower seeds and pepper to taste

Directions:
1. Place a skillet over medium heat add olive oil and let it heat up.
2. Add asparagus, sauté for 5 minutes until browned.
3. Season with sunflower seeds and pepper.
4. Remove heat.
5. Add walnuts and toss.
6. Serve warm!

Nutrition: Calories: 124; Fat: 12g; Carbohydrates: 2g; Protein: 3g

284. Healthy Carrot Chips

Preparation time: 10 minutes
Cooking time: 10 minutes
Servings: 4

Ingredients:
- 3 cups carrots, sliced paper thin rounds
- 2 tablespoons olive oil
- 2 teaspoons ground cumin
- ½ teaspoon smoked paprika
- Pinch of sunflower seeds

Directions:
1. Pre-heat your oven to 400 degrees F.
2. Slice carrot into paper thin shaped coins using a peeler.
3. Place slices in a bowl and toss with oil and spices.
4. Lay out the slices on a parchment paper, lined baking sheet in a single layer.
5. Sprinkle sunflower seeds.
6. Transfer to oven and bake for 8-10 minutes.
7. Remove and serve.
8. Enjoy!

Nutrition: Calories: 434; Fat: 35g; Carbohydrates: 31g; Protein: 2g

285. Beef Soup

Preparation time: 10 minutes
Cooking time: 40 minutes
Servings: 4

Ingredients:
- 1 pound ground beef, lean
- 1 cup mixed vegetables, frozen
- 1 yellow onion, chopped
- 6 cups vegetable broth
- 1 cup low-fat cream
- Pepper to taste

Directions:
1. Take a stockpot and add all the ingredients the except heavy cream, salt, and black pepper.
2. Bring to a boil.
3. Reduce heat to simmer.
4. Cook for 40 minutes.
5. Once cooked, warm the heavy cream.
6. Then add once the soup is cooked.
7. Blend the soup till smooth by using an immersion blender.
8. Season with salt and black pepper.
9. Serve and enjoy!

Nutrition:
Calories: 270; Fat: 14g; Carbohydrates: 6g; Protein: 29g

286. Lime Shrimp and Kale

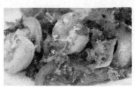

Preparation time: 10 minutes
Cooking time: 20 minutes
Servings: 4

Ingredients:
- 1-pound shrimp, peeled and deveined
- 4 scallions, chopped
- 1 teaspoon sweet paprika
- 1 tablespoon olive oil
- Juice of 1 lime
- Zest of 1 lime, grated
- A pinch of salt and black pepper
- 2 tablespoons parsley, chopped

Directions:
1. Bring the pan to medium heat, add the scallions and sauté for 5 minutes. Add the shrimp and the other ingredients, toss, cook over medium heat for 15 minutes more, divide into bowls and serve.

Nutrition: Calories: 149; Carbs: 12g; Fat: 4g; Protein: 21g; Sodium: 250 mg

287. Parsley Cod Mix

Preparation time: 10 minutes
Cooking time: 20 minutes
Servings: 4

Ingredients:
- 1 tablespoon olive oil
- 2 shallots, chopped
- 4 cod fillets, boneless and skinless
- 2 garlic cloves, minced
- 2 tablespoons lemon juice
- 1 cup chicken stock
- A pinch of salt and black pepper

Directions:
1. Bring the pan to medium heat -high heat, add the shallots and the garlic and sauté for 5 minutes. Add the cod and the other ingredients, cook everything for 15 minutes more, divide between plates and serve for lunch.

Nutrition: Calories: 216; Carbs: 7g; Fat: 5g; Protein: 34g; Sodium: 380 mg

288. Salmon and Cabbage Mix

Preparation time: 5 minutes
Cooking time: 25 minutes
Servings: 4

Ingredients:
- 4 salmon fillets, boneless
- 1 yellow onion, chopped
- 2 tablespoons olive oil
- 1 cup red cabbage, shredded
- 1 red bell pepper, chopped
- 1 tablespoon rosemary, chopped
- 1 tablespoon coriander, ground
- 1 cup tomato sauce
- A pinch of sea salt
- black pepper

Directions:
1. Bring the pan to medium heat, add the onion and sauté for 5 minutes. Put the fish and sear it within 2 minutes on each side. Add the cabbage and the remaining ingredients, toss, cook over medium heat for 20 minutes more, divide between plates and serve.

Nutrition: Calories: 130; Carbs: 8g; Fat: 6g; Protein: 12g; Sodium: 345 mg

289. Decent Beef and Onion Stew

Preparation time: 10 minutes
Cooking time: 1-2 hours
Servings: 4

Ingredients:
- 2 pounds lean beef, cubed
- 3 pounds shallots, peeled
- 5 garlic cloves, peeled, whole
- 3 tablespoons tomato paste
- 1 bay leaves
- ¼ cup olive oil
- 3 tablespoons lemon juice

Directions:
1. Take a stew pot and place it over medium heat.
2. Add olive oil and let it heat up.
3. Add meat and brown.
4. Add remaining ingredients and cover with water.
5. Bring the whole mix to a boil.
6. Reduce heat to low and cover the pot.
7. Simmer for 1-2 hours until beef is cooked thoroughly.
8. Serve hot!

Nutrition: Calories: 136; Fat: 3g; Carbohydrates: 0.9g; Protein: 24g

290. Clean Parsley and Chicken Breast

Preparation time: 10 minutes
Cooking time: 40 minutes
Servings: 2

Ingredients:
- 1/2 tablespoon dry parsley
- 1/2 tablespoon dry basil
- 2 chicken breast halves, boneless and skinless
- 1/4 teaspoon sunflower seeds
- 1/4 teaspoon red pepper flakes, crushed
- 1 tomato, sliced

Directions:
1. Pre-heat your oven to 350 degrees F.
2. Take a 9x13 inch baking dish and grease it up with cooking spray.
3. Sprinkle 1 tablespoon of parsley, 1 teaspoon of basil and spread the mixture over your baking dish.
4. Arrange the chicken breast halves over the dish and sprinkle garlic slices on top.
5. Take a small bowl and add 1 teaspoon parsley, 1 teaspoon of basil, sunflower seeds, basil, and red pepper and mix well. Pour the mixture over the chicken breast.
6. Top with tomato slices and cover, bake for 25 minutes.
7. Remove the cover and bake for 15 minutes more.
8. Serve and enjoy!

Nutrition: Calories: 150; Fat: 4g; Carbohydrates: 4g; Protein: 25g

291. Fruit Shrimp Soup

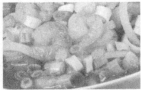

Preparation time: 10 minutes
Cooking time: 25 minutes
Servings: 6
Ingredients:

- 8 ounces shrimp, peeled and deveined
- 1 stalk lemongrass, smashed
- 2 small ginger pieces, grated
- 6 cup chicken stock
- 2 jalapenos, chopped
- 4 lime leaves
- 1 and ½ cups pineapple, chopped
- 1 cup shiitake mushroom caps, chopped
- 1 tomato, chopped
- ½ bell pepper, cubed
- 2 tablespoons fish sauce
- 1 teaspoon sugar
- ¼ cup lime juice
- 1/3 cup cilantro, chopped
- 2 scallions, sliced

Directions:
1. In a pot, mix ginger with lemongrass, stock, jalapenos, and lime leaves, stir, boil over medium heat, cook within 15 minutes. Strain liquid in a bowl and discard solids.
2. Return soup to the pot again, add pineapple, tomato, mushrooms, bell pepper, sugar, and fish sauce, stir, boil over medium heat, cook for 5 minutes, add shrimp and cook for 3 more minutes. Remove from heat, add lime juice, cilantro, and scallions, stir, ladle into soup bowls and serve.

Nutrition: Calories: 290; Carbs: 39g; Fat: 12g; Protein: 7g; Sodium: 21 mg

292. Mussels and Chickpea Soup

Preparation time: 10 minutes
Cooking time: 10 minutes
Servings: 6
Ingredients:

- 3 garlic cloves, minced
- 2 tablespoons olive oil
- A pinch of chili flakes
- 1 and ½ tablespoons fresh mussels, scrubbed
- 1 cup white wine
- 1 cup chickpeas, rinsed
- 1 small fennel bulb, sliced
- Black pepper to the taste
- Juice of 1 lemon
- 3 tablespoons parsley, chopped

Directions:
1. Heat a big saucepan with the olive oil over medium-high heat, add garlic and chili flakes, stir and cook within a couple of minutes. Add white wine and mussels, stir, cover, and cook for 3-4 minutes until mussels open.
2. Transfer mussels to a baking dish, add some of the cooking liquid over them, and fridge until they are cold enough. Take mussels out of the fridge and discard shells.
3. Heat another pan over medium-high heat, add mussels, reserved cooking liquid, chickpeas, and fennel, stir well, and heat them. Add black pepper to the taste, lemon juice, and parsley, stir again, divide between plates and serve.

Nutrition: Calories: 286; Carbs: 49g; Fat: 4g; Protein: 14g; Sodium: 145mg

293. Fish Stew

Preparation time: 10 minutes
Cooking time: 30 minutes
Servings: 4
Ingredients:

- 1 red onion, sliced
- 2 tablespoons olive oil
- 1-pound white fish fillets, boneless, skinless, and cubed
- 1 avocado, pitted and chopped
- 1 tablespoon oregano, chopped
- 1 cup chicken stock
- 2 tomatoes, cubed
- 1 teaspoon sweet paprika
- A pinch of salt and black pepper
- 1 tablespoon parsley, chopped
- Juice of 1 lime

Directions:
1. Warm-up oil in a pot over medium heat, add the onion, and sauté within 5 minutes. Add the fish, the avocado, and the other ingredients, toss, cook over medium heat for 25 minutes more, divide into bowls and serve for lunch.

Nutrition: Calories: 78; Carbs: 8g; Fat: 1g; Protein: 11g; Sodium: 151 mg

294. Shrimp and Broccoli Soup

Preparation time: 5 minutes
Cooking time: 25 minutes
Servings: 4
Ingredients:

- 2 tablespoons olive oil
- 1 yellow onion, chopped
- 4 cups chicken stock
- Juice of 1 lime
- 1-pound shrimp, peeled and deveined
- ½ cup coconut cream
- ½ pound broccoli florets
- 1 tablespoon parsley, chopped

Directions:
1. Heat a pot with the oil over medium heat, add the onion and sauté for 5 minutes. Add the shrimp and the other ingredients, simmer over medium heat for 20 minutes more. Ladle the soup into bowls and serve.

Nutrition: Calories: 220; Carbs: 12g; Fat: 7g; Protein: 26g; Sodium: 577 mg

295. Coconut Turkey Mix

Preparation time: 10 minutes
Cooking time: 30 minutes
Servings: 4
Ingredients:
- 1 yellow onion, chopped
- 1-pound turkey breast, skinless, boneless, and cubed
- 2 tablespoons olive oil
- 2 garlic cloves, minced
- 1 zucchini, sliced
- 1 cup coconut cream
- A pinch of sea salt
- black pepper

Directions:
1. Bring the pan to medium heat, add the onion and the garlic and sauté for 5 minutes. Put the meat and brown within 5 minutes more. Add the rest of the ingredients, toss, bring to a simmer and cook over medium heat for 20 minutes more. Serve for lunch.

Nutrition: Calories 200; Fat 4g; Fiber 2g; Carbs 14g; Protein 7g; Sodium 111mg

296. Shrimp Cocktail

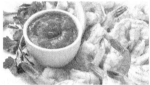

Preparation time: 10 minutes
Cooking time: 5 minutes
Servings: 8
Ingredients:
- 2 pounds big shrimp, deveined
- 4 cups of water
- 2 bay leaves
- 1 small lemon, halved
- Ice for cooling the shrimp
- Ice for serving
- 1 medium lemon sliced for serving
- ¾ cup tomato passata
- 2 and ½ tablespoons horseradish, prepared
- ¼ teaspoon chili powder
- 2 tablespoons lemon juice

Directions:
1. Pour the 4 cups water into a large pot, add lemon and bay leaves. Boil over medium-high heat, reduce temperature, and boil for 10 minutes. Put shrimp, stir and cook within 2 minutes. Move the shrimp to a bowl filled with ice and leave aside for 5 minutes.
2. In a bowl, mix tomato passata with horseradish, chili powder, and lemon juice and stir well. Place shrimp in a serving bowl filled with ice, with lemon slices, and serve with the cocktail sauce you've prepared.

Nutrition: Calories: 276; Carbs: 0g; Fat: 8g; Protein: 25g; Sodium: 182 mg

297. Quinoa and Scallops Salad

Preparation time: 10 minutes
Cooking time: 35 minutes
Servings: 6
Ingredients:
- 12 ounces dry sea scallops
- 4 tablespoons canola oil
- 2 teaspoons canola oil
- 4 teaspoons low sodium soy sauce
- 1 and ½ cup quinoa, rinsed
- 2 teaspoons garlic, minced
- 3 cups of water
- 1 cup snow peas, sliced diagonally
- 1 teaspoon sesame oil
- 1/3 cup rice vinegar
- 1 cup scallions, sliced
- 1/3 cup red bell pepper, chopped
- ¼ cup cilantro, chopped

Directions:
1. In a bowl, mix scallops with 2 teaspoons soy sauce, stir gently, and leave aside for now. Heat a pan with 1 tablespoon canola oil over medium-high heat, add the quinoa, stir and cook for 8 minutes. Put garlic, stir and cook within 1 more minute.
2. Put the water, boil over medium heat, stir, cover, and cook for 15 minutes. Remove from heat and leave aside covered for 5 minutes. Add snow peas, cover again and leave for 5 more minutes.
3. Meanwhile, in a bowl, mix 3 tablespoons canola oil with 2 teaspoons soy sauce, vinegar, and sesame oil and stir well. Add quinoa and snow peas to this mixture and stir again. Add scallions, bell pepper, and stir again.
4. Pat dry the scallops and discard marinade. Heat another pan with 2 teaspoons canola oil over high heat, add scallops, and cook for 1 minute on each side. Add them to the quinoa salad, stir gently, and serve with chopped cilantro.

Nutrition: Calories: 181; Carbs: 12g; Fat: 6g; Protein: 13g; Sodium: 153 mg

298. Squid and Shrimp Salad

Preparation time: 10 minutes
Cooking time: 15 minutes
Servings: 4
Ingredients:
- 8 ounces squid, cut into medium pieces
- 8 ounces shrimp, peeled and deveined
- 1 red onion, sliced
- 1 cucumber, chopped
- 2 tomatoes, cut into medium wedges
- 2 tablespoons cilantro, chopped
- 1 hot jalapeno pepper, cut in rounds
- 3 tablespoons rice vinegar
- 3 tablespoons dark sesame oil
- Black pepper to the taste

Directions:
1. In a bowl, mix the onion with cucumber, tomatoes, pepper, cilantro, shrimp, and squid and stir well. Cut a big

parchment paper in half, fold it in half heart shape and open. Place the seafood mixture in this parchment piece, fold over, seal edges, place on a baking sheet, and introduce in the oven at 400 degrees F for 15 minutes.

2. Meanwhile, in a small bowl, mix sesame oil with rice vinegar and black pepper and stir very well. Take the salad out of the oven, leave to cool down for a few minutes, and transfer to a serving plate. Put the dressing over the salad and serve right away.

Nutrition: Calories: 235; Carbs: 9g; Fat: 8g; Protein: 30g; Sodium: 165 mg

299. Parsley Seafood Cocktail

Preparation time: 2 hours and 10 minutes
Cooking time: 1 hour and 30 minutes
Servings: 4
Ingredients:

- 1 big octopus, cleaned
- 1-pound mussels
- 2 pounds clams
- 1 big squid cut in rings
- 3 garlic cloves, chopped
- 1 celery rib, cut crosswise into thirds
- ½ cup celery rib, sliced
- 1 carrot, cut crosswise into 3 pieces
- 1 small white onion, chopped
- 1 bay leaf
- ¾ cup white wine
- 2 cups radicchio, sliced
- 1 red onion, sliced
- 1 cup parsley, chopped
- 1 cup olive oil
- 1 cup red wine vinegar
- Black pepper to the taste

Directions:

1. Put the octopus in a pot with celery rib cut in thirds, garlic, carrot, bay leaf, white onion, and white wine. Add water to cover the octopus, cover with a lid, bring to a boil over high heat, reduce to low, and simmer within 1 and ½ hours.
2. Drain octopus, reserve boiling liquid, and leave aside to cool down. Put ¼ cup octopus cooking liquid in another pot, add mussels, and heat up over medium-high heat, cook until they open, transfer to a bowl, and leave aside.

3. Add clams to the pan, cover, cook over medium-high heat until they open, transfer to the bowl with mussels, and leave aside. Add squid to the pan, cover and cook over medium-high heat for 3 minutes, transfer to the bowl with mussels and clams.
4. Meanwhile, slice octopus into small pieces and mix with the rest of the seafood. Add sliced celery, radicchio, red onion, vinegar, olive oil, parsley, salt, and pepper, stir gently, and leave aside in the fridge within 2 hours before serving.

Nutrition: Calories: 102; Carbs: 7g; Fat: 1g; Protein: 16g; Sodium: 0mg

300. Shrimp and Onion Ginger Dressing

Preparation time: 10 minutes
Cooking time: 5 minutes
Servings: 2
Ingredients:

- 8 medium shrimp, peeled and deveined
- 12 ounces package mixed salad leaves
- 10 cherry tomatoes, halved
- 2 green onions, sliced
- 2 medium mushrooms, sliced
- 1/3 cup rice vinegar
- ¼ cup sesame seeds, toasted
- 1 tablespoon low-sodium soy sauce
- 2 teaspoons ginger, grated
- 2 teaspoons garlic, minced
- 2/3 cup canola oil
- 1/3 cup sesame oil

Directions:

1. In a bowl, mix rice vinegar with sesame seeds, soy sauce, garlic, ginger, and stir well. Pour this into your kitchen blender, add canola oil and sesame oil, pulse very well, and leave aside. Brush shrimp with 3 tablespoons of the ginger dressing you've prepared.
2. Heat your kitchen grill over high heat, add shrimp and cook for 3 minutes, flipping once. In a salad bowl, mix salad leaves with grilled shrimp, mushrooms, green onions, and tomatoes. Drizzle ginger dressing on top and serve right away!

Nutrition: Calories: 360; Carbs: 14g; Fat: 11g; Protein: 49g; Sodium: 469 mg

MAINS

301. Cauliflower Tabbouleh

Preparation time: 10 minutes
Cooking time: 4 minutes
Servings: 4
Ingredients:

- 1-pound cauliflower head
- 1 cucumber, chopped
- 2 tablespoons lemon juice
- 2 tablespoons olive oil
- ½ cup fresh parsley
- 1 garlic clove, diced
- 1 oz. scallions, chopped
- 1 teaspoon mint

Directions:

1. Trim and chop cauliflower head. Transfer it in the food processor and pulse until you get cauliflower rice.
2. Transfer the cauliflower rice in the glass mixing bowl. Add lemon juice and chopped scallions. Mix up the mixture.
3. Microwave it for 4 minutes.

4. Meanwhile, blend together olive oil, parsley, and diced garlic.
5. Mix up together cooked cauliflower rice with parsley mixture. Add mint and chopped cucumbers.
6. Mix it up and transfer on the serving plates.

Nutrition: Calories 108, Fat 7.3, Fiber 3.7, Carbs 10.2, Protein 3.2

302. Stuffed Artichoke

Preparation time: 10 minutes
Cooking time: 15 minutes
Servings: 4

Ingredients:
- 2 artichokes
- 4 tablespoon Parmesan, grated
- 2 teaspoon almond flour
- 1 teaspoon minced garlic
- 3 tablespoons sour cream
- 1 teaspoon avocado oil
- 1 cup water, for cooking

Directions:
1. Pour water in the saucepan and bring it to boil.
2. When the water is boiling, add artichokes and boil them for 5 minutes.
3. Drain water from artichokes and trim them.
4. Remove the artichoke hearts.
5. Preheat the oven to 365F.
6. Mix up together almond flour, grated Parmesan, minced garlic, sour cream, and avocado oil.
7. Fill the artichokes with cheese mixture and place on the baking tray.
8. Cook the vegetables for 10 minutes.
9. Then cut every artichoke into halves and transfer on the serving plates.

Nutrition: Calories 162, Fat 10.7, Fiber 5.9, Carbs 12.4, Protein 8.2

303. Beef Salpicao

Preparation time: 10 minutes
Cooking time: 18 minutes
Servings: 2

Ingredients:
- 1-pound rib eye, boneless
- 2 garlic cloves, peeled, diced
- 2 tablespoons butter
- 1 tablespoon sour cream
- ½ teaspoon salt
- ½ teaspoon chili pepper
- 1 tablespoon lime juice

Directions:
1. Cut rib eye into the strips.
2. Sprinkle the meat with salt, chili pepper, and lime juice.
3. Toss butter in the skillet. Add diced garlic and roast it for 2 minutes over the medium heat.
4. Then add meat strips and roast them over the high heat for 2 minutes from each side.
5. Add sour cream and close the lid. Cook the meal for 10 minutes more over the medium heat. Stir it from time to time.
6. Transfer cooked beef Salpicao on the serving plates.

Nutrition: Calories 641, Fat 52.8, Fiber 0.1, Carbs 1.9, Protein 42.5

304. Cream Dredged Corn Platter

Preparation Time: 10 minutes
Cooking Time: 4 hours
Servings: 3

Ingredients:
7. 3 cups corn
8. 2 ounces cream cheese, cubed
9. 2 tablespoons milk
10. 2 tablespoons whipping cream
11. 2 tablespoons butter, melted
12. Salt and pepper as needed
13. 1 tablespoon green onion, chopped

Directions:
- Add corn, cream cheese, milk, whipping cream, butter, salt and pepper to your Slow Cooker.
- Give it a nice toss to mix everything well. Place lid and cook on LOW for 4 hours.
- Divide the mix amongst serving platters. Serve and enjoy!

Nutrition: Calories 641, Fat 52.8, Fiber 0.1, Carbs 1.9, Protein 42.5

305. Ethiopian Cabbage Delight

Preparation Time: 15 minutes
Cooking Time: 6- 8 hours
Servings: 6

Ingredients:
10. ½ cup water
11. 1 head green cabbage, cored and chopped
12. 1 pound sweet potatoes, peeled and chopped
13. 3 carrots, peeled and chopped
14. 1 onion, sliced
15. 1 teaspoon extra virgin olive oil
16. ½ teaspoon ground turmeric
17. ½ teaspoon ground cumin
18. ¼ teaspoon ground ginger

Directions:
- Add water to your Slow Cooker. Take a medium bowl and add cabbage, carrots, sweet potatoes, onion and mix.
- Add olive oil, turmeric, ginger, cumin and toss until the veggies are fully coated.
- Transfer veggie mix to your Slow Cooker. Cover and cook on LOW for 6-8 hours. Serve and enjoy!

Nutrition: Calories 641, Fat 52.8, Fiber 0.1, Carbs 1.9, Protein 42.5

306. Mushroom Soup

Preparation time: 10 minutes
Cooking time: 25 minutes
Servings: 4

Ingredients:
- 1 cup of water
- 1 cup of coconut milk
- 1 cup white mushrooms, chopped

- ½ carrot, chopped
- ¼ white onion, diced
- 1 tablespoon butter
- 2 oz. turnip, chopped
- 1 teaspoon dried dill
- ½ teaspoon ground black pepper
- ¾ teaspoon smoked paprika
- 1 oz. celery stalk, chopped

Directions:
1. Pour water and coconut milk in the saucepan. Bring the liquid to boil.
2. Add chopped mushrooms, carrot, and turnip. Close the lid and boil for 10 minutes.
3. Meanwhile, put butter in the skillet. Add diced onion. Sprinkle it with dill, ground black pepper, and smoked paprika. Roast the onion for 3 minutes.
4. Add the roasted onion in the soup mixture.
5. Then add chopped celery stalk. Close the lid.
6. Cook soup for 10 minutes.
7. Then ladle it into the serving bowls.

Nutrition: Calories 181, Fat 17.3, Fiber 2.5, Carbs 6.9, Protein 2.4

307. Stuffed Portobello Mushrooms

Preparation time: 10 minutes
Cooking time: 10 minutes
Servings: 4
Ingredients:
- 2 portobello mushrooms
- 1 cup spinach, chopped, steamed
- 2 oz. artichoke hearts, drained, chopped
- 1 tablespoon coconut cream
- 1 tablespoon cream cheese
- 1 teaspoon minced garlic
- 1 tablespoon fresh cilantro, chopped
- 3 oz. Cheddar cheese, grated
- ½ teaspoon ground black pepper
- 2 tablespoons olive oil
- ½ teaspoon salt

Directions:
1. Sprinkle mushrooms with olive oil and place in the tray.
2. Transfer the tray in the preheated to 360F oven and broil them for 5 minutes.
3. Meanwhile, blend together artichoke hearts, coconut cream, cream cheese, minced garlic, and chopped cilantro.
4. Add grated cheese in the mixture and sprinkle with ground black pepper and salt.
5. Fill the broiled mushrooms with the cheese mixture and cook them for 5 minutes more. Serve the mushrooms only hot.

Nutrition: Calories 183, Fat 16.3, Fiber 1.9, Carbs 3, Protein 7.7

308. Lettuce Salad

Preparation time: 10 minutes
Cooking Time: 10 minutes
Servings: 1
Ingredients:
- 1 cup Romaine lettuce, roughly chopped

- 3 oz. Seitan, chopped
- 1 tablespoon avocado oil
- 1 teaspoon sunflower seeds
- 1 teaspoon lemon juice
- 1 egg, boiled, peeled
- 2 oz. Cheddar cheese, shredded

Directions:
1. Place lettuce in the salad bowl. Add chopped Seitan and shredded cheese.
2. Then chop the egg roughly and add in the salad bowl too.
3. Mix up together lemon juice with the avocado oil.
4. Sprinkle the salad with the oil mixture and sunflower seeds. Don't stir the salad before serving.

Nutrition: Calories 663, Fat 29.5, Fiber 4.7, Carbs 3.8, Protein 84.2

309. Onion Soup

Preparation time: 10 minutes
Cooking time: 25 minutes
Servings: 6
Ingredients:
- 2 cups white onion, diced
- 4 tablespoon butter
- ½ cup white mushrooms, chopped
- 3 cups of water
- 1 cup heavy cream
- 1 teaspoon salt
- 1 teaspoon chili flakes
- 1 teaspoon garlic powder

Directions:
1. Put butter in the saucepan and melt it.
2. Add diced white onion, chili flakes, and garlic powder. Mix it up and sauté for 10 minutes over the medium-low heat.
3. Then add water, heavy cream, and chopped mushrooms. Close the lid.
4. Cook the soup for 15 minutes more.
5. Then blend the soup until you get the creamy texture. Ladle it in the bowls.

Nutrition: Calories 155, Fat 15.1, Fiber 0.9, Carbs 4.7, Protein 1.2

310. Asparagus Salad

Preparation time: 10 minutes
Cooking time: 15 minutes
Servings: 3
Ingredients:
- 10 oz. asparagus
- 1 tablespoon olive oil
- ½ teaspoon white pepper
- 4 oz. Feta cheese, crumbled
- 1 cup lettuce, chopped
- 1 tablespoon canola oil
- 1 teaspoon apple cider vinegar
- 1 tomato, diced

Directions:
1. Preheat the oven to 365F.
2. Place asparagus in the tray, sprinkle with olive oil and white pepper and transfer in the preheated oven. Cook it for 15 minutes.

3. Meanwhile, put crumbled Feta in the salad bowl.
4. Add chopped lettuce and diced tomato.
5. Sprinkle the ingredients with apple cider vinegar.
6. Chill the cooked asparagus to the room temperature and add in the salad.
7. Shake the salad gently before serving.

Nutrition: Calories 207, Fat 17.6, Fiber 2.4, Carbs 6.8, Protein 7.8

311. Prosciutto-Wrapped Asparagus

Preparation time: 15 minutes
Cooking time: 20 minutes
Servings: 6

Ingredients:
- 2-pound asparagus
- 8 oz. prosciutto, sliced
- 1 tablespoon butter, melted
- ½ teaspoon ground black pepper
- 4 tablespoon heavy cream
- 1 tablespoon lemon juice

Directions:
1. Slice prosciutto slices into strips.
2. Wrap asparagus into prosciutto strips and place on the tray.
3. Sprinkle the vegetables with ground black pepper, heavy cream, and lemon juice. Add butter.
4. Preheat the oven to 365F.
5. Place the tray with asparagus in the oven and cook for 20 minutes.
6. Serve the cooked meal only hot.

Nutrition: Calories 138, Fat 7.9, Fiber 3.2, Carbs 6.9, Protein 11.5

312. Stuffed Bell Peppers

Preparation time: 10 minutes
Cooking time: 25 minutes
Servings: 4

Ingredients:
- 4 bell peppers
- 1 ½ cup ground beef
- 1 zucchini, grated
- 1 white onion, diced
- ½ teaspoon ground nutmeg
- 1 tablespoon olive oil
- 1 teaspoon ground black pepper
- ½ teaspoon salt
- 3 oz. Parmesan, grated

Directions:
1. Cut the bell peppers into halves and remove seeds.
2. Place ground beef in the skillet.
3. Add grated zucchini, diced onion, ground nutmeg, olive oil, ground black pepper, and salt.
4. Roast the mixture for 5 minutes.
5. Place bell pepper halves in the tray.
6. Fill every pepper half with ground beef mixture and top with grated Parmesan.
7. Cover the tray with foil and secure the edges.
8. Cook the stuffed bell peppers for 20 minutes at 360F.

Nutrition: Calories 241, Fat 14.6, Fiber 3.4, Carbs 11, Protein 18.6

313. Stuffed Eggplants with Goat Cheese

Preparation time: 15 minutes
Cooking time: 25 minutes
Servings: 4

Ingredients:
- 1 large eggplant, trimmed
- 1 tomato, crushed
- 1 garlic clove, diced
- ½ teaspoon ground black pepper
- ½ teaspoon smoked paprika
- 1 cup spinach, chopped
- 4 oz. goat cheese, crumbled
- 1 teaspoon butter
- 2 oz. Cheddar cheese, shredded

Directions:
1. Cut the eggplants into halves and then cut every half into 2 parts.
2. Remove the flesh from the eggplants to get eggplant boards.
3. Mix up together crushed tomato, diced garlic, ground black pepper, smoked paprika, chopped spinach, crumbled goat cheese, and butter.
4. Fill the eggplants with this mixture.
5. Top every eggplant board with shredded Cheddar cheese.
6. Put the eggplants in the tray.
7. Preheat the oven to 365F.
8. Place the tray with eggplants in the oven and cook for 25 minutes.

Nutrition: Calories 229, Fat 16.1, Fiber 4.6, Carbs 9, Protein 13.8

314. Korma Curry

Preparation time: 10 minutes
Cooking time: 25 minutes
Servings: 6

Ingredients:
- 3-pound chicken breast, skinless, boneless
- 1 teaspoon garam masala
- 1 teaspoon curry powder
- 1 tablespoon apple cider vinegar
- ½ coconut cream
- 1 cup organic almond milk
- 1 teaspoon ground coriander
- ¾ teaspoon ground cardamom
- ½ teaspoon ginger powder
- ¼ teaspoon cayenne pepper
- ¾ teaspoon ground cinnamon
- 1 tomato, diced
- 1 teaspoon avocado oil
- ½ cup of water

Directions:
1. Chop the chicken breast and put it in the saucepan.
2. Add avocado oil and start to cook it over the medium heat.
3. Sprinkle the chicken with garam masala, curry powder, apple cider vinegar, ground coriander, cardamom, ginger

powder, cayenne pepper, ground cinnamon, and diced tomato. Mix up the ingredients carefully. Cook them for 10 minutes.

4. Add water, coconut cream, and almond milk. Sauté the meal for 10 minutes more.

Nutrition: Calories 411, Fat 19.3, Fiber 0.9, Carbs 6, Protein 49.9

315. Zucchini Bars

Preparation time: 10 minutes
Cooking time: 15 minutes
Servings: 8
Ingredients:
- 3 zucchini, grated
- ½ white onion, diced
- 2 teaspoons butter
- 3 eggs, whisked
- 4 tablespoons coconut flour
- 1 teaspoon salt
- ½ teaspoon ground black pepper
- 5 oz. goat cheese, crumbled
- 4 oz. Swiss cheese, shredded
- ½ cup spinach, chopped
- 1 teaspoon baking powder
- ½ teaspoon lemon juice

Directions:
1. In the mixing bowl, mix up together grated zucchini, diced onion, eggs, coconut flour, salt, ground black pepper, crumbled cheese, chopped spinach, baking powder, and lemon juice.
2. Add butter and churn the mixture until homogenous.
3. Line the baking dish with baking paper.
4. Transfer the zucchini mixture in the baking dish and flatten it.
5. Preheat the oven to 365F and put the dish inside.
6. Cook it for 15 minutes. Then chill the meal well.
7. Cut it into bars.

Nutrition: Calories 199, Fat 1316, Fiber 215, Carbs 7.1, Protein 13.1

316. Tuna Tartare

Preparation time: 10 minutes
Servings: 4
Ingredients:
- 1-pound tuna steak
- 1 tablespoon mayonnaise
- 3 oz. avocado, chopped
- 1 cucumber, chopped
- 1 tablespoon lemon juice
- 1 teaspoon cayenne pepper
- 1 teaspoon soy sauce
- 1 teaspoon chives
- ½ teaspoon cumin seeds
- 1 teaspoon canola oil

Directions:
1. Chop tuna steak and place it in the big bowl.
2. Add avocado, cucumber, and chives.

3. Mix up together lemon juice, cayenne pepper, soy sauce, cumin seeds, and canola oil.
4. Add mixed liquid in the tuna mixture and mix up well.
5. Place tuna Tartare in the serving plates.

Nutrition: Calories 292, Fat 13.9, Fiber 2, Carbs 6, Protein 35.1

317. Clam Chowder

Preparation time: 5 minutes
Cooking time: 15 minutes
Servings: 3
Ingredients:
- 1 cup of coconut milk
- 1 cup of water
- 6 oz. clam, chopped
- 1 teaspoon chives
- ½ teaspoon white pepper
- ¾ teaspoon chili flakes
- ½ teaspoon salt
- 1 cup broccoli florets, chopped

Directions:
1. Pour coconut milk and water in the saucepan.
2. Add chopped clams, chives, white pepper, chili flakes, salt, and broccoli florets.
3. Close the lid and cook chowder over the medium-low heat for 15 minutes or until all the ingredients are soft.
4. It is recommended to serve the soup hot.

Nutrition: Calories 139, Fat 9.8, Fiber 1.1, Carbs 10.8, Protein 2.4

318. Asian Beef Salad

Preparation time: 10 minutes
Cooking time: 25 minutes
Servings: 4
Ingredients:
- 14 oz. beef brisket
- 1 teaspoon sesame seeds
- ½ teaspoon cumin seeds
- 1 tablespoon apple cider vinegar
- 1 tablespoon avocado oil
- 1 red bell pepper, sliced
- 1 white onion, sliced
- 1 teaspoon butter
- 1 teaspoon ground black pepper
- 1 teaspoon soy sauce
- 1 garlic clove, sliced
- 1 cup water, for cooking

Directions:
1. Slice beef brisket and place it in the pan. Add water and close the lid.
2. Cook the beef for 25 minutes.
3. Then drain water and transfer beef brisket in the pan.
4. Add butter and roast it for 5 minutes.
5. Put the cooked beef brisket in the salad bowl.
6. Add sesame seeds, cumin seeds, apple cider vinegar, avocado oil, sliced bell pepper, onion, ground black pepper, and soy sauce.
7. Sprinkle the salad with garlic and mix it up.

Nutrition: Calories 227, Fat 8.1, Fiber 1.4, Carbs 6, Protein 31.1

319. Carbonara

Preparation time: 10 minutes
Cooking time: 25 minutes
Servings: 6
Ingredients:
- 3 zucchini, trimmed
- 1 cup heavy cream
- 5 oz. bacon, chopped
- 2 egg yolks
- 4 oz. Cheddar cheese, grated
- 1 tablespoon butter
- 1 teaspoon chili flakes
- 1 teaspoon salt
- ½ cup water, for cooking

Directions:
1. Make the zucchini noodles with the help of the spiralizer.
2. Toss bacon in the skillet and roast it for 5 minutes on the medium heat. Stir it from time to time.
3. Meanwhile, in the saucepan, mix up together heavy cream, butter, salt, and chili flakes.
4. Add egg yolk and whisk the mixture until smooth.
5. Start to preheat the liquid, stir it constantly.
6. When the liquid starts to boil, add grated cheese and fried bacon. Mix it up and close the lid. Sauté it on the low heat for 5 minutes.
7. Meanwhile, place the zucchini noodles in the skillet where bacon was and roast it for 3 minutes.
8. Then pour heavy cream mixture over zucchini and mix up well. Cook it for 1 minute more and transfer on the serving plates.

Nutrition: Calories 324, Fat 27.1, Fiber 1.1, Carbs 4.6, Protein 16

320. Cauliflower Soup with Seeds

Preparation time: 10 minutes
Cooking time: 20 minutes
Servings: 4
Ingredients:
- 2 cups cauliflower
- 1 tablespoon pumpkin seeds
- 1 tablespoon chia seeds
- ½ teaspoon salt
- 1 teaspoon butter
- ¼ white onion, diced
- ½ cup coconut cream
- 1 cup of water
- 4 oz. Parmesan, grated
- 1 teaspoon paprika
- 1 tablespoon dried cilantro

Directions:
1. Chop cauliflower and put in the saucepan.
2. Add salt, butter, diced onion, paprika, and dried cilantro.
3. Cook the cauliflower over the medium heat for 5 minutes.
4. Then add coconut cream and water.
5. Close the lid and boil soup for 15 minutes.
6. Then blend the soup with the help of hand blender.
7. Dring to boil it again.
8. Add grated cheese and mix up well.
9. Ladle the soup into the serving bowls and top every bowl with pumpkin seeds and chia seeds.

Nutrition: Calories 214, Fat 16.4, Fiber 3.6, Carbs 8.1, Protein 12.1

321. Crepe Pie

Preparation time: 10 minutes
Cooking time: 15 minutes
Servings: 8
Ingredients:
- 1 cup almond flour
- 1 cup coconut flour
- ½ cup heavy cream
- 1 teaspoon baking powder
- ½ teaspoon salt
- 10 oz. ham, sliced
- ½ cup cream cheese
- 1 teaspoon chili flakes
- 1 tablespoon fresh cilantro, chopped
- 4 oz. Cheddar cheese, shredded

Directions:
1. Make crepes: in the mixing bowl, mix up together almond flour, coconut flour, heavy cream, salt, and baking powder. Whisk the mixture.
2. Preheat the non-sticky skillet well and ladle 1 ladle of the crepe batter in it.
3. Make the crepes: cook them for 1 minute from each side over the medium heat.
4. Mix up together cream cheese, chili flakes, cilantro, and shredded Cheddar cheese.
5. After this, transfer 1st crepe in the plate. Spread it with cream cheese mixture. Add ham.
6. Repeat the steps until you use all the ingredients.
7. Bake the crepe pie for 5 minutes in the preheated to the 365F oven.
8. Cut it into the serving and serve hot.

Nutrition: Calories 272, Fat 18.8, Fiber 6.9, Carbs 13.2, Protein 13.4

322. Coconut Soup

Preparation time: 15 minutes
Cooking time: 25 minutes
Servings: 4
Ingredients:
- 1 cup of coconut milk
- 2 cups of water
- 1 teaspoon curry paste
- 4 chicken thighs
- ½ teaspoon fresh ginger, grated
- 1 garlic clove, diced
- 1 teaspoon butter
- 1 teaspoon chili flakes
- 1 tablespoon lemon juice

Directions:
1. Toss the butter in the skillet and melt it.
2. Add diced garlic and grated ginger. Cook the ingredients for 1 minute. Stir them constantly.
3. Pour water in the saucepan. Add coconut milk and curry paste. Mix up the liquid until homogenous.

4. Add chicken thighs, chili flakes, and cooked ginger mixture.
5. Close the lid and cook soup for 15 minutes.
6. Then start to whisk soup with the hand whisker and add lemon juice.
7. When all lemon juice is added, stop to whisk it.
8. Close the lid and cook soup for 5 minutes more over the medium heat.
9. Then remove soup from the heat and let it rest for 15 minutes.

Nutrition: Calories 318, Fat 26, Fiber 1.4, Carbs 4.2, Protein 20.6

323. Fish Tacos

Preparation time: 10 minutes
Cooking time: 5 minutes
Servings: 4
Ingredients:
- 4 lettuce leaves
- ½ red onion, diced
- ½ jalapeno pepper, minced
- 1 tablespoon olive oil
- 1-pound cod fillet
- 1 tablespoon lemon juice
- ¼ teaspoon ground coriander

Directions:
1. Sprinkle cod fillet with a ½ tablespoon of olive oil and ground coriander.
2. Preheat the grill well.
3. Grill the fish for 2 minutes from each side. The cooked fish has a light brown color.
4. After this, mix up together diced red onion, minced jalapeno pepper, remaining olive oil, and lemon juice.
5. Cut the grilled cod fillet into 4 pieces.
6. Place the fish in the lettuce leaves. Add mixed red onion mixture over the fish and transfer the tacos on the serving plates.

Nutrition: Calories 157, Fat 4.5, Fiber 0.4, Carbs 1.6, Protein 26.1

324. Cobb Salad

Preparation time: 10 minutes
Cooking time: 5 minutes
Servings: 2
Ingredients:
- 2 oz. bacon, sliced
- 1 egg, boiled, peeled
- ½ tomato, chopped
- 1 oz. Blue cheese
- 1 teaspoon chives
- 1/3 cup lettuce, chopped
- 1 tablespoon mayonnaise
- 1 tablespoon lemon juice

Directions:
1. Place the bacon in the preheated skillet and roast it 1.5 minutes from each side.
2. When the bacon is cooked, chop it roughly and transfer in the salad bowl.
3. Chop the eggs roughly and add them in the salad bowl too.
4. After this, add chopped tomato, chives, and lettuce.

5. Chop Blue cheese and add it in the salad.
6. Then make seasoning: whisk together mayonnaise with lemon juice.
7. Pour the mixture over the salad and shake little.

Nutrition: Calories 270, Fat 20.7, Fiber 0.3, Carbs 3.7, Protein 16.6

325. Cheese Soup

Preparation time: 10 minutes
Cooking time: 15 minutes
Servings: 3
Ingredients:
- 2 white onion, peeled, diced
- 1 cup Cheddar cheese, shredded
- ½ cup heavy cream
- ½ cup of water
- 1 teaspoon ground black pepper
- 1 tablespoon butter
- ½ teaspoon salt

Directions:
1. Pour water and heavy cream in the saucepan.
2. Bring it to boil.
3. Meanwhile, toss the butter in the pan, add diced onions and sauté them.
4. When the onions are translucent, transfer them in the boiling liquid.
5. Add ground black pepper, salt, and cheese. Cook the soup for 5 minutes.
6. Then let it chill little and ladle it into the bowls.

Nutrition: Calories 286, Fat 23.8, Fiber 1.8, Carbs 8.3, Protein 10.7

326. Veggie Wrap

Preparation time: 15 minutes
Cooking time: 0 minutes
Servings: 2
Ingredients:
- 2 Homemade wraps or any flour tortillas
- ½ cup spinach
- 1/2 cup alfalfa sprouts
- ½ cup avocado, sliced thinly
- 1 medium tomato, sliced thinly
- ½ cup cucumber, sliced thinly
- Pinch of salt and pepper

Directions:
1. Put 2 tablespoons of cream cheese on each tortilla. Layer each veggie according to your liking. Pinch of salt and pepper. Roll and cut into half. Serve and Enjoy!

Nutrition: Calories 249, Carbohydrates 12.3g, Protein 5.7g, Fat 21.5g, Sodium 169mg

327. Salmon Wrap

Preparation time: 15 minutes
Cooking time: 0 minutes
Servings: 1
Ingredients:
- 2 oz. Smoke Salmon
- 2 teaspoon low-fat cream cheese

- ½ medium-size red onion, finely sliced
- ½ teaspoon fresh basil or dried basil
- Pinch of pepper
- Arugula leaves
- 1 Homemade wrap or any whole-meal tortilla

Directions:
1. Warm wraps or tortilla into a heated pan or oven. Combine cream cheese, basil, pepper, and spread into the tortilla. Top with salmon, arugula, and sliced onion. Roll up and slice. Serve and Enjoy!

Nutrition: Calories 151, Carbohydrates 19.2g, Protein 10.4g, Fat 3.4g, Sodium 316mg

328. Dill Chicken Salad

Preparation time: 15 minutes
Cooking time: 15 minutes
Servings: 3
Ingredients:
- 1 tablespoon unsalted butter
- 1 small onion, diced
- 2 cloves garlic, minced
- 500g boneless skinless chicken breasts
- Salad:
- 2/3 cup Fat-free yogurt
- ¼ cup mayonnaise light
- 2 large shallots, minced
- ½ cup fresh dill, finely chopped

Directions:
1. Dissolve the butter over medium heat in a wide pan. Sauté onion and garlic in the butter and chicken breasts. Put water to cover the chicken breasts by 1 inch. Bring to boil. Cover and reduce the heat to a bare simmer.
2. Cook within 8 to 10 minutes or until the chicken is cooked through. Cool thoroughly. The shred chicken finely using 2 forks. Set aside. Whisk yogurt and mayonnaise. Then toss with the chicken. Add shallots and dill. Mix again all. Serve and Enjoy!

Nutrition: Calories 253, Carbohydrates 9g, Protein 33.1g, Fat 9.5g, Sodium 236mg

329. Spinach Rolls

Preparation time: 10 minutes
Cooking time: 10 minutes
Servings: 4
Ingredients:
- 4 eggs, whisked
- 1/3 cup organic almond milk
- ½ teaspoon salt
- ½ teaspoon white pepper
- 1 teaspoon butter
- 9 oz. chicken breast, boneless, skinless, cooked
- 2 cups spinach
- 2 tablespoon heavy cream

Directions:
1. Mix up together whisked eggs with almond milk and salt.
2. Preheat the skillet well and toss the butter in it.
3. Melt it.
4. Cook 4 crepes in the preheated skillet.
5. Meanwhile, chop the spinach and chicken breast.
6. Fill every egg crepe with chopped spinach, chicken breast, and heavy cream.
7. Roll the crepes and transfer on the serving plate.

Nutrition: Calories 220, Fat 14.5, Fiber 0.8, Carbs 2.4, Protein 20.1

330. Goat Cheese Fold-Overs

Preparation time: 15 minutes
Cooking time: 8 minutes
Servings: 4
Ingredients:
- 8 oz. goat cheese, crumbled
- 5 oz. ham, sliced
- 1 cup almond flour
- ¼ cup of coconut milk
- 1 teaspoon olive oil
- ½ teaspoon dried dill
- 1 teaspoon Italian seasoning
- ½ teaspoon salt

Directions:
1. In the mixing bowl, mix up together almond flour, coconut milk, olive oil, and salt. You will get a smooth batter.
2. Preheat the non-stick skillet.
3. Separate batter into 4 parts. Pour 1st batter part in the preheated skillet and cook it for 1 minute from each side.
4. Repeat the same steps with all batter.
5. After this, mix up together crumbled goat cheese, dried dill, and Italian seasoning.
6. Spread every almond flour pancake with goat cheese mixture. Add sliced ham and fold them.

Nutrition: Calories 402 Fat 31.8, Fiber 1.6, Carbs 5.1, Protein 25.1

331. Sweet and Sour Vegetable Noodles

Preparation time: 15 minutes
Cooking time: 30 minutes
Servings: 4
Ingredients:
- 4 chicken fillets (75 g each)
- 300g of whole-wheat spaghetti
- 750g carrots
- ½ liter clear chicken broth (instant)
- 1 tablespoon sugar
- 1 tbsp. of green peppercorns
- 2-3 tbsp. balsamic vinegar
- Capuchin flowers
- Pinch of salt

Directions:
1. Cook spaghetti in boiling water for about 8 minutes. Then drain. In the meantime, peel and wash carrots. Cut into long strips (best with a special grater). Blanch within 2 minutes in boiling salted water, drain. Wash chicken fillets. Add to the boiling chicken soup and cook for about 15 minutes.
2. Melt the sugar until golden brown. Measure 1/4 liter of chicken stock and deglaze the sugar with it. Add peppercorns, cook for 2 minutes. Season with salt and

vinegar. Add the fillets, then cut into thin slices. Then turn the pasta and carrots in the sauce and serve garnished with capuchin blossoms. Serve and enjoy.

Nutrition: Calories 374, Fat 21g, Protein 44g, Sodium 295mg, Carbohydrate 23.1

332. Tuna Sandwich

Preparation time: 15 minutes
Cooking time: 0 minutes
Servings: 1
Ingredients:

- 2 slices whole-grain bread
- 1 6-oz. can low sodium tuna in water, in its juice
- 2 tsp. Yogurt (1.5% fat) or low-fat mayonnaise
- 1 medium tomato, diced
- ½ small sweet onion, finely diced
- Lettuce leaves

Directions:
1. Toast whole grain bread slices. Mix tuna, yogurt, or mayonnaise, diced tomato, and onion. Cover a toasted bread with lettuce leaves and spread the tuna mixture on the sandwich. Spread tuna mixed on toasted bread with lettuce leaves. Place another disc as a cover on top. Enjoy the sandwich.

Nutrition: Calories 235, Fat 3g, Protein 27.8g, Sodium 350mg, Carbohydrate 25.9

333. Fruited Quinoa Salad

Preparation time: 15 minutes
Cooking time: 0 minutes
Servings: 2
Ingredients:

- 2 cups cooked quinoa
- 1 mango, sliced and peeled
- 1 cup strawberry, quartered
- ½ cup blueberries
- 2 tablespoon pine nuts
- Chopped mint leave for garnish
- Lemon vinaigrette:
- ¼ cup olive oil
- ¼ cup apple cider vinegar
- Zest of lemon
- 3 tablespoon lemon juice
- 1 teaspoon sugar

Directions:
1. For the Lemon Vinaigrette, whisk olive oil, apple cider vinegar, lemon zest and juice, and sugar to a bowl; set aside. Combine quinoa, mango strawberries, blueberries, and pine nuts in a large bowl. Stir the lemon vinaigrette and garnish with mint. Serve and enjoy!

Nutrition: Calories 425, Carbohydrates 76.1g, Proteins 11.3g, Fat 10.9, Sodium 16mg

334. Turkey Wrap

Preparation time: 15 minutes
Cooking time: 0 minutes

Servings: 2
Ingredients:

- 2 slices of low-fat Turkey breast (deli-style)
- 4 tablespoon non-fat cream cheese
- ½ cup lettuce leaves
- ½ cup carrots, slice into a stick
- 2 Homemade wraps or store-bought whole-wheat tortilla wrap

Directions:
1. Prepare all the ingredients. Spread 2 tablespoons of non-fat cream cheese on each wrap. Arrange lettuce leaves, then add a slice of turkey breast; a slice of carrots stick on top. Roll and cut into half. Serve and enjoy!

Nutrition: Calories 224, Carbohydrates 35g, Protein 10.3g, Fat 3.8g, Sodium 293mg

335. Chicken Wrap

Preparation time: 15 minutes
Cooking time: 15 minutes
Servings: 2
Ingredients:

- 1 tablespoon extra- virgin olive oil
- Lemon juice, divided into 3 parts
- 2 cloves garlic, minced
- 1 lb. boneless skinless chicken breasts
- ½ cup non- fat plain Greek yogurt
- ½ teaspoon paprika
- Pinch of salt and pepper
- Hot sauce to taste
- Pita bread
- Tomato slice

Directions:
1. For the marinade, whisk 1 tablespoon olive oil, juice of 2 lemons, garlic, salt, and pepper in a bowl. Add chicken breasts to the marinade and place it into a large Ziploc. Let marinate for 30 mins. To 4 hours.
2. For the yogurt sauce, mix yogurt, hot sauce, and the remaining lemon juice season with paprika and a pinch of salt and pepper.
3. Warm skillet over medium heat and coat it with oil. Add chicken breast and cook until golden brown and cook about 8 minutes per side. Remove from pan and rest for few minutes, then slice.
4. To a piece of pita bread, add lettuce, tomato, and chicken slices. Drizzle with the prepared spicy yogurt sauce. Serve and enjoy!

Nutrition: Calories 348, Carbohydrates 8.7g, Proteins 56g, Fat 10.2g, Sodium 198mg

336. Veggie Variety

Preparation time: 15 minutes
Cooking time: 15 minutes
Servings: 2
Ingredients:

- ½ onion, diced
- 1 teaspoon vegetable oil (corn or sunflower oil)
- 200 g Tofu/ bean curd
- 4 cherry tomatoes, halved

- 30ml vegetable milk (soy or oat milk)
- ½ tsp. curry powder
- 0.25 tsp. paprika
- Pinch of Salt & Pepper
- 2 slices of Vegan protein bread/ Whole grain bread
- Chives for garnish

Directions:
1. Dice the onion and fry in a frying pan with the oil. Break the tofu by hand into small pieces and put them in the pan. Sauté 7-8 min. Season with curry, paprika, salt, and pepper. The cherry tomatoes and milk and cook it all over roast a few minutes. Serve with bread as desired and sprinkle with chopped chives.

Nutrition: Calories 216, Fat 8.4g, Protein 14.1g, Sodium 140mg, Carbohydrate 24.8g

337. Vegetable Pasta

Preparation time: 15 minutes
Cooking time: 15 minutes
Servings: 4
Ingredients:
- 1 kg of thin zucchini
- 20 g of fresh ginger
- 350g smoked tofu
- 1 lime
- 2 cloves of garlic
- 2 tbsp. sunflower oil
- 2 tablespoons of sesame seeds
- Pinch of salt and pepper
- 4 tablespoons fried onions

Directions:
1. Wash and clean the zucchini and, using a julienne cutter, cut the pulp around the kernel into long thin strips (noodles). Ginger peel and finely chop. Crumble tofu. Halve lime, squeeze juice. Peel and chop garlic.
2. Warm-up 1 tbsp. of oil in a large pan and fry the tofu for about 5 minutes. After about 3 minutes, add ginger, garlic, and sesame. Season with soy sauce. Remove from the pan and keep warm.
3. Wipe out the pan, then warm 2 tablespoons of oil in it. Stir fry zucchini strips for about 4 minutes while turning. Season with salt, pepper, and lime juice. Arrange pasta and tofu. Sprinkle with fried onions.

Nutrition: Calories 262, Fat 17.7g, Protein 15.4g, Sodium 62mg, Carbohydrate 17.1g

338. Vegetable Noodles with Bolognese

Preparation time: 15 minutes
Cooking time: 15 minutes
Servings: 4
Ingredients:
- kg of small zucchini (e.g., green and yellow)
- 600g of carrots
- 1 onion
- 1 tbsp. olive oil
- 250g of beef steak
- Pinch of Salt and pepper

- 2 tablespoons tomato paste
- 1 tbsp. flour
- 1 teaspoon vegetable broth (instant)
- 40g pecorino or parmesan
- 1 small potty of basil

Directions:
1. Clean and peel zucchini and carrots and wash. Using a sharp, long knife, cut first into thin slices, then into long, fine strips. Clean or peel the soup greens, wash and cut into tiny cubes. Peel the onion and chop finely. Heat the Bolognese oil in a large pan. Fry hack in it crumbly. Season with salt and pepper.
2. Briefly sauté the prepared vegetable and onion cubes. Stir in tomato paste. Dust the flour, sweat briefly. Pour in 400 ml of water and stir in the vegetable stock. Boil everything, simmer for 7-8 minutes.
3. Meanwhile, cook the vegetable strips in plenty of salted water for 3-5 minutes. Drain, collecting some cooking water. Add the vegetable strips to the pan and mix well. If the sauce is not liquid enough, stir in some vegetable cooking water and season everything again.
4. Slicing cheese into fine shavings. Wash the basil, shake dry, peel off the leaves, and cut roughly. Arrange vegetable noodles, sprinkle with parmesan and basil

Nutrition: Calories 269, Fat 9.7g, Protein 25.6g, Sodium 253mg, Carbohydrate 21.7g

339. Harissa Bolognese with Vegetable Noodles

Preparation time: 15 minutes
Cooking time: 30 minutes
Servings: 4
Ingredients:
- 2 onions
- 1 clove of garlic
- 3-4 tbsp. oil
- 400g ground beef
- Pinch salt, pepper, cinnamon
- 1 tsp. Harissa (Arabic seasoning paste, tube)
- 1 tablespoon tomato paste
- 2 sweet potatoes
- 2 medium Zucchini
- 3 stems/basil
- 100g of feta

Directions:
1. Peel onions and garlic, finely dice. Warm-up 1 tbsp. of oil in a wide saucepan. Fry hack in it crumbly. Fry onions and garlic for a short time. Season with salt, pepper, and ½ teaspoon cinnamon. Stir in harissa and tomato paste.
2. Add tomatoes and 200 ml of water, bring to the boil and simmer for about 15 minutes with occasional stirring. Peel sweet potatoes and zucchini or clean and wash. Cut vegetables into spaghetti with a spiral cutter.
3. Warm-up 2-3 tablespoons of oil in a large pan. Braise sweet potato spaghetti in it for about 3 minutes. Add the zucchini spaghetti and continue to simmer for 3-4 minutes while turning.
4. Season with salt and pepper. Wash the basil, shake dry and peel off the leaves. Garnish vegetable spaghetti and Bolognese on plates. Feta crumbles over. Sprinkle with basil.

Nutrition: Calories 452, Fat 22.3g, Protein 37.1g, Sodium 253mg, Carbohydrate 27.6g

340. Curry Vegetable Noodles with Chicken

Preparation time: 15 minutes
Cooking time: 15 minutes
Servings: 2
Ingredients:

- 600g of zucchini
- 500g chicken fillet
- Pinch of salt and pepper
- 2 tbsp. oil
- 150 g of red and yellow cherry tomatoes
- 1 teaspoon curry powder
- 150g fat-free cheese
- 200 ml vegetable broth
- 4 stalk (s) of fresh basil

Directions:
1. Wash the zucchini, clean, and cut into long thin strips with a spiral cutter. Wash meat, pat dry, and season with salt. Heat 1 tbsp. oil in a pan. Roast chicken in it for about 10 minutes until golden brown.
2. Wash cherry tomatoes and cut in half. Approximately 3 minutes before the end of the cooking time to the chicken in the pan. Heat 1 tbsp. oil in another pan. Sweat curry powder into it then stirs in cream cheese and broth. Flavor the sauce with salt plus pepper and simmer for about 4 minutes.
3. Wash the basil, shake it dry and pluck the leaves from the stems. Cut small leaves of 3 stems. Remove meat from the pan and cut it into strips. Add tomatoes, basil, and zucchini to the sauce and heat for 2-3 minutes. Serve vegetable noodles and meat on plates and garnish with basil.

Nutrition: Calories 376, Fat 17.2g, Protein 44.9g, Sodium 352mg, Carbohydrate 9.5, Cholesterol 53mg

341. Mushroom Cakes

Preparation time: 15 minutes
Cooking time: 10 minutes
Servings: 4
Ingredients:

- 2 cups mushrooms, chopped
- 3 garlic cloves, chopped
- 1 tablespoon dried dill
- 1 egg, beaten
- ¼ cup of rice, cooked
- 1 tablespoon sesame oil
- 1 teaspoon chili powder

Directions:
1. Grind the mushrooms in the food processor. Add garlic, dill, egg, rice, and chili powder. Blend the mixture for 10 seconds. After this, heat sesame oil for 1 minute.
2. Make the medium size mushroom cakes and put in the hot sesame oil. Cook the mushroom cakes for 5 minutes per side on medium heat.

Nutrition: Calories 103, Protein 3.7g, Carbohydrates 12g, Fat 4.8g, Sodium 27mg

342. Glazed Eggplant Rings

Preparation time: 15 minutes
Cooking time: 10 minutes
Servings: 4
Ingredients:

- 3 eggplants, sliced
- 1 tablespoon liquid honey
- 1 teaspoon minced ginger
- 2 tablespoons lemon juice
- 3 tablespoons avocado oil
- ½ teaspoon ground coriander
- 3 tablespoons water

Directions:
1. Rub the eggplants with ground coriander. Then heat the avocado oil in the skillet for 1 minute. When the oil is hot, add the sliced eggplant and arrange it in one layer.
2. Cook the vegetables for 1 minute per side. Transfer the eggplant to the bowl. Then add minced ginger, liquid honey, lemon juice, and water in the skillet. Bring it to boil and add cooked eggplants. Coat the vegetables in the sweet liquid well and cook for 2 minutes more.

Nutrition: Calories 136, Protein 4.3g, Carbohydrates 29.6g, Fat 2.2g, Sodium 11mg

343. Sweet Potato Balls

Preparation time: 15 minutes
Cooking time: 10 minutes
Servings: 4
Ingredients:

- 1 cup sweet potato, mashed, cooked
- 1 tablespoon fresh cilantro, chopped
- 1 egg, beaten
- 3 tablespoons ground oatmeal
- 1 teaspoon ground paprika
- ½ teaspoon ground turmeric
- 2 tablespoons coconut oil

Directions:
1. Mix mashed sweet potato, fresh cilantro, egg, ground oatmeal, paprika, and turmeric in a bowl. Stir the mixture until smooth and make the small balls. Heat the coconut oil in the saucepan. Put the sweet potato balls, then cook them until golden brown.

Nutrition: Calories 133, Protein 2.8g, Carbohydrates 13.1g, Fat 8.2g, Sodium 44mg

344. Chickpea Curry

Preparation time: 15 minutes
Cooking time: 10 minutes
Servings: 4
Ingredients:

- 1 ½ cup chickpeas, boiled
- 1 teaspoon curry powder
- ½ teaspoon garam masala
- 1 cup spinach, chopped

- 1 teaspoon coconut oil
- ¼ cup of soy milk
- 1 tablespoon tomato paste
- ½ cup of water

Directions:
1. Heat coconut oil in the saucepan. Add curry powder, garam masala, tomato paste, and soy milk. Whisk the mixture until smooth and bring it to boil.
2. Add water, spinach, and chickpeas. Stir the meal and close the lid. Cook it within 5 minutes over medium heat.

Nutrition: Calories 298, Protein 15.4g, Carbohydrates 47.8g, Fat 6.1g, Sodium 37mg

345. Pan-Fried Salmon with Salad

Preparation time: 15 minutes
Cooking time: 20 minutes
Servings: 4
Ingredients:
- Pinch of salt and pepper
- 1 tablespoon extra-virgin olive oil
- 2 tablespoon unsalted butter
- ½ teaspoon fresh dill
- 1 tablespoon fresh lemon juice
- 100g salad leaves, or bag of mixed leaves
- Salad Dressing:
- 3 tablespoons olive oil
- 2 tablespoons balsamic vinaigrette
- 1/2 teaspoon maple syrup (honey)

Directions:
1. Pat-dry the salmon fillets with a paper towel and season with a pinch of salt and pepper. In a skillet, warm-up oil over medium-high heat and add fillets. Cook each side within 5 to 7 minutes until golden brown.
2. Dissolve butter, dill, and lemon juice in a small saucepan. Put the butter mixture onto the cooked salmon. Lastly, combine all the salad dressing ingredients and drizzle to mixed salad leaves in a large bowl. Toss to coat. Serve with fresh salads on the side. Enjoy!

Nutrition: Calories 307, Fat 22g, Protein 34.6g, Sodium 80mg, Carbohydrate 1.7g

346. Vegan Chili

Preparation time: 15 minutes
Cooking time: 25 minutes
Servings: 4
Ingredients:
- ½ cup bulgur
- 1 cup tomatoes, chopped
- 1 chili pepper, chopped
- 1 cup red kidney beans, cooked
- 2 cups low-sodium vegetable broth
- 1 teaspoon tomato paste
- ½ cup celery stalk, chopped

Directions:
1. Put all ingredients in the big saucepan and stir well. Close the lid and simmer the chili for 25 minutes over medium-low heat.

Nutrition: Calories 234, Protein 13.1g, Carbohydrates 44.9g, Fat 0.9g, Sodium 92mg

347. Aromatic Whole Grain Spaghetti

Preparation time: 15 minutes
Cooking time: 10 minutes
Servings: 2
Ingredients:
- 1 teaspoon dried basil
- ¼ cup of soy milk
- 6 oz. whole-grain spaghetti
- 2 cups of water
- 1 teaspoon ground nutmeg

Directions:
1. Bring the water to boil, add spaghetti, and cook them for 8-10 minutes. Meanwhile, bring the soy milk to boil. Drain the cooked spaghetti and mix them up with soy milk, ground nutmeg, and dried basil. Stir the meal well.

Nutrition: Calories 128, Protein 5.6g, Carbohydrates 25g, Fat 1.4g, Sodium 25mg

348. Chunky Tomatoes

Preparation time: 15 minutes
Cooking time: 15 minutes
Servings: 3
Ingredients:
- 2 cups plum tomatoes, roughly chopped
- ½ cup onion, diced
- ½ teaspoon garlic, diced
- 1 teaspoon Italian seasonings
- 1 teaspoon canola oil
- 1 chili pepper, chopped

Directions:
1. Heat canola oil in the saucepan. Add chili pepper and onion. Cook the vegetables for 5 minutes. Stir them from time to time. After this, add tomatoes, garlic, and Italian seasonings. Close the lid and sauté the dish for 10 minutes.

Nutrition: Calories 550, Protein 1.7g, Carbohydrates 8.4g, Fat 2.3g, Sodium 17mg

349. Baked Falafel

Preparation time: 15 minutes
Cooking time: 25 minutes
Servings: 6
Ingredients:
- 2 cups chickpeas, cooked
- 1 yellow onion, diced
- 3 tablespoons olive oil
- 1 cup fresh parsley, chopped
- 1 teaspoon ground cumin
- ½ teaspoon coriander
- 2 garlic cloves, diced

Directions:

1. Blend all fixing in the food processor. Preheat the oven to 375F. Then line the baking tray with the baking paper. Make the balls from the chickpeas mixture and press them gently in the shape of the falafel. Put the falafel in the tray and bake in the oven for 25 minutes.

Nutrition: Calories 316, Protein 13.5g, Carbohydrates 43.3g, Fat 11.2g, Fiber 12.4g, Sodium 23mg

350. Paella

Preparation time: 15 minutes
Cooking time: 25 minutes
Servings: 6
Ingredients:
- 1 teaspoon dried saffron
- 1 cup short-grain rice
- 1 tablespoon olive oil
- 2 cups of water
- 1 teaspoon chili flakes
- 6 oz. artichoke hearts, chopped
- ½ cup green peas
- 1 onion, sliced
- 1 cup bell pepper, sliced

Directions:
1. Pour water into the saucepan. Add rice and cook it for 15 minutes. Meanwhile, heat olive oil in the skillet. Add dried saffron, chili flakes, onion, and bell pepper. Roast the vegetables for 5 minutes.
2. Add them to the cooked rice. Then add artichoke hearts and green peas. Stir the paella well and cook it for 10 minutes over low heat.

Nutrition: Calories 170, Protein 4.2g, Carbohydrates 32.7g, Fat 2.7g, Sodium 33mg

351. Hassel back Eggplant

Preparation time: 15 minutes
Cooking time: 25 minutes
Servings: 2
Ingredients:
- 2 eggplants, trimmed
- 2 tomatoes, sliced
- 1 tablespoon low-fat yogurt
- 1 teaspoon curry powder
- 1 teaspoon olive oil

Directions:
1. Make the cuts in the eggplants in the shape of the Hassel back. Then rub the vegetables with curry powder and fill with sliced tomatoes. Sprinkle the eggplants with olive oil and yogurt and wrap in the foil (each Hassel back eggplant wrap separately). Bake the vegetables at 375F for 25 minutes.

Nutrition: Calories 188, Protein 7g, Carbohydrates 38.1g, Fat 3g, Sodium 23mg

352. Vegetarian Kebabs

Preparation time: 15 minutes
Cooking time: 6 minutes
Servings: 4

Ingredients:
- 2 tablespoons balsamic vinegar
- 1 tablespoon olive oil
- 1 teaspoon dried parsley
- 2 tablespoons water
- 2 sweet peppers
- 2 red onions, peeled
- 2 zucchinis, trimmed

Directions:
1. Cut the sweet peppers and onions into medium size squares. Then slice the zucchini. String all vegetables into the skewers. After this, in the shallow bowl, mix up olive oil, dried parsley, water, and balsamic vinegar.
2. Sprinkle the vegetable skewers with olive oil mixture and transfer in the preheated to 390F grill. Cook the kebabs within 3 minutes per side or until the vegetables are light brown.

Nutrition: Calories 88, Protein 2.4g, Carbohydrates 13g, Fat 3.9g, Sodium 14mg

353. White Beans Stew

Preparation time: 15 minutes
Cooking time: 55 minutes
Servings: 4
Ingredients:
- 1 cup white beans, soaked
- 1 cup low-sodium vegetable broth
- 1 cup zucchini, chopped
- 1 teaspoon tomato paste
- 1 tablespoon avocado oil
- 4 cups of water
- ½ teaspoon peppercorns
- ½ teaspoon ground black pepper
- ¼ teaspoon ground nutmeg

Directions:
1. Heat avocado oil in the saucepan, add zucchinis, and roast them for 5 minutes. After this, add white beans, vegetable broth, tomato paste, water, peppercorns, ground black pepper, and ground nutmeg. Simmer the stew within 50 minutes on low heat.

Nutrition: Calories 184, Protein 12.3g, Carbohydrates 32.6g, Fat 1g, Sodium 55mg

354. Vegetarian Lasagna

Preparation time: 15 minutes
Cooking time: 30 minutes
Servings: 6
Ingredients:
- 1 cup carrot, diced
- ½ cup bell pepper, diced
- 1 cup spinach, chopped
- 1 tablespoon olive oil
- 1 teaspoon chili powder
- 1 cup tomatoes, chopped
- 4 oz. low-fat cottage cheese
- 1 eggplant, sliced
- 1 cup low-sodium vegetable broth

Directions:

1. Put carrot, bell pepper, and spinach in the saucepan. Add olive oil and chili powder and stir the vegetables well. Cook them for 5 minutes.
2. Make the sliced eggplant layer in the casserole mold and top it with vegetable mixture. Add tomatoes, vegetable stock, and cottage cheese. Bake the lasagna for 30 minutes at 375F.

Nutrition: Calories 77, Protein 4.1g, Carbohydrates 9.7g, Fat 3g, Sodium 124mg

355. Carrot Cakes

Preparation time: 15 minutes
Cooking time: 10 minutes
Servings: 4
Ingredients:
- 1 cup carrot, grated
- 1 tablespoon semolina
- 1 egg, beaten
- 1 teaspoon Italian seasonings
- 1 tablespoon sesame oil

Directions:
1. In the mixing bowl, mix up grated carrot, semolina, egg, and Italian seasonings. Heat sesame oil in the skillet. Make the carrot cakes with the help of 2 spoons and put in the skillet. Roast the cakes for 4 minutes per side.

Nutrition: Calories 70, Protein 1.9g, Carbohydrates 4.8g, Fat 4.9g, Sodium 35mg

356. Gnocchi with Tomato Basil Sauce

Preparation time: 15 minutes
Cooking time: 25 minutes
Servings: 6
Ingredients:
- 2 tablespoons olive oil
- ½ yellow onion, peeled and diced
- 3 cloves garlic, peeled and minced
- 1 (32-ounce) can no-salt-added crushed San Marzano tomatoes
- ¼ cup fresh basil leaves
- 2 teaspoons Italian seasoning
- ½ teaspoon kosher or sea salt
- 1 teaspoon granulated sugar
- ½ teaspoon ground black pepper
- 1/8 teaspoon crushed red pepper flakes
- 1 tablespoon heavy cream (optional)
- 12 ounces gnocchi
- ¼ cup freshly grated Parmesan cheese

Directions:
1. Heat-up the olive oil in a Dutch oven or stockpot over medium heat. Add the onion and sauté for 5 to 6 minutes, until soft. Stir in the garlic and stir until fragrant, 30 to 60 seconds. Then stir in the tomatoes, basil, Italian seasoning, salt, sugar, black pepper, and crushed red pepper flakes.
2. Bring to a simmer for 15 minutes. Stir in the heavy cream, if desired. For a smooth, puréed sauce, use an immersion blender or transfer sauce to a blender and

purée until smooth. Taste and adjust the seasoning, if necessary.
3. While the sauce simmers, cook the gnocchi according to the package instructions, remove with a slotted spoon, and transfer to 6 bowls. Pour the sauce over the gnocchi and top with the Parmesan cheese.

Nutrition: Calories: 287, Fat: 7g, Sodium: 527mg, Carbohydrate: 41g, Protein: 10g

357. Creamy Pumpkin Pasta

Preparation time: 15 minutes
Cooking time: 30 minutes
Servings: 6
Ingredients:
- 1-pound whole-grain linguine
- 1 tablespoon olive oil
- 3 garlic cloves, peeled and minced
- 2 tablespoons chopped fresh sage
- 1½ cups pumpkin purée
- 1 cup unsalted vegetable stock
- ½ cup low-fat evaporated milk
- ¾ teaspoon kosher or sea salt
- ½ teaspoon ground black pepper
- ½ teaspoon ground nutmeg
- ¼ teaspoon ground cayenne pepper
- ½ cup freshly grated Parmesan cheese, divided

Directions:
1. Cook the whole-grain linguine in a large pot of boiled water. Reserve ½ cup of pasta water and drain the rest. Set the pasta aside.
2. Warm-up olive oil over medium heat in a large skillet. Add the garlic and sage and sauté for 1 to 2 minutes, until soft and fragrant. Whisk in the pumpkin purée, stock, milk, and reserved pasta water and simmer for 4 to 5 minutes, until thickened.
3. Whisk in the salt, black pepper, nutmeg, and cayenne pepper and half of the Parmesan cheese. Stir in the cooked whole-grain linguine. Evenly divide the pasta among 6 bowls and top with the remaining Parmesan cheese.

Nutrition: Calories: 381, Fat: 8g, Sodium: 175mg, Carbohydrate: 63g, Protein: 15g

358. Mexican-Style Potato Casserole

Preparation time: 15 minutes
Cooking time: 60 minutes
Servings: 8
Ingredients:
- Cooking spray
- 2 tablespoons canola oil
- ½ yellow onion, peeled and diced
- 4 garlic cloves, peeled and minced
- 2 tablespoons all-purpose flour
- 1¼ cups milk
- 1 tablespoon chili powder
- ½ tablespoon ground cumin
- 1 teaspoon kosher salt or sea salt

- ½ teaspoon ground black pepper
- ¼ teaspoon ground cayenne pepper
- 1½ cups shredded Mexican-style cheese, divided
- 1 (4-ounce) can green chilies, drained
- 1½ pounds baby Yukon Gold or red potatoes, thinly sliced
- 1 red bell pepper, thinly sliced

Directions:

1. Preheat the oven to 400°F. Oiled a 9-by-13-inch baking dish with cooking spray. In a large saucepan, warm canola oil on medium heat. Add the onion and sauté for 4 to 5 minutes, until soft. Mix in the garlic, then cook until fragrant, 30 to 60 seconds.
2. Mix in the flour, then put in the milk while whisking. Slow simmer for about 5 minutes, until thickened. Whisk in the chili powder, cumin, salt, black pepper, and cayenne pepper.
3. Remove from the heat and whisk in half of the shredded cheese and the green chilies. Taste and adjust the seasoning, if necessary. Line up one-third of the sliced potatoes and sliced bell pepper in the baking dish and top with a quarter of the remaining shredded cheese.
4. Repeat with 2 more layers. Pour the cheese sauce over the top and sprinkle with the remaining shredded cheese. Cover it with aluminum foil and bake within 45 to 50 minutes, until the potatoes are tender.
5. Remove the foil and bake again within 5 to 10 minutes, until the topping is slightly browned. Let cool within 20 minutes before slicing into 8 pieces. Serve.

Nutrition: Calories: 195, Fat: 10g, Sodium: 487mg, Carbohydrate: 19g, Protein: 8g

359. Black Bean Stew with Cornbread

Preparation time: 15 minutes
Cooking time: 55 minutes
Servings: 6

Ingredients:

- For the black bean stew:
- 2 tablespoons canola oil
- 1 yellow onion, peeled and diced
- 4 garlic cloves, peeled and minced
- 1 tablespoon chili powder
- 1 tablespoon ground cumin
- ¼ teaspoon kosher or sea salt
- ½ teaspoon ground black pepper
- 2 cans no-salt-added black beans, drained
- 1 (10-ounce) can fire-roasted diced tomatoes
- ½ cup fresh cilantro leaves, chopped
- For the cornbread topping:
- 1¼ cups cornmeal
- ½ cup all-purpose flour
- ½ teaspoon baking powder
- ¼ teaspoon baking soda
- 1/8 teaspoon kosher or sea salt
- 1 cup low-fat buttermilk
- 2 tablespoons honey
- 1 large egg

Directions:

1. Warm-up canola oil over medium heat in a large Dutch oven or stockpot. Add the onion and sauté for 4 to 6 minutes, until the onion is soft. Stir in the garlic, chili powder, cumin, salt, and black pepper.
2. Cook within 1 to 2 minutes, until fragrant. Add the black beans and diced tomatoes. Bring to a simmer and cook for 15 minutes. Remove, then stir in the fresh cilantro. Taste and adjust the seasoning, if necessary.
3. Preheat the oven to 375°F. While the stew simmers, prepare the cornbread topping. Mix the cornmeal, baking soda, flour, baking powder, plus salt in a bowl. In a measuring cup, whisk the buttermilk, honey, and egg until combined. Put the batter into the dry fixing until just combined.
4. In oven-safe bowls or dishes, spoon out the black bean soup. Distribute dollops of the cornbread batter on top and then spread it out evenly with a spatula. Bake within 30 minutes, until the cornbread is just set.

Nutrition: Calories: 359, Fat: 7g, Sodium: 409mg, Carbohydrate: 61g, Protein: 14g

360. Mushroom Florentine

Preparation time: 15 minutes
Cooking time: 20 minutes
Servings: 4

Ingredients:

- 5 oz. whole-grain pasta
- ¼ cup low-sodium vegetable broth
- 1 cup mushrooms, sliced
- ¼ cup of soy milk
- 1 teaspoon olive oil
- ½ teaspoon Italian seasonings

Directions:

1. Cook the pasta according to the direction of the manufacturer. Then pour olive oil into the saucepan and heat it. Add mushrooms and Italian seasonings. Stir the mushrooms well and cook for 10 minutes.
2. Then add soy milk and vegetable broth. Add cooked pasta and mix up the mixture well. Cook it for 5 minutes on low heat.

Nutrition: Calories 287, Protein 12.4g, Carbohydrates 50.4g, Fat 4.2g, Sodium 26mg

361. Eggplant Parmesan Stacks

Preparation time: 15 minutes
Cooking time: 20 minutes
Servings: 4

Ingredients:

- 1 large eggplant, cut into thick slices
- 2 tablespoons olive oil, divided
- ¼ teaspoon kosher or sea salt
- ¼ teaspoon ground black pepper
- 1 cup panko bread crumbs
- ¼ cup freshly grated Parmesan cheese
- 5 to 6 garlic cloves, minced
- ½ pound fresh mozzarella, sliced
- 1½ cups lower-sodium marinara

- ½ cup fresh basil leaves, torn

Directions:
1. Preheat the oven to 425°F. Coat the eggplant slices in 1 tablespoon olive oil and sprinkle with the salt and black pepper. Put on a large baking sheet, then roast for 10 to 12 minutes, until soft with crispy edges. Remove the eggplant and set the oven to a low broil.
2. In a bowl, stir the remaining tablespoon of olive oil, bread crumbs, Parmesan cheese, and garlic. Remove the cooled eggplant from the baking sheet and clean it.
3. Create layers on the same baking sheet by stacking a roasted eggplant slice with a slice of mozzarella, a tablespoon of marinara, and a tablespoon of the bread crumb mixture, repeating with 2 layers of each ingredient. Cook under the broiler within 3 to 4 minutes until the cheese is melted and bubbly.

Nutrition: Calories: 377, Fat: 22g, Sodium: 509mg, Carbohydrate: 29g, Protein: 16g

362. Roasted Vegetable Enchiladas

Preparation time: 15 minutes
Cooking time: 45 minutes
Servings: 8
Ingredients:
- 2 zucchinis, diced
- 1 red bell pepper, seeded and sliced
- 1 red onion, peeled and sliced
- 2 ears corn
- 2 tablespoons canola oil
- 1 can no-salt-added black beans, drained
- 1½ tablespoons chili powder
- 2 teaspoon ground cumin
- 1/8 teaspoon kosher or sea salt
- ½ teaspoon ground black pepper
- 8 (8-inch) whole-wheat tortillas
- 1 cup Enchilada Sauce or store-bought enchilada sauce
- ½ cup shredded Mexican-style cheese
- ½ cup plain nonfat Greek yogurt
- ½ cup cilantro leaves, chopped

Directions:
1. Preheat oven to 400°F. Place the zucchini, red bell pepper, and red onion on a baking sheet. Place the ears of corn separately on the same baking sheet. Drizzle all with the canola oil and toss to coat. Roast for 10 to 12 minutes, until the vegetables are tender. Remove and reduce the temperature to 375°F.
2. Cut the corn from the cob. Transfer the corn kernels, zucchini, red bell pepper, and onion to a bowl and stir in the black beans, chili powder, cumin, salt, and black pepper until combined.
3. Oiled a 9-by-13-inch baking dish with cooking spray. Line up the tortillas in the greased baking dish. Evenly distribute the vegetable bean filling into each tortilla. Pour half of the enchilada sauce and sprinkle half of the shredded cheese on top of the filling.
4. Roll each tortilla into enchilada shape and place them seam-side down. Pour the remaining enchilada sauce and sprinkle the remaining cheese over the enchiladas. Bake for 25 minutes until the cheese is melted and bubbly.

Serve the enchiladas with Greek yogurt and chopped cilantro.
Nutrition: Calories: 335, Fat: 15g, Sodium: 557mg, Carbohydrate: 42g, Protein: 13g

363. Lentil Avocado Tacos

Preparation time: 15 minutes
Cooking time: 35 minutes
Servings: 6
Ingredients:
- 1 tablespoon canola oil
- ½ yellow onion, peeled and diced
- 2-3 garlic cloves, minced
- 1½ cups dried lentils
- ½ teaspoon kosher or sea salt
- 3 to 3½ cups unsalted vegetable or chicken stock
- 2½ tablespoons Taco Seasoning or store-bought low-sodium taco seasoning
- 16 (6-inch) corn tortillas, toasted
- 2 ripe avocados, peeled and sliced

Directions:
1. Heat-up the canola oil in a large skillet or Dutch oven over medium heat. Cook the onion within 4 to 5 minutes, until soft. Mix in the garlic and cook within 30 seconds until fragrant. Then add the lentils, salt, and stock. Bring to a simmer for 25 to 35 minutes, adding additional stock if needed.
2. When there's only a small amount of liquid left in the pan, and the lentils are al dente, stir in the taco seasoning and let simmer for 1 to 2 minutes. Taste and adjust the seasoning, if necessary. Spoon the lentil mixture into tortillas and serve with the avocado slices.

Nutrition: Calories: 400, Fat: 14g, Sodium: 336mg, Carbohydrate: 64g, Fiber: 15g, Protein: 16g

364. Tomato & Olive Orecchiette with Basil Pesto

Preparation time: 15 minutes
Cooking time: 25 minutes
Servings: 6
Ingredients:
- 12 ounces orecchiette pasta
- 2 tablespoons olive oil
- 1-pint cherry tomatoes, quartered
- ½ cup Basil Pesto or store-bought pesto
- ¼ cup Kalamata olives, sliced
- 1 tablespoon dried oregano leaves
- ¼ teaspoon kosher or sea salt
- ½ teaspoon freshly cracked black pepper
- ¼ teaspoon crushed red pepper flakes
- 2 tablespoons freshly grated Parmesan cheese

Directions:
1. Boil a large pot of water. Cook the orecchiette, drain and transfer the pasta to a large nonstick skillet.
2. Put the skillet over medium-low heat, then heat the olive oil. Stir in the cherry tomatoes, pesto, olives, oregano,

salt, black pepper, and crushed red pepper flakes. Cook within 8 to 10 minutes, until heated throughout. Serve the pasta with the freshly grated Parmesan cheese.

Nutrition: Calories: 332, Fat: 13g, Sodium: 389mg, Carbohydrate: 44g, Protein: 9g

365. Italian Stuffed Portobello Mushroom Burgers

Preparation time: 15 minutes
Cooking time: 25 minutes
Servings: 4
Ingredients:

- 1 tablespoon olive oil
- 4 large portobello mushrooms, washed and dried
- ½ yellow onion, peeled and diced
- 4 garlic cloves, peeled and minced
- 1 can cannellini beans, drained
- ½ cup fresh basil leaves, torn
- ½ cup panko bread crumbs
- 1/8 teaspoon kosher or sea salt
- ¼ teaspoon ground black pepper
- 1 cup lower-sodium marinara, divided
- ½ cup shredded mozzarella cheese
- 4 whole-wheat buns, toasted
- 1 cup fresh arugula

Directions:
1. Heat-up the olive oil in a large skillet to medium-high heat. Sear the mushrooms for 4 to 5 minutes per side, until slightly soft. Place on a baking sheet. Preheat the oven to a low broil.
2. Put the onion in the skillet and cook for 4 to 5 minutes, until slightly soft. Mix in the garlic then cooks within 30 to 60 seconds. Move the onions plus garlic to a bowl. Add the cannellini beans and smash with the back of a fork to form a chunky paste. Stir in the basil, bread crumbs, salt, and black pepper and half of the marinara. Cook for 5 minutes.
3. Remove the bean mixture from the stove and divide among the mushroom caps. Spoon the remaining marinara over the stuffed mushrooms and top each with the mozzarella cheese. Broil within 3 to 4 minutes, until the cheese is melted and bubbly. Transfer the burgers to the toasted whole-wheat buns and top with the arugula.

Nutrition: Calories: 407, Fat: 9g, Sodium: 575mg, Carbohydrate: 63g, Protein: 25g

366. Tofu & Green Bean Stir-Fry

Preparation time: 15 minutes
Cooking time: 20 minutes
Servings: 4
Ingredients:

- 1 (14-ounce) package extra-firm tofu
- 2 tablespoons canola oil
- 1-pound green beans, chopped
- 2 carrots, peeled and thinly sliced

- ½ cup Stir-Fry Sauce or store-bought lower-sodium stir-fry sauce
- 2 cups Fluffy Brown Rice
- 2 scallions, thinly sliced
- 2 tablespoons sesame seeds

Directions:
1. Put the tofu on your plate lined with a kitchen towel, put separate kitchen towel over the tofu, and place a heavy pot on top, changing towels every time they become soaked. Let sit within 15 minutes to remove the moisture. Cut the tofu into 1-inch cubes.
2. Heat the canola oil in a large wok or skillet to medium-high heat. Add the tofu cubes and cook, flipping every 1 to 2 minutes, so all sides become browned. Remove from the skillet and place the green beans and carrots in the hot oil. Stir-fry for 4 to 5 minutes, occasionally tossing, until crisp and slightly tender.
3. While the vegetables are cooking, prepare the Stir-Fry Sauce (if using homemade). Place the tofu back in the skillet. Put the sauce over the tofu and vegetables and let simmer for 2 to 3 minutes. Serve over rice, then top with scallions and sesame seeds.

Nutrition: Calories: 380, Fat: 15g, Sodium: 440mg, Potassium: 454mg, Carbohydrate: 45g, Protein: 16g

367. Peanut Vegetable Pad Thai

Preparation time: 15 minutes
Cooking time: 20 minutes
Servings: 6
Ingredients:

- 8 ounces brown rice noodles
- 1/3 cup natural peanut butter
- 3 tablespoons unsalted vegetable broth
- 1 tablespoon low-sodium soy sauce
- 2 tablespoons of rice wine vinegar
- 1 tablespoon honey
- 2 teaspoons sesame oil
- 1 teaspoon sriracha (optional)
- 1 tablespoon canola oil
- 1 red bell pepper, thinly sliced
- 1 zucchini, cut into matchsticks
- 2 large carrots, cut into matchsticks
- 3 large eggs, beaten
- ¾ teaspoon kosher or sea salt
- ½ cup unsalted peanuts, chopped
- ½ cup cilantro leaves, chopped

Directions:
1. Boil a large pot of water. Cook the rice noodles as stated in package directions. Mix the peanut butter, vegetable broth, soy sauce, rice wine vinegar, honey, sesame oil, and sriracha in a bowl. Set aside.
2. Warm-up canola oil over medium heat in a large nonstick skillet. Add the red bell pepper, zucchini, and carrots, and sauté for 2 to 3 minutes, until slightly soft. Stir in the eggs and fold with a spatula until scrambled. Add the cooked rice noodles, sauce, and salt. Toss to combine. Spoon into bowls and evenly top with the peanuts and cilantro.

Nutrition: Calories: 393, Fat: 19g, Sodium: 561mg, Carbohydrate: 45g, Protein: 13g

368. Spicy Tofu Burrito Bowls with Cilantro Avocado Sauce

Preparation time: 15 minutes
Cooking time: 15 minutes
Servings: 4
Ingredients:

- For the sauce:
- ¼ cup plain nonfat Greek yogurt
- ½ cup fresh cilantro leaves
- ½ ripe avocado, peeled
- Zest and juice of 1 lime
- 2 garlic cloves, peeled
- ¼ teaspoon kosher or sea salt
- 2 tablespoons water
- For the burrito bowls:
- 1 (14-ounce) package extra-firm tofu
- 1 tablespoon canola oil
- 1 yellow or orange bell pepper, diced
- 2 tablespoons Taco Seasoning
- ¼ teaspoon kosher or sea salt
- 2 cups Fluffy Brown Rice
- 1 (15-ounce) can black beans, drained

Directions:

1. Place all the sauce ingredients in the bowl of a food processor or blender and purée until smooth. Taste and adjust the seasoning, if necessary. Refrigerate until ready for use.
2. Put the tofu on your plate lined with a kitchen towel. Put another kitchen towel over the tofu and place a heavy pot on top, changing towels if they become soaked. Let it stand within 15 minutes to remove the moisture. Cut the tofu into 1-inch cubes.
3. Warm-up canola oil in a large skillet over medium heat. Add the tofu and bell pepper and sauté, breaking up the tofu into smaller pieces for 4 to 5 minutes. Stir in the taco seasoning, salt, and ¼ cup of water. Evenly divide the rice and black beans among 4 bowls. Top with the tofu/bell pepper mixture and top with the cilantro avocado sauce.

Nutrition: Calories: 383, Fat: 13g, Sodium: 438mg, Carbohydrate: 48g, Protein: 21g

369. Sweet Potato Cakes with Classic Guacamole

Preparation time: 15 minutes
Cooking time: 20 minutes
Servings: 4
Ingredients:

- For the guacamole:
- 2 ripe avocados, peeled and pitted
- ½ jalapeño, seeded and finely minced
- ¼ red onion, peeled and finely diced
- ¼ cup fresh cilantro leaves, chopped
- Zest and juice of 1 lime
- ¼ teaspoon kosher or sea salt
- For the cakes:
- 3 sweet potatoes, cooked and peeled
- ½ cup cooked black beans
- 1 large egg
- ½ cup panko bread crumbs
- 1 teaspoon ground cumin
- 1 teaspoon chili powder
- ½ teaspoon kosher or sea salt
- ¼ teaspoon ground black pepper
- 2 tablespoons canola oil

Directions:

1. Mash the avocado, then stir in the jalapeño, red onion, cilantro, lime zest and juice, and salt in a bowl. Taste and adjust the seasoning, if necessary.
2. Put the cooked sweet potatoes plus black beans in a bowl and mash until a paste form. Stir in the egg, bread crumbs, cumin, chili powder, salt, and black pepper until combined.
3. Warm-up canola oil in a large skillet at medium heat. Form the sweet potato mixture into 4 patties, place them in the hot skillet, and cook within 3 to 4 minutes per side, until browned and crispy. Serve the sweet potato cakes with guacamole on top.

Nutrition: Calories: 369, Fat: 22g, Sodium: 521mg, Carbohydrate: 38g, Protein: 8g

370. Chickpea Cauliflower Tikka Masala

Preparation time: 15 minutes
Cooking time: 40 minutes
Servings: 6
Ingredients:

- 2 tablespoons olive oil
- 1 yellow onion, peeled and diced
- 4 garlic cloves, peeled and minced
- 1-inch piece fresh ginger, peeled and minced
- 2 tablespoons Garam Masala
- 1 teaspoon kosher or sea salt
- ½ teaspoon ground black pepper
- ¼ teaspoon ground cayenne pepper
- ½ small head cauliflower, small florets
- 2 (15-ounce) cans no-salt-added chickpeas, rinsed and drained
- 1 (15-ounce) can no-salt-added petite diced tomatoes, drained
- 1½ cups unsalted vegetable broth
- ½ (15-ounce) can coconut milk
- Zest and juice of 1 lime
- ½ cup fresh cilantro leaves, chopped, divided
- 1½ cups cooked Fluffy Brown Rice, divided

Directions:

1. Warm-up olive oil over medium heat, then put the onion and sauté within 4 to 5 minutes in a large Dutch oven or stockpot. Stir in the garlic, ginger, garam masala, salt, black pepper, and cayenne pepper and toast for 30 to 60 seconds, until fragrant.
2. Stir in the cauliflower florets, chickpeas, diced tomatoes, and vegetable broth and increase to medium-high. Simmer within 15 minutes, until the cauliflower is fork-tender.
3. Remove, then stir in the coconut milk, lime juice, lime zest, and half of the cilantro. Taste and adjust the

seasoning, if necessary. Serve over the rice and the remaining chopped cilantro.

Nutrition: Calories: 323, Fat: 12g, Sodium: 444mg, Carbohydrate: 44g, Protein: 11g

371. Roasted Sweet Potato and Red Beets

Preparation time: 5 minutes
Cooking time: 20 minutes
Servings: 6
Ingredients
- 1 ½ cups Brussels sprouts, trimmed
- 1 cup large sweet potato chunks
- 1 cup large carrot chunks
- 1 ½ cup broccoli florets
- 1 cup cubed red beets
- 1/2 cup yellow onion chunks
- 2 tablespoons sesame seed oil
- salt and ground black pepper to taste

Directions:
1. Preheat your oven to 425 degrees F (220 degrees C). Set the rack to the second-lowest level in the oven.
2. Pour some lightly salted water in a bowl. Submerge the Brussels sprouts in salted water for 15 minutes and drain.
3. Place the rest of the ingredients together in a bowl. Spread the vegetables in a single layer onto a baking pan.
4. Roast in the oven until the vegetables start to brown and cook through, for about 45 minutes.

Nutrition: 156 Calories, 9.4g Protein, 12.2g Carbohydrates, 7.1g Fat, 0.8g Fiber, 7mg Cholesterol, 86mg Sodium, 365mg Potassium

372. Sichuan Style Baked Chioggia Beets and Broccoli Florets

Preparation time: 5 minutes
Cooking time: 20 minutes
Servings: 6
Ingredients
- 1 ½ cups Brussels sprouts, trimmed
- 1 cup broccoli florets
- 1 cup Chioggia beets, cut into chunks
- 1 ½ cup cauliflower florets
- 1 cup button mushrooms, sliced
- 1/2 cup red onion chunks
- 2 tablespoons sesame oil
- ½ tsp. Sichuan peppercorns
- salt ground black pepper to taste

Directions:
1. Preheat your oven to 425 degrees F (220 degrees C). Set the rack to the second-lowest level in the oven.
2. Pour some lightly salted water in a bowl. Submerge the Brussels sprouts in salted water for 15 minutes and drain.
3. Place the rest of the ingredients together in a bowl. Spread the vegetables in a single layer onto a baking pan.
4. Roast in the oven until the vegetables start to brown and cook through, for about 45 minutes.

Nutrition: 156 Calories, 9.4g Protein, 12.2g Carbohydrates, 7.1g Fat, 0.8g Fiber, 7mg Cholesterol, 86mg Sodium, 365mg Potassium

373. Baked Enoki and Mini Cabbage

Preparation time: 5 minutes
Cooking time: 20 minutes
Servings: 6
Ingredients
- 1 ½ cups mini cabbage, trimmed
- 1 cup broccoli florets
- 1 cup enoki mushrooms, sliced
- 1 ½ cup cauliflower florets
- 1 cup oyster mushrooms
- 1/2 cup red onion chunks
- 2 tablespoons olive oil
- salt and ground black pepper to taste

Directions:
1. Preheat your oven to 425 degrees F (220 degrees C). Set the rack to the second-lowest level in the oven.
2. Pour some lightly salted water in a bowl. Submerge the Brussels sprouts in salted water for 15 minutes and drain.
3. Place the rest of the ingredients together in a bowl. Spread the vegetables in a single layer onto a baking pan.
4. Roast in the oven until the vegetables start to brown and cook through, for about 45 minutes.

Nutrition: 156 Calories, 9.4g Protein, 12.2g Carbohydrates, 7.1g Fat, 0.8g Fiber, 7mg Cholesterol, 86mg Sodium, 365mg Potassium

374. Roasted Triple Mushrooms

Preparation time: 5 minutes
Cooking time: 20 minutes
Servings: 6
Ingredients
- 2 cups Spinach, rinsed
- 1 cup oyster mushrooms
- 1 cup button mushrooms, sliced
- 1 ½ cup enoki mushrooms
- 1/2 cup red onion chunks
- 2 tablespoons extra-virgin olive oil
- salt and ground black pepper to taste
- 1/4 cup Ricotta cheese

Directions:
1. Preheat your oven to 425 degrees F (220 degrees C). Set the rack to the second-lowest level in the oven.
2. Pour some lightly salted water in a bowl. Submerge the spinach in salted water for 15 minutes and drain.
3. Place the rest of the ingredients together in a bowl. Spread the vegetables in a single layer onto a baking pan.
4. Roast in the oven until the vegetables start to brown and cook through, for about 45 minutes.

Nutrition: 156 Calories, 9.4g Protein, 12.2g Carbohydrates, 7.1g Fat, 0.8g Fiber, 7mg Cholesterol, 86mg Sodium, 365mg Potassium

375. Roasted Mini Cabbage and Sweet Potato

Preparation time: 5 minutes
Cooking time: 20 minutes
Servings: 6
Ingredients

- 1 ½ cups mini cabbage, trimmed
- 1 cup large potato chunks
- 1 cup large rainbow carrot chunks
- 1 ½ cup potato chunks
- 1 cup parsnips
- 1/2 cup red onion chunks
- 2 tablespoons extra-virgin olive oil
- Sea salt
- Rainbow peppercorns to taste
- 1/4 cup cottage cheese

Directions:

1. Preheat your oven to 425 degrees F (220 degrees C). Set the rack to the second-lowest level in the oven.
2. Pour some lightly salted water in a bowl. Submerge the mini cabbage in salted water for 15 minutes and drain.
3. Place the rest of the ingredients together in a bowl. Spread the vegetables in a single layer onto a baking pan.
4. Roast in the oven until the vegetables start to brown and cook through, for about 45 minutes.

Nutrition: 156 Calories, 9.4g Protein, 12.2g Carbohydrates, 7.1g Fat, 0.8g Fiber, 7mg Cholesterol, 86mg Sodium, 365mg Potassium

376. Roasted Soy Beans and Winter Squash

Preparation time: 5 minutes
Cooking time: 20 minutes
Servings: 6
Ingredients

- 2 (15 ounce) cans soy beans, rinsed and drained
- 1/2 winter squash - peeled, seeded, and cut into 1-inch pieces
- 1 red onion, diced 1 sweet potato, peeled and cut into 1-inch cubes
- 2 large carrots, cut into 1 inch pieces
- 3 medium potatoes, cut into 1-inch pieces
- 4 tablespoons extra virgin oil
- Seasoning ingredients
- 1 teaspoon salt
- 1/2 teaspoon ground black pepper
- 1 teaspoon onion powder
- 1 teaspoon dried basil
- 1 teaspoon Italian seasoning
- Garnishing Ingredients
- 2 green onions, chopped (optional)

Directions:

1. Preheat your oven to 350 degrees F. Grease your baking pan.
2. Combine the beans, squash, onion, sweet potato, carrots, and russet potatoes on the prepared sheet pan. Drizzle with the oil and toss to coat.
3. Combine the seasoning ingredients in a bowl Sprinkle them over the vegetables on the pan and toss to coat with seasonings. Bake in the oven for 25 minutes.
4. Stir frequently until vegetables are soft and lightly browned and beans are crisp, for about 20 to 25 minutes more. Season with more salt and black pepper to taste, top with the green onion before serving.

Nutrition: 156 Calories, 9.4g Protein, 12.2g Carbohydrates, 7.1g Fat, 0.8g Fiber, 7mg Cholesterol, 86mg Sodium, 365mg Potassium

377. Roasted Button Mushrooms and Squash

Preparation time: 5 minutes
Cooking time: 20 minutes
Servings: 6
Ingredients

- 2 (15 ounce) cans button mushrooms, rinsed and drained
- 1/2 summer squash - peeled, seeded, and cut into 1-inch pieces
- 1 red onion, diced
- 2 large turnips, cut into 1 inch pieces
- 2 large parsnips, cut into 1 inch pieces
- 1 medium potatoes, cut into 1-inch pieces
- 3 tablespoons butter Seasoning ingredients
- 1 teaspoon salt
- 1/2 teaspoon ground black pepper
- 1 teaspoon onion powder
- 2 teaspoon garlic powder
- 1 teaspoon Herbs de Provence
- Garnishing Ingredients
- 2 sprigs of thyme, chopped (optional)

Directions:

1. Preheat your oven to 350 degrees F. Grease your baking pan.
2. Combine the main ingredients on the prepared sheet pan. Drizzle with the melted butter or margarine and toss to coat.
3. Combine the seasoning ingredients in a bowl Sprinkle them over the vegetables on the pan and toss to coat with seasonings.
4. Bake in the oven for 25 minutes. Stir frequently until vegetables are soft and lightly browned and chickpeas are crisp, for about 20 to 25 minutes more.
5. Season with more salt and black pepper to taste, top with thyme before serving.

Nutrition: 156 Calories, 9.4g Protein, 12.2g Carbohydrates, 7.1g Fat, 0.8g Fiber, 7mg Cholesterol, 86mg Sodium, 365mg Potassium

378. Roasted Tomatoes Rutabaga and Kohlrabi Main

Preparation time: 5 minutes
Cooking time: 20 minutes
Servings: 6
Ingredients

- 3 large tomatoes, cut into 1-inch pieces
- 3 red onion, diced

- 1 rutabaga, peeled and cut into 1-inch cubes
- 2 large carrots, cut into 1 inch pieces
- 3 medium kohlrabi, cut into 1-inch pieces
- 3 tablespoons extra virgin olive oil
- Seasoning ingredients
- 1 teaspoon salt
- 1/2 teaspoon ground black pepper
- 1 teaspoon onion powder
- 2 teaspoon garlic powder
- 1 teaspoon Spanish paprika
- 1 teaspoon cumin
- Garnishing Ingredients
- 2 sprigs parsley, chopped (optional)

Directions:
1. Preheat your oven to 350 degrees F. Grease your baking pan.
2. Combine the main ingredients on the prepared sheet pan. Drizzle with the oil and toss to coat.
3. Combine the seasoning ingredients in a bowl Sprinkle them over the vegetables on the pan and toss to coat with seasonings.
4. Bake in the oven for 25 minutes. Stir frequently until vegetables are soft, for about 20 to 25 minutes more. Season with more salt and black pepper to taste, top with the parsley before serving.

Nutrition:156 Calories, 9.4g Protein, 12.2g Carbohydrates, 7.1g Fat, 0.8g Fiber, 7mg Cholesterol, 86mg Sodium, 365mg Potassium

379. Roasted Brussels sprouts and Broccoli

Preparation time: 5 minutes
Cooking time: 20 minutes
Servings: 6
Ingredients
- 1 large broccoli, sliced
- 1 cup bean sprouts
- 1 red onion, diced
- 3 large kohlrabi, cut into 1 inch pieces
- 2 large carrots, cut into 1 inch pieces
- 3 medium potatoes, cut into 1-inch pieces
- 3 tablespoons extra virgin olive oil
- Seasoning ingredients
- 1 teaspoon salt
- 1/2 teaspoon ground black pepper
- 1 teaspoon onion powder
- 2 teaspoon garlic powder
- 1 teaspoon ground fennel seeds
- 1 teaspoon dried rubbed sage
- Garnishing Ingredients
- 2 green onions, chopped (optional)

Directions:
1. Preheat your oven to 350 degrees F. Grease your baking pan.
2. Combine the main ingredients on the prepared sheet pan. Drizzle with the oil and toss to coat.
3. Combine the seasoning ingredients in a bowl Sprinkle them over the vegetables on the pan and toss to coat with seasonings.

4. Bake in the oven for 25 minutes. Stir frequently until vegetables are soft and lightly browned and chickpeas are crisp, for about 20 to 25 minutes more.
5. Season with more salt and black pepper to taste, top with the green onion before serving.

Nutrition: 156 Calories, 9.4g Protein, 12.2g Carbohydrates, 7.1g Fat, 0.8g Fiber, 7mg Cholesterol, 86mg Sodium, 365mg Potassium

380. Roasted Broccoli Sweet Potatoes & Bean Sprouts

Preparation time: 5 minutes
Cooking time: 20 minutes
Servings: 6
Ingredients
- 1 large broccoli, sliced
- 1 cup bean sprouts
- 1 yellow onion, diced
- 1 sweet potato, peeled and cut into 1-inch cubes
- 2 large carrots, cut into 1 inch pieces
- 3 medium potatoes, cut into 1-inch pieces
- 3 tablespoons canola oil
- Seasoning ingredients
- 1 teaspoon salt
- 1/2 teaspoon ground black pepper
- 1 teaspoon onion powder
- 2 teaspoon garlic powder
- ½ cup grated gouda cheese
- ¼ cup parmesan cheese
- Garnishing Ingredients
- 2 green onions, chopped (optional)

Directions:
1. Preheat your oven to 350 degrees F. Grease your baking pan.
2. Combine the main ingredients on the prepared sheet pan. Drizzle with the oil and toss to coat.
3. Combine the seasoning ingredients in a bowl Sprinkle them over the vegetables on the pan and toss to coat with seasonings.
4. Bake in the oven for 25 minutes. Stir frequently until vegetables are soft and lightly browned and chickpeas are crisp, for about 20 to 25 minutes more.
5. Season with more salt and black pepper to taste, top with the green onion before serving.

Nutrition: 156 Calories, 9.4g Protein, 12.2g Carbohydrates, 7.1g Fat, 0.8g Fiber, 7mg Cholesterol, 86mg Sodium, 365mg Potassium

381. Thai Roasted Spicy Black Beans and Choy Sum

Preparation time: 5 minutes
Cooking time: 20 minutes
Servings: 6
Ingredients
- Cooking spray
- 1 tablespoon sesame oil
- 3 cloves garlic, minced
- 1/2 teaspoon sea salt
- 1 tbsp. Thai chili paste

- 1/4 teaspoon ground black pepper
- 3 1/2 cups Choy Sum, coarsely chopped
- 2 1/2 cups cherry tomatoes
- 1 (15 ounce) can black beans, drained
- 1 lime, cut into wedges
- 1 tablespoon chopped fresh cilantro

Directions:
7. Preheat your oven to 450 degrees F.
8. Line a baking sheet with foil and grease with sesame oil. Mix the olive oil, garlic, salt, Thai chili paste, and pepper in a bowl.
9. Add in the Choy sum, tomatoes, and black beans Combine until well coated.
10. Spread them out in a single layer on the baking sheet.
11. Add the lime wedges.
12. Roast in the oven until vegetables become caramelized, for about 25 minutes.
13. Take out the lime wedges and top with the cilantro.

Nutrition: 156 Calories, 9.4g Protein, 12.2g Carbohydrates, 7.1g Fat, 0.8g Fiber, 7mg Cholesterol, 86mg Sodium, 365mg Potassium

382. Simple Roasted Broccoli and Cauliflower

Preparation time: 5 minutes
Cooking time: 20 minutes
Servings: 6
Ingredients
- Cooking spray
- 1 tablespoon extra-virgin olive oil
- 3 cloves garlic, minced
- 1/2 teaspoon sea salt
- 1/4 teaspoon ground black pepper
- 3 1/2 cups broccoli florets
- 2 1/2 cups cauliflower florets
- 1 tablespoon chopped fresh thyme

Directions:
10. Preheat your oven to 450 degrees F.
11. Line a baking sheet with foil and grease with olive oil.
12. Mix the olive oil, garlic, salt, and pepper in a bowl.
13. Add in the cauliflower and tomatoes Combine until well coated.
14. Spread them out in a single layer on the baking sheet.
15. Roast in the oven until vegetables become caramelized, for about 25 minutes.
16. Top with the thyme. Simple

Nutrition: 156 Calories, 9.4g Protein, 12.2g Carbohydrates, 7.1g Fat, 0.8g Fiber, 7mg Cholesterol, 86mg Sodium, 365mg Potassium

383. Roasted Napa Cabbage and Turnips Extra

Preparation time: 5 minutes
Cooking time: 20 minutes
Servings: 6
Ingredients
- Cooking spray
- 1 tablespoon extra-virgin olive oil
- 1/2 teaspoon sea salt
- 1/4 teaspoon ground black pepper
- 1/2 medium Napa cabbage, sliced thinly
- 1 medium turnip, sliced thinly

Directions:
7. Preheat your oven to 450 degrees F.
8. Line a baking sheet with foil and grease with olive oil.
9. Mix the extra ingredients thoroughly. Add in the main ingredients
10. Combine until well coated. Spread them out in a single layer on the baking sheet.
11. Roast in the oven until vegetables become caramelized, for about 25 minutes.

Nutrition: 156 Calories, 9.4g Protein, 12.2g Carbohydrates, 7.1g Fat, 0.8g Fiber, 7mg Cholesterol, 86mg Sodium, 365mg Potassium

384. Simple Roasted Kale Artichoke Heart and Choy Sum Extra

Preparation time: 5 minutes
Cooking time: 20 minutes
Servings: 6
Ingredients
- Cooking spray
- 1 tablespoon extra-virgin olive oil
- 1/2 teaspoon sea salt
- 1/4 teaspoon ground black pepper
- 1 bunch of kale, rinsed and drained
- 1 cup canned artichoke hearts
- 1/2 medium Chinese flowery cabbage (Choy sum), coarsely chopped

Directions:
1. Preheat your oven to 450 degrees F.
2. Line a baking sheet with foil and grease with olive oil. Mix the extra ingredients thoroughly. Add in the main ingredients
3. Combine until well coated. Spread them out in a single layer on the baking sheet.
4. Roast in the oven until vegetables become caramelized, for about 25 minutes.

Nutrition: 156 Calories, 9.4g Protein, 12.2g Carbohydrates, 7.1g Fat, 0.8g Fiber, 7mg Cholesterol, 86mg Sodium, 365mg Potassium

385. Roasted Kale and Bok Choy Extra

Preparation time: 5 minutes
Cooking time: 20 minutes
Servings: 6
Ingredients
- Cooking spray
- 1 tablespoon extra-virgin olive oil
- 1/2 teaspoon sea salt
- 1/4 teaspoon ground black pepper
- 1 bunch of kale, rinsed and drained
- 1 bunch of bok Choy, rinsed ,drained and coarsely chopped

Directions:
1. Preheat your oven to 450 degrees F. Line a baking sheet with foil and grease with olive oil.

2. Mix the extra ingredients thoroughly. Add in the main ingredients
3. Combine until well coated. Spread them out in a single layer on the baking sheet.
4. Roast in the oven until vegetables become caramelized, for about 25 minutes.

Nutrition: 156 Calories, 9.4g Protein, 12.2g Carbohydrates, 7.1g Fat, 0.8g Fiber, 7mg Cholesterol, 86mg Sodium, 365mg Potassium

386. Very Wild Mushroom Pilaf

Preparation time: 10 minutes
Cooking time: 3 hours
Servings: 4
Ingredients:
- 1 cup wild rice
- 2 garlic cloves, minced
- 6 green onions, chopped
- 2 tablespoons olive oil
- ½ pound baby Bella mushrooms
- 2 cups water

Directions:
1. Add rice, garlic, onion, oil, mushrooms and water to your Slow Cooker.
2. Stir well until mixed.
3. Place lid and cook on LOW for 3 hours.
4. Stir pilaf and divide between serving platters.
5. Enjoy!

Nutrition: 156 Calories, 9.4g Protein, 12.2g Carbohydrates, 7.1g Fat, 0.8g Fiber, 7mg Cholesterol, 86mg Sodium, 365mg Potassium

387. Sporty Baby Carrots

Preparation time: 5 minutes
Cooking time: 5 minutes
Servings: 4
Ingredients:
- 1 pound baby carrots
- 1 cup water
- 1 tablespoon clarified ghee
- 1 tablespoon chopped up fresh mint leaves
- Sea flavored vinegar as needed

Directions:
1. Place a steamer rack on top of your pot and add the carrots.
2. Add water.
3. Lock the lid and cook at HIGH pressure for 2 minutes.
4. Do a quick release.
5. Pass the carrots through a strainer and drain them.
6. Wipe the insert clean.
7. Return the insert to the pot and set the pot to Sauté mode.
8. Add clarified butter and allow it to melt.
9. Add mint and sauté for 30 seconds.
10. Add carrots to the insert and sauté well.
11. Remove them and sprinkle with bit of flavored vinegar on top. Enjoy

Nutrition: 156 Calories, 9.4g Protein, 12.2g Carbohydrates, 7.1g Fat, 0.8g Fiber, 7mg Cholesterol, 86mg Sodium, 365mg Potassium

388. Garden Salad

Preparation time: 5 minutes
Cooking time: 20 minutes
Servings: 6
Ingredients:
- 1 pound raw peanuts in shell
- 1 bay leaf
- 2 medium-sized chopped up tomatoes
- ½ cup diced up green pepper
- ½ cup diced up sweet onion
- ¼ cup finely diced hot pepper
- ¼ cup diced up celery
- 2 tablespoons olive oil
- ¾ teaspoon flavored vinegar
- ¼ teaspoon freshly ground black pepper

Directions:
1. Boil your peanuts for 1 minute and rinse them.
2. The skin will be soft, so discard the skin.
3. Add 2 cups of water to the Instant Pot.
4. Add bay leaf and peanuts.
5. Lock the lid and cook on HIGH pressure for 20 minutes.
6. Drain the water.
7. Take a large bowl and add the peanuts, diced up vegetables.
8. Whisk in olive oil, lemon juice, pepper in another bowl.
9. Pour the mixture over the salad and mix. Enjoy!

Nutrition: 156 Calories, 9.4g Protein, 12.2g Carbohydrates, 7.1g Fat, 0.8g Fiber, 7mg Cholesterol, 86mg Sodium, 365mg Potassium

389. Baked Smoky Broccoli and Garlic

Preparation time: 5 minutes
Cooking time: 20 minutes
Servings: 6
Ingredients
- Cooking spray
- 1 tablespoon extra-virgin olive oil
- 3 cloves garlic, minced
- 1/2 teaspoon sea salt
- 1/4 teaspoon ground black pepper
- ½ tsp. cumin
- ½ tsp. annatto seeds
- 3 1/2 cups sliced broccoli
- 1 lime, cut into wedges
- 1 tablespoon chopped fresh cilantro

Directions:
1. Preheat your oven to 450 degrees F.
2. Line a baking sheet with foil and grease with olive oil.
3. Mix the olive oil, garlic, cumin, annatto seeds, salt, and pepper in a bowl.
4. Add in the cauliflower, carrots, and broccoli.
5. Combine until well coated.
6. Spread them out in a single layer on the baking sheet.
7. Add the lime wedges.
8. Roast in the oven until vegetables become caramelized, for about 25 minutes.
9. Take out the lime wedges and top with the cilantro.

Nutrition: 156 Calories, 9.4g Protein, 12.2g Carbohydrates, 7.1g Fat, 0.8g Fiber, 7mg Cholesterol, 86mg Sodium, 365mg Potassium

390. Roasted Cauliflower and Lima Beans

Preparation time: 5 minutes
Cooking time: 20 minutes
Servings: 6
Ingredients
- Cooking spray
- 1 tablespoon melted vegan butter/margarine
- 9 cloves garlic, minced
- 1/2 teaspoon sea salt
- 1/4 teaspoon ground black pepper
- 1 1/2 cups sliced cauliflower
- 3 1/2 cups cherry tomatoes
- 1 (15 ounce) can lima beans, drained
- 1 lemon , cut into wedges

Directions:
1. Preheat your oven to 450 degrees F.
2. Line a baking sheet with foil and grease with melted vegan butter or margarine.
3. Mix the olive oil, garlic, salt, and pepper in a bowl.
4. Add in the cauliflower, tomatoes, and lima beans
5. Combine until well coated.
6. Spread them out in a single layer on the baking sheet.
7. Add the lemon wedges.
8. Roast in the oven until vegetables become caramelized, for about 25 minutes.
9. Take out the lemon wedges.

Nutrition: 156 Calories, 9.4g Protein, 12.2g Carbohydrates, 7.1g Fat, 0.8g Fiber, 7mg Cholesterol, 86mg Sodium, 365mg Potassium

391. The Delish Turkey Wrap

Preparation time: 10 minutes
Cooking time: 10 minutes
Servings: 6
Ingredients:
- 1 ¼ pounds ground turkey, lean
- 4 green onions, minced
- 1 tablespoon olive oil
- 1 garlic clove, minced
- 2 teaspoons chili paste
- 8-ounce water chestnut, diced
- 3 tablespoons hoisin sauce
- 2 tablespoon coconut aminos
- 1 tablespoon rice vinegar
- 12 almond butter lettuce leaves
- 1/8 teaspoon sunflower seeds

Directions:
1. Take a pan and place it over medium heat, add turkey and garlic to the pan.
2. Heat for 6 minutes until cooked.
3. Take a bowl and transfer turkey to the bowl.
4. Add onions and water chestnuts.
5. Stir in hoisin sauce, coconut aminos, and vinegar and chili paste.
6. Toss well and transfer mix to lettuce leaves.

7. Serve and enjoy!
Nutrition: 156 Calories, 9.4g Protein, 12.2g Carbohydrates, 7.1g Fat, 0.8g Fiber, 7mg Cholesterol, 86mg Sodium, 365mg Potassium

392. Zucchini Zoodles with Chicken and Basil

Preparation time: 10 minutes
Cooking time: 10 minutes
Servings: 3
Ingredients:
- 2 chicken fillets, cubed
- 2 tablespoons ghee
- 1 pound tomatoes, diced
- ½ cup basil, chopped
- ¼ cup almond milk
- 1 garlic clove, peeled, minced
- 1 zucchini, shredded

Directions:
1. Sauté cubed chicken in ghee until no longer pink.
2. Add tomatoes and season with sunflower seeds.
3. Simmer and reduce liquid.
4. Prepare your zucchini Zoodles by shredding zucchini in a food processor.
5. Add basil, garlic, coconut almond milk to the chicken and cook for a few minutes.
6. Add half of the zucchini Zoodles to a bowl and top with creamy tomato basil chicken.
7. Enjoy!

Nutrition: 156 Calories, 9.4g Protein, 12.2g Carbohydrates, 7.1g Fat, 0.8g Fiber, 7mg Cholesterol, 86mg Sodium, 365mg Potassium

393. Parmesan Baked Chicken

Preparation time: 5 minutes
Cooking time: 20 minutes
Servings: 2
Ingredients:
- 2 tablespoons ghee
- 2 boneless chicken breasts, skinless
- Pink sunflower seeds
- Freshly ground black pepper
- ½ cup mayonnaise, low fat
- ¼ cup parmesan cheese, grated
- 1 tablespoon dried Italian seasoning, low fat, low sodium
- ¼ cup crushed pork rinds

Directions:
1. Preheat your oven to 425 degrees F.
2. Take a large baking dish and coat with ghee.
3. Pat chicken breasts dry and wrap with a towel.
4. Season with sunflower seeds and pepper.
5. Place in baking dish.
6. Take a small bowl and add mayonnaise, parmesan cheese, Italian seasoning.
7. Slather mayo mix evenly over chicken breast.
8. Sprinkle crushed pork rinds on top.
9. Bake for 20 minutes until topping is browned.
10. Serve and enjoy!

Nutrition: 156 Calories, 9.4g Protein, 12.2g Carbohydrates, 7.1g Fat, 0.8g Fiber, 7mg Cholesterol, 86mg Sodium, 365mg Potassium

394. Crazy Japanese Potato and Beef Croquettes

Preparation time: 10 minutes
Cooking time: 20 minutes
Servings: 10
Ingredients:

- 3 medium russet potatoes, peeled and chopped
- 1 tablespoon almond butter
- 1 tablespoon vegetable oil
- 3 onions, diced
- ¾ pound ground beef
- 4 teaspoons light coconut aminos
- All-purpose flour for coating
- 2 eggs, beaten
- Panko bread crumbs for coating
- ½ cup oil, frying

Directions:

1. Take a saucepan and place it over medium-high heat; add potatoes and sunflower seeds water, boil for 16 minutes.
2. Remove water and put potatoes in another bowl, add almond butter and mash the potatoes.
3. Take a frying pan and place it over medium heat, add 1 tablespoon oil and let it heat up. Add onions and stir fry until tender.
4. Add coconut aminos to beef to onions.
5. Keep frying until beef is browned.
6. Mix the beef with the potatoes evenly.
7. Take another frying pan and place it over medium heat; add half a cup of oil.
8. Form croquettes using the mashed potato mixture and coat them with flour, then eggs and finally breadcrumbs.
9. Fry patties until golden on all sides.
10. Enjoy!

Nutrition: 156 Calories, 9.4g Protein, 12.2g Carbohydrates, 7.1g Fat, 0.8g Fiber, 7mg Cholesterol, 86mg Sodium, 365mg Potassium

395. Golden Eggplant Fries

Preparation time: 10 minutes
Cooking time: 15 minutes
Servings: 8
Ingredients:

- 2 eggs
- 2 cups almond flour
- 2 tablespoons coconut oil, spray
- 2 eggplant, peeled and cut thinly
- Sunflower seeds and pepper

Directions:

1. Preheat your oven to 400 degrees F.
2. Take a bowl and mix with sunflower seeds and black pepper.
3. Take another bowl and beat eggs until frothy.
4. Dip the eggplant pieces into the eggs.
5. Then coat them with the flour mixture.
6. Add another layer of flour and egg.
7. Then, take a baking sheet and grease with coconut oil on top.
8. Bake for about 15 minutes.

9. Serve and enjoy!

Nutrition: 156 Calories, 9.4g Protein, 12.2g Carbohydrates, 7.1g Fat, 0.8g Fiber, 7mg Cholesterol, 86mg Sodium, 365mg Potassium

396. Juicy and Peppery Tenderloin

Preparation time: 10 minutes
Cooking time: 20 minutes
Servings: 4
Ingredients:

- 2 teaspoons sage, chopped
- Sunflower seeds
- Pepper
- 2 1/2 pounds beef tenderloin
- 2 teaspoons thyme, chopped
- 2 garlic cloves, sliced
- 2 teaspoons rosemary, chopped
- 4 teaspoons olive oil

Directions:

1. Preheat your oven to 425 degrees F.
2. Take a small knife and cut incisions in the tenderloin; insert one slice of garlic into the incision.
3. Rub meat with oil.
4. Take a bowl and add sunflower seeds, sage, thyme, rosemary, pepper and mix well.
5. Rub the spice mix over tenderloin.
6. Put rubbed tenderloin into the roasting pan and bake for 10 minutes.
7. Lower temperature to 350 degrees F and cook for 20 minutes more until an internal thermometer reads 145 degrees F.
8. Transfer tenderloin to a cutting board and let sit for 15 minutes; slice into 20 pieces and enjoy!

Nutrition: 156 Calories, 9.4g Protein, 12.2g Carbohydrates, 7.1g Fat, 0.8g Fiber, 7mg Cholesterol, 86mg Sodium, 365mg Potassium

397. Ravaging Beef Pot Roast

Preparation time: 10 minutes
Cooking time: 75 minutes
Servings: 4
Ingredients:

- 3 ½ pounds beef roast
- 4 ounces mushrooms, sliced
- 12 ounces beef stock
- 1-ounce onion soup mix
- ½ cup Italian dressing, low sodium, and low fat

Directions:

1. Take a bowl and add the stock, onion soup mix and Italian dressing.
2. Stir.
3. Put beef roast in pan.
4. Add mushrooms, stock mix to the pan and cover with foil.
5. Preheat your oven to 300 degrees F.
6. Bake for 1 hour and 15 minutes.
7. Let the roast cool.
8. Slice and serve.

Nutrition: 156 Calories, 9.4g Protein, 12.2g Carbohydrates, 7.1g Fat, 0.8g Fiber, 7mg Cholesterol, 86mg Sodium, 365mg Potassium

398. Epic Mango Chicken

Preparation time: 10 minutes
Cooking time: 25 minutes
Servings: 4
Ingredients:
- 2 medium mangoes, peeled and sliced
- 10-ounce coconut almond milk
- 4 teaspoons vegetable oil
- 4 teaspoons spicy curry paste
- 14-ounce chicken breast halves, skinless and boneless, cut in cubes
- 4 medium shallots
- 1 large English cucumber, sliced and seeded

Directions:
1. Slice half of the mangoes and add the halves to a bowl.
2. Add mangoes and coconut almond milk to a blender and blend until you have a smooth puree.
3. Keep the mixture on the side.
4. Take a large-sized pot and place it over medium heat, add oil and allow the oil to heat up.
5. Add curry paste and cook for 1 minute until you have a nice fragrance, add shallots and chicken to the pot and cook for 5 minutes.
6. Pour mango puree in to the mix and allow it to heat up.
7. Serve the cooked chicken with mango puree and cucumbers.
8. Enjoy

Nutrition: 156 Calories, 9.4g Protein, 12.2g Carbohydrates, 7.1g Fat, 0.8g Fiber, 7mg Cholesterol, 86mg Sodium, 365mg Potassium

399. Hearty Chicken Liver Stew

Preparation time: 10 minutes
Cooking time: 25 minutes
Servings: 2
Ingredients:

- 10 ounces chicken livers
- 1-ounce onion, chopped
- 2 ounces sour cream
- 1 tablespoon olive oil
- Sunflower seeds to taste

Directions:
1. Take a pan and place it over medium heat.
2. Add oil and let it heat up.
3. Add onions and fry until just browned.
4. Add livers and season with sunflower seeds.
5. Cook until livers are half cooked.
6. Transfer the mix to a stew pot.
7. Add sour cream and cook for 20 minutes.
8. Serve and enjoy!

Nutrition: 156 Calories, 9.4g Protein, 12.2g Carbohydrates, 7.1g Fat, 0.8g Fiber, 7mg Cholesterol, 86mg Sodium, 365mg Potassium

400. Mustard Chicken

Preparation time: 10 minutes
Cooking time: 40 minutes
Servings: 2
Ingredients:
- 2 chicken breasts
- 1/4 cup chicken broth
- 2 tablespoons mustard
- 1 1/2 tablespoons olive oil
- 1/2 teaspoon paprika
- 1/2 teaspoon chili powder
- 1/2 teaspoon garlic powder

Directions:
1. Take a small bowl and mix mustard, olive oil, paprika, chicken broth, garlic powder, chicken broth, and chili.
2. Add chicken breast and marinate for 30 minutes.
3. Take a lined baking sheet and arrange the chicken.
4. Bake for 35 minutes at 375 degrees F.
5. Serve and enjoy!

Nutrition: 156 Calories, 9.4g Protein, 12.2g Carbohydrates, 7.1g Fat, 0.8g Fiber, 7mg Cholesterol, 86mg Sodium, 365mg Potassium

SIDES & APPETIZERS

401. Mediterranean Pop Corn Bites

Preparation time: 5 minutes + 20 minutes chill
Cooking time: 2-3 minutes
Servings: 4
Ingredients:
1. 3 cups Medjool dates, chopped
2. 12 ounces brewed coffee
3. cup pecan, chopped
4. ½ cup coconut, shredded
5. ½ cup cocoa powder

Directions:
4. Soak dates in warm coffee for 5 minutes.

5. Remove dates from coffee and mash them, making a fine smooth mixture.
6. Stir in remaining ingredients (except cocoa powder) and form small balls out of the mixture.
7. Coat with cocoa powder, serve and enjoy!

Nutrition: Calories: 265; Fat: 12g; Carbohydrates: 43g; Protein 3g

402. Hearty Buttery Walnuts

Preparation time: 10 minutes
Cooking time: 20 minutes
Servings: 4
Ingredients:
- 4 walnut halves

- ½ tablespoon almond butter

Directions:
- Spread butter over two walnut halves.
- Top with other halves.
- Serve and enjoy!

Nutrition: Calories: 90; Fat: 10g; Carbohydrates: 0g; Protein: 1g

403. Refreshing Watermelon Sorbet

Preparation time: 20 minutes + 20 hours chill time
Cooking time: 20 minutes
Servings: 4

Ingredients:
3. 4 cups watermelon, seedless and chunked
4. ¼ cup coconut sugar
5. 2 tablespoons lime juice

Directions:
- Add the listed ingredients to a blender and puree.
- Transfer to a freezer container with a tight-fitting lid.
- Freeze the mix for about 4-6 hours until you have gelatin-like consistency.
- Puree the mix once again in batches and return to the container.
- Chill overnight.
- Allow the sorbet to stand for 5 minutes before serving and enjoy!

Nutrition: Calories: 91; Fat: 0g; Carbohydrates: 25g; Protein: 1g

404. Lovely Faux Mac and Cheese

Preparation time: 15 minutes
Cooking time: 45 minutes
Servings: 4

Ingredients:
2. 5 cups cauliflower florets
3. Salt and pepper to taste
4. cup coconut milk
5. ½ cup vegetable broth
6. tablespoons coconut flour, sifted
7. organic egg, beaten
8. cups cheddar cheese

Directions:
- Pre-heat your oven to 350 degrees F.
- Season florets with salt and steam until firm.
- Place florets in greased ovenproof dish.
- Heat coconut milk over medium heat in a skillet, make sure to season the oil with salt and pepper.
- Stir in broth and add coconut flour to the mix, stir.
- Cook until the sauce begins to bubble.
- Remove heat and add beaten egg.
- Pour the thick sauce over cauliflower and mix in cheese.
- Bake for 30-45 minutes.
- Serve and enjoy!

Nutrition: Calories: 229; Fat: 14g; Carbohydrates: 9g; Protein: 15g

405. Beautiful Banana Custard

Preparation time: 10 minutes
Cooking time: 25 minutes
Servings: 3

Ingredients:
2. 2 ripe bananas, peeled and mashed finely
3. ½ teaspoon of vanilla extract
4. 14-ounce unsweetened almond milk
5. 3 eggs

Directions:
- Pre-heat your oven to 350 degrees F.
- Grease 8 custard glasses lightly.
- Arrange the glasses in a large baking dish.
- Take a large bowl and mix all of the ingredients and mix them well until combined nicely.
- Divide the mixture evenly between the glasses.
- Pour water in the baking dish.
- Bake for 25 minutes.
- Take out and serve.
- Enjoy!

Nutrition: Calories: 59; Fat: 2.4g; Carbohydrates: 7g; Protein: 3g

406. Pumpkin Pie Fat Bombs

Preparation time: 35 minutes
Cooking time: 5 minutes
Servings: 12

Ingredients:
- 2 tablespoons coconut oil
- 1/3 cup pumpkin puree
- 1/3 cup almond oil
- ¼ cup almond oil
- 3 ounces sugar-free dark chocolate
- ½ teaspoons pumpkin pie spice mix
- Stevia to taste

Direct
1. Melt almond oil and dark chocolate over a double boiler.
2. Take this mixture and layer the bottom of 12 muffin cups.
3. Freeze until the crust has set.
4. Meanwhile, take a saucepan and combine the rest of the ingredients.
5. Put the saucepan on low heat.
6. Heat until softened and mix well.
7. Pour this over the initial chocolate mixture.
8. Let it chill for at least 1 hour.

Nutrition: Total Carbs: 3g; Fiber: 1g; Protein: 3g; Fat: 13g; Calories: 124

407. Sensational Lemonade Fat Bomb

Preparation time: 2 hours
Cooking time: 20 minutes
Servings: 2

Ingredients:
- ½ lemon
- 4 ounces cream cheese

- 2 ounces almond butter
- Salt to taste
- 2 teaspoons natural sweetener

Directions:
1. Take a fine grater and zest lemon.
2. Squeeze lemon juice into bowl with zest.
3. Add butter, cream cheese in a bowl and add zest, juice, salt, and sweetener.
4. Mix well using a hand mixer until smooth.
5. Spoon mixture into molds and let them freeze for 2 hours.
6. Serve and enjoy!

Nutrition: Calories: 404; Fat: 43g; Carbohydrates: 4g; Protein: 4g

408. Sweet Almond and Coconut Fat Bombs

Preparation time: 10 minutes
Cooking time: 20 minutes
Servings: 6
Ingredients:
- ¼ cup melted coconut oil
- 9 ½ tablespoons almond butter
- 90 drops liquid stevia
- 3 tablespoons cocoa
- 9 tablespoons melted butter, salted

Directions:
1. Take a bowl and add all of the listed ingredients.
2. Mix them well.
3. Pour scant 2 tablespoons of the mixture into as many muffin molds as you like.
4. Chill for 20 minutes and pop them out.
5. Serve and enjoy!

Nutrition: Total Carbs: 2g; Fiber: 0g; Protein: 2.53g; Fat: 14g

409. Almond and Tomato Balls

Preparation time: 10 minutes
Cooking time: 20 minutes
Servings: 6
Ingredients:
- 1/3 cup pistachios, de-shelled
- 10 ounces cream cheese
- 1/3 cup sun dried tomatoes, diced

Directions:
1. Chop pistachios into small pieces.
2. Add cream cheese, tomatoes in a bowl and mix well.
3. Chill for 15-20 minutes and turn into balls.
4. Roll into pistachios.
5. Serve and enjoy!

Nutrition: Carb: 183; Fat: 18g; Carb: 5g; Protein: 5g

410. Avocado Tuna Bites

Preparation time: 10 minutes
Cooking time: 20 minutes
Servings: 4
Ingredients:
- 1/3 cup coconut oil
- avocado, cut into cubes

- 10 ounces canned tuna, drained
- ¼ cup parmesan cheese, grated
- ¼ teaspoon garlic powder
- 1/4 teaspoon onion powder
- 1/3 cup almond flour
- ¼ teaspoon pepper
- ¼ cup low fat mayonnaise
- Pepper as needed

Directions:
1. Take a bowl and add tuna, mayo, flour, parmesan, spices and mix well.
2. Fold in avocado and make 12 balls out of the mixture.
3. Melt coconut oil in pan and cook over medium heat, until all sides are golden.
4. Serve and enjoy!

Nutrition: Calories: 185; Fat: 18g; Carbohydrates: 1g; Protein: 5g

411. Juicy Simple Lemon Fat Bombs

Preparation time: 10 minutes
Cooking time: 20 minutes
Servings: 3
Ingredients:
- 1 whole lemon
- 4 ounces cream cheese
- 2 ounces butter
- 2 teaspoons natural sweetener

Directions:
1. Take a fine grater and zest your lemon.
2. Squeeze lemon juice into a bowl alongside the zest.
3. Add butter, cream cheese to a bowl and add zest, salt, sweetener and juice.
4. Stir well using a hand mixer until smooth.
5. Spoon mix into molds and freeze for 2 hours.
6. Serve and enjoy!

Nutrition: Total Carbs: 4g; Fiber: 1g; Protein: 4g; Fat: 43g; Calories: 404

412. Chocolate Coconut Bombs

Preparation time: 20 minutes
Cooking time: 20 minutes
Servings: 12
Ingredients:
- ½ cup dark cocoa powder
- ½ tablespoon vanilla extract
- 5 drops stevia
- 1 cup coconut oil, solid
- tablespoon peppermint extract

Directions:
1. Take a high speed food processor and add all the ingredients.
2. Blend until combined.
3. Take a teaspoon and drop a spoonful onto parchment paper.
4. Refrigerate until solidified and keep refrigerated.

Nutrition: Total Carbs: 0g; Fiber: 0g; Protein: 0g; Fat: 14g; Calories: 126

413. Terrific Jalapeno Bacon Bombs

Preparation time: 15 minutes
Cooking time: 10 minutes
Servings: 2
Ingredients:
- 12 large jalapeno peppers
- 16 bacon strips
- 6 ounces full fat cream cheese
- 2 teaspoon garlic powder
- teaspoon chili powder

Directions:
1. Pre-heat your oven to 350 degrees F.
2. Place a wire rack over a roasting pan and keep it on the side.
3. Make a slit lengthways across jalapeno pepper and scrape out the seeds, discard them.
4. Place a nonstick skillet over high heat and add half of your bacon strips, cook until crispy.
5. Drain them.
6. Chop the cooked bacon strips and transfer to large bowl.
7. Add cream cheese and mix.
8. Season the cream cheese and bacon mix with garlic and chili powder.
9. Mix well.
10. Stuff the mix into the jalapeno peppers with and wrap a raw bacon strip all around.
11. Arrange the stuffed wrapped jalapeno on prepared wire rack.
12. Roast for 10 minutes.
13. Transfer to cooling rack and serve!

Nutrition: Calories: 209; Fat: 9g; Net Carbohydrates: 15g; Protein: 9g

414. Yummy Espresso Fat Bombs

Preparation time: 20 minutes
Cooking time: 20 minutes
Servings: 24
Ingredients:
- 5 tablespoons butter, tender
- 3 ounces cream cheese, soft
- 2 ounces espresso
- 4 tablespoons coconut oil
- 2 tablespoons coconut whipping cream
- 2 tablespoons stevia

Directions
1. Prepare your double boiler and melt all ingredients (except stevia) for 3-4 minutes and mix.
2. Add sweetener and mix using hand mixer.
3. Spoon mixture into silicone muffin molds and freeze for 4 hours.
4. Remove fat bombs and enjoy!

Nutrition: Total Carbs: 1.3g; Fiber: 0.2g; Protein: 0.3g; Fat: 7g

415. Crispy Coconut Bombs

Preparation time: 10 minutes
Cooking time: 20 minutes
Servings: 6
Ingredients:
- 14 ½ ounces coconut milk
- ¾ cup coconut oil
- cup unsweetened coconut flakes
- 20 drops stevia

Directions:
1. Microwave your coconut oil for 20 seconds in microwave.
2. Mix in coconut milk and stevia in the hot oil.
3. Stir in coconut flakes and pour the mixture into molds.
4. Let it chill for 60 minutes in fridge.
5. Serve and enjoy!

Nutrition: Total Carbs: 2g; Fiber: 0.5g; Protein: 1g; Fat: 13g; Calories: 123; Net Carbs: 1g

416. Spiced Up Pumpkin Seeds Bowls

Preparation time: 10 minutes
Cooking time: 20 minutes
Servings: 4
Ingredients:
- ½ tablespoon chili powder
- ½ teaspoon cayenne
- 2 cups pumpkin seeds
- 2 teaspoons lime juice

Direction:
1. Spread pumpkin seeds over lined baking sheet, add lime juice, cayenne and chili powder.
2. Toss well.
3. Pre-heat your oven to 275 degrees F.
4. Roast in your oven for 20 minutes and transfer to small bowls.
5. Serve and enjoy!

Nutrition: Calories: 170; Fat: 3g; Carbohydrates: 10g; Protein: 6g

417. Mozzarella Cauliflower Bars

Preparation time: 10 minutes
Cooking time: 40 minutes
Servings: 4
Ingredients:
- 1 cauliflower head, riced
- 12 cup low-fat mozzarella cheese, shredded
- ¼ cup egg whites
- 1 teaspoon Italian dressing, low fat
- Pepper to taste

Directions:
1. Spread cauliflower rice over lined baking sheet.
2. Pre-heat your oven to 375 degrees F.
3. Roast for 20 minutes.
4. Transfer to bowl and spread pepper, cheese, seasoning, egg whites and stir well.

5. Spread in a rectangular pan and press.
6. Transfer to oven and cook for 20 minutes more.
7. Serve and enjoy!

Nutrition: Calories: 140; Fat: 2g; Carbohydrates: 6g; Protein: 6g

418. Tomato Pesto Crackers

Preparation time: 10 minutes
Cooking time: 15 minutes
Servings: 4

Ingredients:
- 1 ¼ cups almond flour
- ½ teaspoon garlic powder
- ½ teaspoon baking powder
- 2 tablespoons sun-dried tomato Pesto
- 3 tablespoons ghee
- ½ teaspoon dried basil
- ¼ teaspoon pepper

Directions:
1. Pre-heat your oven to 325 degrees F.
2. Take a bowl and add listed ingredients.
3. Mix well and combine.
4. Take a baking sheet lined with parchment paper and spread the dough.
5. Transfer to oven and bake for 15 minutes.
6. Break into small sized crackers and serve.
7. Enjoy!

Nutrition: Calories: 204; Fat: 20g; Carbohydrates: 3g; Protein: 3g

419. Garlic Cottage Cheese Crispy

Preparation time: 5 minutes
Cooking time: 2 minutes
Servings: 4

Ingredients:
- 1 cup cottage cheese
- ½ teaspoon Garlic powder
- Pinch of pepper
- Pinch of onion powder

Direction:
1. Take a skillet and place it over medium heat.
2. Take a bowl and mix in cheese and spices.
3. Scoop half a teaspoon of the cheese mix and place in the pan.
4. Cook for 1 minute per side.
5. Repeat until done.
6. Enjoy!

Nutrition: Calories: 70; Fat: 6g; Carbohydrates: 1g; Protein: 6g

420. Tasty Cucumber Bites

Preparation time: 5 minutes
Cooking time: 20 minutes
Servings: 4

Ingredients:
- 1 (8 ounce) cream cheese container, low fat
- 1 tablespoon bell pepper, diced
- 1 tablespoon shallots, diced
- 1 tablespoon parsley, chopped
- 2 cucumbers
- Pepper to taste

Directions:
1. Take a bowl and add cream cheese, onion, pepper, parsley.
2. Peel cucumbers and cut in half.
3. Remove seeds and stuff with cheese mix.
4. Cut into bite sized portions and enjoy!

Nutrition: Calories: 85; Fat: 4g; Carbohydrates: 2g; Protein: 3g

421. Hearty Almond Crackers

Preparation time: 10 minutes
Cooking time: 20 minutes
Servings: 40 crackers

Ingredients:
- 1 cup almond flour
- ¼ teaspoon baking soda
- 1/8 teaspoon black pepper
- 3 tablespoons sesame seeds
- 1 egg, beaten
- Salt and pepper to taste

Directions:
1. Pre-heat your oven to 350 degrees F.
2. Line two baking sheets with parchment paper and keep them on the side.
3. Mix the dry ingredients in a large bowl and add egg, mix well and form dough.
4. Divide dough into two balls.
5. Roll out the dough between two pieces of parchment paper.
6. Cut into crackers and transfer them to prepared baking sheet.
7. Bake for 15-20 minutes.
8. Repeat until all the dough has been used up.
9. Leave crackers to cool and serve.
10. Enjoy!

Nutrition: Total Carbs: 8g; Fiber: 2g; Protein: 9g; Fat: 28g

422. Black Bean Salsa

Preparation time: 10 minutes
Cooking time: 20 minutes
Servings: 4

Ingredients:
- 1 tablespoon coconut aminos
- ½ teaspoon cumin, ground
- 1 cup canned black beans, no salt
- 1 cup salsa
- 6 cups romaine lettuce, torn
- ½ cup avocado, peeled, pitted and cubed

Directions:
1. Take a bowl and add beans, alongside other ingredients.
2. Toss well and serve.
3. Enjoy!

Nutrition: Calories: 181; Fat: 5g; Carbohydrates: 14g; Protein: 7g

423. Corn Spread

Preparation time: 10 minutes
Cooking time: 10 minutes
Servings: 4
Ingredients:
- 30 ounce canned corn, drained
- 2 green onions, chopped
- ½ cup coconut cream
- 1 jalapeno, chopped
- ½ teaspoon chili powder

Direction:
1. Take a pan and add corn, green onions, jalapeno, and chili powder, stir well.
2. Bring to a simmer over medium heat and cook for 10 minutes.
3. Let it chill and add coconut cream.
4. Stir well.
5. Serve and enjoy!

Nutrition: Calories: 192; Fat: 5g; Carbohydrates: 11g; Protein: 8g

424. Moroccan Leeks Snack

Preparation time: 10 minutes
Cooking time: 20 minutes
Servings: 4
Ingredients:
- 1 bunch radish, sliced
- 3 cups leeks, chopped
- 1 ½ cups olives, pitted and sliced
- Pinch turmeric powder
- 2 tablespoons essential olive oil
- 1 cup cilantro, chopped

Directions:
1. Take a bowl and mix in radishes, leeks, olives and cilantro.
2. Mix well.
3. Season with pepper, oil, turmeric and toss well.
4. Serve and enjoy!

Nutrition: Calories: 120; Fat: 1g; Carbohydrates: 1g; Protein: 6g

425. The Bell Pepper Fiesta

Preparation time: 10 minutes
Cooking time: 20 minutes
Servings: 4
Ingredients:
- 2 tablespoons dill, chopped
- 1 yellow onion, chopped
- 1 pound multi colored peppers, cut, halved, seeded and cut into thin strips
- 3 tablespoons organic olive oil
- 2 ½ tablespoons white wine vinegar
- Black pepper to taste

Directions:
1. Take a bowl and mix in sweet pepper, onion, dill, pepper, oil, vinegar and toss well.
2. Divide between bowls and serve.
3. Enjoy!

Nutrition: Calories: 120; Fat: 3g; Carbohydrates: 1g; Protein: 6g

426. Hearty Cashew and Almond Butter

Preparation time: 5 minutes
Cooking time: 10 minutes
Servings: 1 and ½ cup
Ingredients:
- 1 cup almonds, blanched
- 1/3 cup cashew nuts
- 2 tablespoons coconut oil
- ½ teaspoon cinnamon

Directions:
1. Pre-heat your oven to 350 degrees F.
2. Bake almonds and cashews for 12 minutes.
3. Let them cool.
4. Transfer to food processor and add remaining ingredients.
5. Add oil and keep blending until smooth.
6. Serve and enjoy!

Nutrition: Calories: 205; Fat: 19g; Carbohydrates: g; Protein: 2.8g

427. Red Coleslaw

Preparation time: 10 minutes
Cooking time: 0 minutes
Servings: 4
Ingredients:
- 1 2/3 pounds red cabbage
- 2 tablespoons ground caraway seeds
- 1 tablespoon whole grain mustard
- 1 1/4 cups mayonnaise, low fat, low sodium
- Salt and black pepper

Directions:
1. Cut the red cabbage into small slices.
2. Take a large-sized bowl and add all the ingredients alongside cabbage.
3. Mix well, season with salt and pepper.
4. Serve and enjoy!

Nutrition: Calories: 406; Fat: 40.8g; Carbohydrates: 10g; Protein: 2.2g

428. Avocado Mayo Medley

Preparation time: 5 minutes
Cooking time: 10 minutes
Servings: 4
Ingredients:
- 1 medium avocado, cut into chunks
- ½ teaspoon ground cayenne pepper
- 2 tablespoons fresh cilantro
- ¼ cup olive oil
- ½ cup mayo, low fat and los sodium

Directions:
1. Take a food processor and add avocado, cayenne pepper, lime juice, salt and cilantro.
2. Mix until smooth.

3. Slowly incorporate olive oil, add 1 tablespoon at a time and keep processing between additions.
4. Store and use as needed!

Nutrition: Calories: 231; Fat: 20g; Carbohydrates: 5g; Protein: 3g

429. Amazing Garlic Aioli

Preparation time: 5 minutes
Cooking time: 10 minutes
Servings: 4
Ingredients:
- ½ cup mayonnaise, low fat and low sodium
- 2 garlic cloves, minced
- Juice of 1 lemon
- 1 tablespoon fresh-flat leaf Italian parsley, chopped
- 1 teaspoon chives, chopped
- Salt and pepper to taste

Directions:
1. Add mayonnaise, garlic, parsley, lemon juice, chives and season with salt and pepper.
2. Blend until combined well.
3. Pour into refrigerator and chill for 30 minutes.
4. Serve and use as needed!

Nutrition: Calories: 813; Fat: 88g; Carbohydrates: 9g; Protein: 2g

430. Easy Seed Crackers

Preparation time: 10 minutes
Cooking time: 60 minutes
Servings: 72 crackers
Ingredients:
- 1 cup boiling water
- 1/3 cup chia seeds
- 1/3 cup sesame seeds
- 1/3 cup pumpkin seeds
- 1/3 cup Flaxseeds
- 1/3 cup sunflower seeds
- 1 tablespoon Psyllium powder
- 1 cup almond flour
- 1 teaspoon salt
- ¼ cup coconut oil, melted

Directions:
1. Pre-heat your oven to 300 degrees F.
2. Line a cookie sheet with parchment paper and keep it on the side.
3. Add listed ingredients (except coconut oil and water) to food processor and pulse until ground.
4. Transfer to a large mixing bowl and pour melted coconut oil and boiling water, mix.
5. Transfer mix to prepared sheet and spread into a thin layer.
6. Cut dough into crackers and bake for 60 minutes.
7. Cool and serve.
8. Enjoy!

Nutrition: Total Carbs: 10.6g; Fiber: 3g; Protein: 5g; Fat: 14.6g

431. Chickpeas and Curried Veggies

Preparation time: 15 minutes
Cooking time: 4 hours
Servings: 2
Ingredients:
- ½ tbsp. Canola Oil
- 2 sliced Celery Ribs
- 1/8 tsp. Cayenne Pepper
- ¼ cup Water
- 2 sliced Carrots
- 2 sliced red Potatoes (sliced)
- ½ tbsp. Curry Powder
- ½ cup of Coconut Milk (light)
- ¼ cup drained Chickpeas (low sodium)
- Chopped Cilantro
- ¼ cup Yogurt (low fat)

Directions:
1. Sauté potatoes for 5 mins in oil. Add the carrots, celery, and onion. Sauté for 5 more mins. Sprinkle on the curry powder and cayenne pepper. Stir well to combine.
2. In a slow cooker, pour water and coconut milk. Add in the potatoes. Cook on "low" for 3 hrs. Add chickpeas and cook for 30 more mins. Serve in bowls along with the yogurt and cilantro garnish.

Nutrition: Calories 271, Fats 11 g, Sodium 207 mg, Carbohydrates 39 g, Protein 7 g

432. Brussels sprouts Casserole

Preparation time: 15 minutes
Cooking time: 4 hours & 15 minutes
Servings: 3
Ingredients:
- ¾ lb. Brussels Sprouts
- 1 diced slice Pancetta
- 1 minced clove Garlic
- 1 tbsp. chopped Shallot
- ¼ cup pine nuts (toasted)
- ¼ tsp. Black Pepper (cracked)
- 4 tbsp. Water

Directions:
1. Slice sprouts and place them in the slow cooker along with the water. Cook on "high" for 1 hr. Drain well. Remove the fat from the pancetta. Sauté the pancetta for 4 mins. Add the shallots, garlic, and 1/8 cup of Pine Nuts to the sauté.
2. Now, add the sprouts. Cook for 3 mins. Transfer the prepared mixture to the slow cooker. Add black pepper. 4 tbsp. of water, and cook again on "low" for 2 hrs. Serve immediately.

Nutrition: Calories 128; Fats 9 g; Sodium 56 mg; Carbohydrates 5 g; Protein 5 g

433. Tasty Cauliflower

Preparation time: 15 minutes

Cooking time: 6 hours & 15 minutes
Servings: 4
Ingredients:
- 2 minced cloves Garlic
- 2 cups Cauliflower florets
- 2 tbsp. Olive Oil
- Pinch of Sea Salt
- ¼ tsp. Pepper Flakes (chili)
- Pinch of Black Pepper (cracked)
- 4 tbsp. Water
- Zest of ½ lemon

Directions:
1. In a slow cooker, place cauliflower and oil. Add vinegar. Toss well to coat thoroughly. Put in the rest of the ingredients and toss again. Cook on "low" for 2 hrs. Serve immediately.

Nutrition: Calories 150; Fats 14 g; Sodium 69 mg; Carbohydrates 6 g; Protein 2.2 g

434. Artichoke and Spinach Dip

Preparation time: 15 minutes
Cooking time: 2 hours & 10 minutes
Servings: 2
Ingredients:
- 1/8 tsp. Basil (dried)
- 14 oz. chopped Artichoke Hearts
- 1 ½ cups spinach
- ½ minced clove Garlic
- ¼ cup Sour Cream (low fat)
- ¼ cup shredded Cheese (Parmesan)
- ¼ cup Mozzarella Cheese (shredded)
- 1/8 tsp. Parsley (dried)
- ½ cup Yogurt (Greek)
- Pinch of Black Pepper
- Pinch of Kosher Salt

Directions:
1. Boil spinach in water for 1 min. Drain the water. Set the spinach aside to cool and then chop. Puree all the ingredients, including spinach, in a blender.
2. Transfer the mixture to the slow cooker. Add cheeses and cook for 1 hour on "low." Serve with sliced vegetables.

Nutrition: Calories 263; Fats 14 g; Sodium 537 mg; Carbohydrates 18 g; Protein 20 g

435. Apple Salsa

Preparation time: 15 minutes
Cooking time: 2 hours
Servings: 3
Ingredients:
- 7 ½ oz. drained Black Beans
- ¼ cubed Apples (Granny Smith)
- ¼ chopped Chili Pepper (Serrano)
- 1/8 cup chopped onion (red)
- 1 ½ tbsp. chopped cilantro
- ¼ Lemon
- ¼ Orange

- Pinch of Sea Salt
- Pinch of Black Pepper (cracked)

Directions:
1. Mix all the ingredients in the cooker (slow cooker). Cook on "low" for an hour. Transfer to a covered container and allow to cool for 1 hr. Serve.

Nutrition: Calories 100; Fats 0.4 g; Sodium 50 mg; Carbohydrates 20 g; Protein 5 g

436. Quinoa Curry

Preparation time: 15 minutes
Cooking time: 4 hours
Servings: 8
Ingredients:
- 1 chopped Sweet Potato
- 2 cups Green Beans
- ½ diced onion (white)
- 1 diced Carrot
- 15 oz. Chick Peas (organic and drained)
- 28 oz. Tomatoes (diced)
- 29 oz. Coconut Milk
- 2 minced cloves of garlic
- ¼ cup Quinoa
- 1 tbs. Turmeric (ground)
- 1 tbsp. Ginger (grated)
- 1 ½ cups Water
- 1 tsp. of Chili Flakes
- 2 tsp. of Tamari Sauce

Directions:
1. Put all the listed fixing in the slow cooker. Add 1 cup of water. Stir well. Cook on "high" for 4 hrs. Serve with rice.

Nutrition: Calories 297; Fat 18 g; Sodium 364 mg; Carbohydrates 9 mg; Protein 28 g

437. Lemon and Cilantro Rice

Preparation time: 15 minutes
Cooking time: 6 hours
Servings: 4
Ingredients:
- 3 cups Vegetable Broth (low sodium)
- 1 ½ cups Brown Rice (uncooked)
- Juice of 2 lemons
- 2 tbsp. chopped cilantro

Directions:
1. In a slow cooker, place broth and rice. Cook on "low" for 5 hrs. Check the rice for doneness with a fork. Add the lemon juice and cilantro before serving.

Nutrition: Calories 56; Fats 0.3 g; Sodium 174 mg; Carbohydrates 12 g; Protein 1 g

438. Chili Beans

Preparation time: 15 minutes
Cooking time: 4 hours
Servings: 5
Ingredients:

- 1 ½ cup chopped Bell Pepper
- 1 ½ cup sliced Mushrooms (white)
- 1 cup chopped Onion
- 1 tbsp. Olive Oil
- 1 tbsp. Chili Powder
- 2 chopped cloves Garlic
- 1 tsp. chopped Chipotle Chili
- ½ tsp. Cumin
- oz. drained Black Beans
- 1 cup diced tomatoes (no salt)
- 2 tbsp. chopped cilantro

Directions:
1. Put all the fixing above in the slow cooker. Cook on "high" for 4 hrs. Serve

Nutrition: Calories 343; Fat 11 g; Sodium 308 mg; Carbohydrates 9 mg; Protein 29 g

439. Bean Spread

Preparation time: 15 minutes
Cooking time: 4 hours
Servings: 20
Ingredients:
- 30 ounces Cannellini Beans
- ½ cup Broth (chicken or veg)
- 1 tbsp. Olive Oil
- 3 minced cloves Garlic
- ½ tsp. Marjoram
- ½ tsp. Rosemary
- 1/8 tsp. Pepper
- Pita Chips
- 1 tbsp. Olive Oil

Directions:
1. Place olive oil, beans, broth, marjoram, garlic, rosemary, and pepper in the slow cooker. Cook on "low" for 4 hrs. Mash the mixture and transfer to a bowl. Serve with Pita.

Nutrition: Calories 298; Fat 18 g; Sodium 298 mg; Carbohydrates 30 mg; Protein 19 g

440. Stir-Fried Steak, Shiitake, and Asparagus

Preparation time: 15 minutes
Cooking time: 2 hours & 20 minutes
Servings: 4
Ingredients:
- 1 tbsp. Sherry (dry)
- 1 tbsp. Vinegar (rice)
- ½ tbsp. Soy Sauce (low sodium)
- ½ tbsp. Cornstarch
- 2 tsp. Canola Oil
- ¼ tsp. Black Pepper (ground)
- 1 minced clove Garlic
- ½ lb. sliced Sirloin Steak
- 3 oz. Shiitake Mushrooms
- ½ tbsp. minced Ginger
- 6 oz. sliced Asparagus
- 3 oz. Peas (sugar snap)

- 2 sliced scallions
- ¼ cup Water

Directions:
1. Combine cornstarch, soy sauce, sherry vinegar, broth, and pepper. Place the steaks in 1 tsp. hot oil in the slow cooker for 2 mins. Transfer the steaks to a plate. Sauté ginger and garlic in the remaining oil. Add in the mushrooms, peas, and asparagus.
2. Add water and cook on "low" for 1 hr. add the scallions and cook again for 30 mins on low. Change the heat to "high" and add the vinegar. When the sauce has thickened, transfer the steaks to the slow cooker. Stir well and serve immediately.

Nutrition: Calories 182, Fats 7 g, Sodium 157 mg, Carbohydrates 10 mg, Protein 20 g

441. Jalapeno Black-Eyed Peas Mix

Preparation time: 10 minutes
Cooking time: 5 hours
Servings: 12
Ingredients:
- 17 ounces black-eyed peas
- 1 sweet red pepper, chopped
- ½ cup sausage, chopped
- 1 yellow onion, chopped
- 1 jalapeno, chopped
- 2 garlic cloves minced
- 6 cups of water
- ½ teaspoon cumin, ground
- A pinch of black pepper
- 2 tablespoons cilantro, chopped

Directions:
1. In your slow cooker, mix the peas with the sausage, onion, red pepper, jalapeno, garlic, cumin, black pepper, water, cilantro, cover, and cook low for 5 hours. Serve.

Nutrition: Calories 75; Fat 3.5g; Sodium 94mg; Carbohydrate 7.2g; Fiber 1.7g; Sugars 0.9g; Protein 4.3g

442. Sour Cream Green Beans

Preparation time: 10 minutes
Cooking time: 4 hours
Servings: 8
Ingredients:
- 15 ounces green beans
- 14 ounces corn
- 4 ounces mushrooms, sliced
- 11 ounces cream of mushroom soup, low-fat and sodium-free
- ½ cup low-fat sour cream
- ½ cup almonds, chopped
- ½ cup low-fat cheddar cheese, shredded

Directions:
1. In your slow cooker, mix the green beans with the corn, mushrooms soup, mushrooms, almonds, cheese, sour cream, toss, cover, and cook on Low for 4 hours. Stir one more time, divide between plates and serve as a side dish.

Nutrition: Calories360; Fat 12.7g; Sodium 220mg; Carbohydrate 58.3g; Fiber 10g; Sugars 10.3g; Protein 14g

443. Cumin Brussels sprouts

Preparation time: 10 minutes
Cooking time: 3 hours
Servings: 4
Ingredients:

- 1 cup low-sodium veggie stock
- 1-pound Brussels sprouts, trimmed and halved
- 1 teaspoon rosemary, dried
- 1 teaspoon cumin, ground
- 1 tablespoon mint, chopped

Directions:
1. In your slow cooker, combine the sprouts with the stock and the other ingredients, cook on Low within 3 hours. Serve.

Nutrition: Calories 56; Fat 0.6g; Sodium 65mg; Carbohydrate 11.4g; Fiber 4.5g; Sugars 2.7g; Protein 4g

444. Peach and Carrots

Preparation time: 10 minutes
Cooking time: 6 hours
Servings: 6
Ingredients:

- 2 pounds small carrots, peeled
- ½ cup low-fat butter, melted
- ½ cup canned peach, unsweetened
- 2 tablespoons cornstarch
- 3 tablespoons stevia
- 2 tablespoons water
- ½ teaspoon cinnamon powder
- 1 teaspoon vanilla extract
- A pinch of nutmeg, ground

Directions:
1. In your slow cooker, mix the carrots with the butter, peach, stevia, cinnamon, vanilla, nutmeg, and cornstarch mixed with water, toss, cover, and cook on Low for 6 hours. Toss the carrots one more time, divide between plates and serve as a side dish.

Nutrition: Calories139; Fat 10.7g; Sodium 199mg; Carbohydrate 35.4g; Fiber 4.2g; Sugars 6.9g; Protein 3.8g

445. Baby Spinach and Grains Mix

Preparation time: 10 minutes
Cooking time: 4 hours
Servings: 12
Ingredients:

- 1 butternut squash, peeled and cubed
- 1 cup whole-grain blend, uncooked
- 12 ounces low-sodium veggie stock
- 6 ounces baby spinach
- 1 yellow onion, chopped

- 3 garlic cloves, minced
- ½ cup of water
- 2 teaspoons thyme, chopped
- A pinch of black pepper

Directions:
1. In your slow cooker, mix the squash with whole grain, onion, garlic, water, thyme, black pepper, stock, spinach, cover, and cook on Low for 4 hours. Serve.

Nutrition: Calories78; Fat 0.6g; Sodium 259mg; Carbohydrate 16.4g; Fiber 1.8g; Sugars 2g; Protein 2.5g

446. Pilaf with Bella Mushrooms

Preparation time: 10 minutes
Cooking time: 3 hours
Servings: 6
Ingredients:

- 1 cup wild rice
- 6 green onions, chopped
- ½ pound baby Bella mushrooms
- 2 cups of water
- 2 tablespoons olive oil
- 2 garlic cloves, minced

Directions:
1. In your slow cooker, mix the rice with garlic, onions, oil, mushrooms, water, toss, cover, and cook on Low for 3 hours. Stir the pilaf one more time, divide between plates and serve.

Nutrition: Calories 151; Fat 5.1g; Sodium 9mg; Carbohydrate 23.3g; Fiber 2.6g; Sugars 1.7g; Protein 5.2g

447. Parsley Fennel

Preparation time: 10 minutes
Cooking time: 2 hours and 30 minutes
Servings: 4
Ingredients:

- 2 fennel bulbs, sliced
- Juice and zest of 1 lime
- 2 teaspoons avocado oil
- ½ teaspoon turmeric powder
- 1 tablespoon parsley, chopped
- ¼ cup veggie stock, low-sodium

Directions:
1. In a slow cooker, combine the fennel with the lime juice, zest, and the other ingredients, cook on Low within 2 hours and 30 minutes. Serve.

Nutrition: Calories 47; Fat 0.6g; Sodium 71mg; Carbohydrate 10.8g; Protein 1.7g

448. Sweet Butternut

Preparation time: 10 minutes
Cooking time: 4 hours
Servings: 8
Ingredients:

- 1 cup carrots, chopped
- 1 tablespoon olive oil
- 1 yellow onion, chopped
- ½ teaspoon stevia
- 1 garlic clove, minced
- ½ teaspoon curry powder
- 1 butternut squash, cubed
- 2 and ½ cups low-sodium veggie stock
- ½ cup basmati rice
- ¾ cup of coconut milk
- ½ teaspoon cinnamon powder
- ¼ teaspoon ginger, grated

Directions:
1. Heat-up, a pan with the oil over medium-high heat, add the oil, onion, garlic, stevia, carrots, curry powder, cinnamon, ginger, stir, and cook 5 minutes and transfer to your slow cooker.
2. Add squash, stock, and coconut milk, stir, cover, and cook on Low for 4 hours. Divide the butternut mix between plates and serve as a side dish.

Nutrition: Calories 134; Fat 7.2g; Sodium 59mg; Carbohydrate 16.5g; Fiber 1.7g; Sugars 2.7g; Protein 1.8g

449. Mushroom Sausages

Preparation time: 10 minutes
Cooking time: 2 hours
Servings: 12
Ingredients:
- 6 celery ribs, chopped
- 1 pound no-sugar, beef sausage, chopped
- 2 tablespoons olive oil
- ½ pound mushrooms, chopped
- ½ cup sunflower seeds, peeled
- 1 cup low-sodium veggie stock
- 1 cup cranberries, dried
- 2 yellow onions, chopped
- 2 garlic cloves, minced
- 1 tablespoon sage, dried
- 1 whole-wheat bread loaf, cubed

Directions:
1. Heat-up a pan with the oil over medium-high heat, add beef, stir and brown for a few minutes. Add mushrooms, onion, celery, garlic, and sage, stir, cook for a few more minutes and transfer to your slow cooker.
2. Add stock, cranberries, sunflower seeds, and the bread cubes; cover and cook on High for 2 hours. Stir the whole mix, divide between plates and serve as a side dish.

Nutrition: Calories 188; Fat 13.8g; Sodium 489mg; Carbohydrate 8.2g; Fiber 1.9g; Protein 7.6g

450. Parsley Red Potatoes

Preparation time: 10 minutes
Cooking time: 6 hours
Servings: 8
Ingredients:
- 16 baby red potatoes, halved
- 2 cups low-sodium chicken stock
- 1 carrot, sliced
- 1 celery rib, chopped
- ¼ cup yellow onion, chopped
- 1 tablespoon parsley, chopped
- 2 tablespoons olive oil
- A pinch of black pepper
- 1 garlic clove minced

Directions:
1. In your slow cooker, mix the potatoes with the carrot, celery, onion, stock, parsley, garlic, oil, and black pepper, toss, cover, and cook on Low for 6 hours. Serve.

Nutrition: Calories 257; Fat 9.5g; Sodium 845mg; Carbohydrate 43.4g; Protein 4.4g

451. Spiced Broccoli Florets

Preparation time: 10 minutes
Cooking time: 3 hours
Servings: 10
Ingredients:
- 6 cups broccoli florets
- 1 and ½ cups low-fat cheddar cheese, shredded
- ½ teaspoon cider vinegar
- ¼ cup yellow onion, chopped
- 10 ounces tomato sauce, sodium-free
- 2 tablespoons olive oil
- A pinch of black pepper

Directions:
1. Grease your slow cooker with the oil, add broccoli, tomato sauce, cider vinegar, onion, and black pepper, cook on High within 2 hours, and 30 minutes. Sprinkle the cheese all over, cover, cook on High for 30 minutes more, divide between plates, and serve as a side dish.

Nutrition: Calories 119; Fat 8.7g; Sodium 272mg; Carbohydrate 5.7g; Fiber 1.9g; Sugars 2.3g; Protein 6.2g

452. Lima Beans Dish

Preparation time: 10 minutes
Cooking time: 5 hours
Servings: 10
Ingredients:
- 1 green bell pepper, chopped
- 1 sweet red pepper, chopped
- 1 and ½ cups tomato sauce, salt-free
- 1 yellow onion, chopped
- ½ cup of water
- 16 ounces canned kidney beans, no-salt-added, drained and rinsed
- 16 ounces canned black-eyed peas, no-salt-added, drained and rinsed
- 15 ounces corn
- 15 ounces canned lima beans, no-salt-added, drained and rinsed
- 15 oz. canned black beans, no-salt-added, drained
- 2 celery ribs, chopped
- 2 bay leaves
- 1 teaspoon ground mustard
- 1 tablespoon cider vinegar

Directions:

1. In your slow cooker, mix the tomato sauce with the onion, celery, red pepper, green bell pepper, water, bay leaves, mustard, vinegar, kidney beans, black-eyed peas, corn, lima beans, and black beans, cook on Low within 5 hours. Discard bay leaves, divide the whole mix between plates, and serve.

Nutrition: Calories 602; Fat 4.8g; Sodium 255mg; Carbohydrate 117.7g; Fiber 24.6g; 13.4g; Protein 33g

453. Soy Sauce Green Beans

Preparation time: 10 minutes
Cooking time: 2 hours
Servings: 12
Ingredients:
- 3 tablespoons olive oil
- 16 ounces green beans
- ½ teaspoon garlic powder
- ½ cup of coconut sugar
- 1 teaspoon low-sodium soy sauce

Directions:
1. In your slow cooker, mix the green beans with the oil, sugar, soy sauce, and garlic powder, cover, and cook on Low for 2 hours. Toss the beans, divide them between plates, and serve as a side dish.

Nutrition: Calories 46; Fat 3.6g; Sodium 29mg; Carbohydrate 3.6g; Fiber 1.3g; Sugars 0.6g; Protein 0.8g

454. Butter Corn

Preparation time: 10 minutes
Cooking time: 4 hours
Servings: 12
Ingredients:
- 20 ounces fat-free cream cheese
- 10 cups corn
- ½ cup low-fat butter
- ½ cup fat-free milk
- A pinch of black pepper
- 2 tablespoons green onions, chopped

Directions:
1. In your slow cooker, mix the corn with cream cheese, milk, butter, and black pepper, and onions, cook on Low within 4 hours. Toss one more time, divide between plates and serve as a side dish.

Nutrition: Calories 279; Fat 18g; Cholesterol 52mg; Sodium 165mg; Carbohydrate 26g; Fiber 3.5g; Sugars 4.8g; Protein 8.1g

455. Stevia Peas with Marjoram

Preparation time: 10 minutes
Cooking time: 5 hours
Servings: 12
Ingredients:
- 1-pound carrots, sliced
- 1 yellow onion, chopped
- 16 ounces peas

- 2 tablespoons stevia
- 2 tablespoons olive oil
- 4 garlic cloves, minced
- ¼ cup of water
- 1 teaspoon marjoram, dried
- A pinch of white pepper

Directions:
1. In your slow cooker, mix the carrots with water, onion, oil, stevia, garlic, marjoram, white pepper, peas, toss, cover, and cook on High for 5 hours. Divide between plates and serve as a side dish.

Nutrition: Calories 71; Fat 2.5g; Sodium 29mg; Carbohydrate 12.1g; Fiber 3.1g; Sugars 4.4g; Protein 2.5g; Potassium 231mg

456. Colored Iceberg Salad

Preparation time: 10 minutes
Cooking time: 0 minutes
Servings: 4
Ingredients:
- 1 iceberg lettuce head, leaves torn
- 6 bacon slices, cooked and halved
- 2 green onions, sliced
- 3 carrots, shredded
- 6 radishes, sliced
- ¼ cup red vinegar
- ¼ cup olive oil
- 3 garlic cloves, minced
- A pinch of black pepper

Directions:
1. Mix the lettuce leaves with the bacon, green onions, carrots, radishes, vinegar, oil, garlic, and black pepper in a large salad bowl, toss, divide between plates and serve as a side dish.

Nutrition: Calories: 15; Carbs: 3g; Fat: 0g; Protein: 1g; Sodium: 15 mg

457. Fennel Salad with Arugula

Preparation time: 10 minutes
Cooking time: 0 minutes
Servings: 4
Ingredients:
- 2 fennel bulbs, trimmed and shaved
- 1 and ¼ cups zucchini, sliced
- 2/3 cup dill, chopped
- ¼ cup lemon juice
- ¼ cup olive oil
- 6 cups arugula
- ½ cups walnuts, chopped
- 1/3 cup low-fat feta cheese, crumbled

Directions:
1. Mix the fennel with the zucchini, dill, lemon juice, arugula, oil, walnuts, and cheese in a large bowl, toss, and then serve.

Nutrition: Calories: 65; Carbs: 6g; Fat: 5g; Protein: 1g; Sodium: 140 mg

458. Corn Mix

Preparation time: 10 minutes
Cooking time: 0 minutes
Servings: 4
Ingredients:

- ½ cup cider vinegar
- ¼ cup of coconut sugar
- A pinch of black pepper
- 4 cups corn
- ½ cup red onion, chopped
- ½ cup cucumber, sliced
- ½ cup red bell pepper, chopped
- ½ cup cherry tomatoes halved
- 3 tablespoons parsley, chopped
- 1 tablespoon basil, chopped
- 1 tablespoon jalapeno, chopped
- 2 cups baby arugula leaves

Directions:

1. Mix the corn with onion, cucumber, bell pepper, cherry tomatoes, parsley, basil, jalapeno, and arugula in a large bowl. Add vinegar, sugar, and black pepper, toss well, divide between plates and serve as a side dish.

Nutrition: Calories: 110; Carbs: 25g; Fat: 0g; Protein: 2g; Sodium: 120 mg

459. Persimmon Salad

Preparation time: 10 minutes
Cooking time: 0 minutes
Servings: 4
Ingredients:

- Seeds from 1 pomegranate
- 2 persimmons, cored and sliced
- 5 cups baby arugula
- 6 tablespoons green onions, chopped
- 4 navel oranges, cut into segments
- ¼ cup white vinegar
- 1/3 cup olive oil
- 3 tablespoons pine nuts
- 1 and ½ teaspoons orange zest, grated
- 2 tablespoons orange juice
- 1 tablespoon coconut sugar
- ½ shallot, chopped
- A pinch of cinnamon powder

Directions:

1. In a salad bowl, combine the pomegranate seeds with persimmons, arugula, green onions, and oranges and toss. In another bowl, combine the vinegar with the oil, pine nuts, orange zest, orange juice, sugar, shallot, and cinnamon, whisk well, add to the salad, toss and serve as a side dish.

Nutrition: Calories: 310; Carbs: 33g; Fat: 16g; Protein: 7g; Sodium: 320 mg

460. Avocado Side Salad

Preparation time: 10 minutes
Cooking time: 0 minutes

Servings: 4
Ingredients:

- 4 blood oranges, slice into segments
- 2 tablespoons olive oil
- A pinch of red pepper, crushed
- 2 avocados, peeled, cut into wedges
- 1 and ½ cups baby arugula
- ¼ cup almonds, toasted and chopped
- 1 tablespoon lemon juice

Directions:

1. Mix. the oranges with the oil, red pepper, avocados, arugula, almonds, and lemon juice in a bowl, then serve

Nutrition: Calories: 146; Carbs: 8g; Fat: 7g; Protein: 15g; Sodium: 320 mg

461. Spicy Brussels sprouts

Preparation time: 10 minutes
Cooking time: 20 minutes
Servings: 6
Ingredients:

- 2 pounds Brussels sprouts, halved
- 2 tablespoons olive oil
- A pinch of black pepper
- 1 tablespoon sesame oil
- 2 garlic cloves, minced
- ½ cup coconut aminos
- 2 teaspoons apple cider vinegar
- 1 tablespoon coconut sugar
- 2 teaspoons chili sauce
- A pinch of red pepper flakes
- Sesame seeds for serving

Directions:

1. Spread the sprouts on a lined baking dish, add the olive oil, the sesame oil, black pepper, garlic, aminos, vinegar, coconut sugar, chili sauce, and pepper flakes, toss well, introduce in the oven and bake within 20 minutes at 425 degrees F. Divide the sprouts between plates, sprinkle sesame seeds on top and serve as a side dish.

Nutrition: Calories: 64; Carbs: 13g; Fat: 0g; Protein: 4g; Sodium: 314 mg

462. Baked Cauliflower with Chili

Preparation time: 10 minutes
Cooking time: 30 minutes
Servings: 4
Ingredients:

- 3 tablespoons olive oil
- 2 tablespoons chili sauce
- Juice of 1 lime
- 3 garlic cloves, minced
- 1 cauliflower head, florets separated
- A pinch of black pepper
- 1 teaspoon cilantro, chopped

Directions:

1. In a bowl, combine the oil with the chili sauce, lime juice, garlic, and black pepper and whisk. Add cauliflower

florets, toss, spread on a lined baking sheet, introduce in the oven and bake at 425 degrees F for 30 minutes. Divide the cauliflower between plates, sprinkle cilantro on top, and serve as a side dish.

Nutrition: Calories: 31; Carbs: 3g; Fat: 0g; Protein: 3g; Sodium: 4 mg

463. Baked Broccoli

Preparation time: 10 minutes
Cooking time: 15 minutes
Servings: 4
Ingredients:
- 1 tablespoon olive oil
- 1 broccoli head, florets separated
- 2 garlic cloves, minced
- ½ cup coconut cream
- ½ cup low-fat mozzarella, shredded
- ¼ cup low-fat parmesan, grated
- A pinch of pepper flakes, crushed

Directions:
1. In a baking dish, combine the broccoli with oil, garlic, cream, pepper flakes, mozzarella, and toss. Sprinkle the parmesan on top, introduce in the oven and bake at 375 degrees F for 15 minutes. Serve.

Nutrition: Calories: 90; Carbs: 6g; Fat: 7g; Protein: 3g; Sodium: 30 mg

464. Slow Cooked Potatoes with Cheddar

Preparation time: 10 minutes
Cooking time: 6 hours
Servings: 6
Ingredients:
- Cooking spray
- 2 pounds baby potatoes, quartered
- 3 cups low-fat cheddar cheese, shredded
- 2 garlic cloves, minced
- 8 bacon slices, cooked and chopped
- ¼ cup green onions, chopped
- 1 tablespoon sweet paprika
- A pinch of black pepper

Directions:
1. Spray a slow cooker with the cooking spray, add baby potatoes, cheddar, garlic, bacon, green onions, paprika, and black pepper, toss, cover, and cook on High for 6 hours. Serve.

Nutrition: Calories: 112; Carbs: 26g; Fat: 4g; Protein: 8g; Sodium: 234 mg

465. Squash Salad with Orange

Preparation time: 10 minutes
Cooking time: 30 minutes
Servings: 6
Ingredients:

- 1 cup of orange juice
- 3 tablespoons coconut sugar
- 1 and ½ tablespoons mustard
- 1 tablespoon ginger, grated
- 1 and ½ pounds butternut squash, peeled and roughly cubed
- Cooking spray
- A pinch of black pepper
- 1/3 cup olive oil
- 6 cups salad greens
- 1 radicchio, sliced
- ½ cup pistachios, roasted

Directions:
1. Mix the orange juice with the sugar, mustard, ginger, black pepper, squash in a bowl, toss well, spread on a lined baking sheet, spray everything with cooking oil, and bake for 30 minutes 400 degrees F.
2. In a salad bowl, combine the squash with salad greens, radicchio, pistachios, and oil, toss well, and then serve.

Nutrition: Calories: 17; Carbs: 2g; Fat: 0g; Protein: 0g; Sodium: 0 mg

466. Easy Carrots Mix

Preparation time: 10 minutes
Cooking time: 40 minutes
Servings: 6
Ingredients:
- 15 carrots, halved lengthwise
- 2 tablespoons coconut sugar
- ¼ cup olive oil
- ½ teaspoon rosemary, dried
- ½ teaspoon garlic powder
- A pinch of black pepper

Directions:
1. In a bowl, combine the carrots with the sugar, oil, rosemary, garlic powder, and black pepper, toss well, spread on a lined baking sheet, introduce in the oven and bake at 400 degrees F for 40 minutes. Serve.

Nutrition: Calories: 60; Carbs: 9g; Fat: 0g; Protein: 2g; Sodium: 0 mg

467. Tasty Grilled Asparagus

Preparation time: 10 minutes
Cooking time: 6 minutes
Servings: 4
Ingredients:
- 2 pounds asparagus, trimmed
- 2 tablespoons olive oil
- A pinch of salt and black pepper

Directions:
1. In a bowl, combine the asparagus with salt, pepper, and oil and toss well. Place the asparagus on a preheated grill over medium-high heat, cook for 3 minutes on each side, then serve.

Nutrition: Calories: 50; Carbs: 8g; Fat: 1g; Protein: 5g; Sodium: 420 mg

468. Roasted Carrots

Preparation time: 10 minutes
Cooking time: 30 minutes
Servings: 4
Ingredients:
- 2 pounds carrots, quartered
- A pinch of black pepper
- 3 tablespoons olive oil
- 2 tablespoons parsley, chopped

Directions:
1. Arrange the carrots on a lined baking sheet, add black pepper and oil, toss, introduce in the oven, and cook within 30 minutes at 400 degrees F. Add parsley, toss, divide between plates and serve as a side dish.

Nutrition: Calories: 89; Carbs: 10g; Fat: 6g; Protein: 1g; Sodium: 0 mg

469. Oven Roasted Asparagus

Preparation time: 10 minutes
Cooking time: 25 minutes
Servings: 4
Ingredients:
- 2 pounds asparagus spears, trimmed
- 3 tablespoons olive oil
- A pinch of black pepper
- 2 teaspoons sweet paprika
- 1 teaspoon sesame seeds

Directions:
1. Arrange the asparagus on a lined baking sheet, add oil, black pepper, and paprika, toss, introduce in the oven and bake within 25 minutes at 400 degrees F. Divide the asparagus between plates, sprinkle sesame seeds on top, and serve as a side dish.

Nutrition: Calories: 45; Carbs: 5g; Fat: 2g; Protein: 2g; Sodium: 0 mg

470. Baked Potato with Thyme

Preparation time: 10 minutes
Cooking time: 1 hour and 15 minutes
Servings: 8
Ingredients:
- 6 potatoes, peeled and sliced
- 2 garlic cloves, minced
- 2 tablespoons olive oil
- 1 and ½ cups of coconut cream
- ¼ cup of coconut milk
- 1 tablespoon thyme, chopped
- ¼ teaspoon nutmeg, ground
- A pinch of red pepper flakes
- 1 and ½ cups low-fat cheddar, shredded
- ½ cup low-fat parmesan, grated

Directions:
1. Heat-up a pan with the oil over medium heat, add garlic, stir and cook for 1 minute. Add coconut cream, coconut milk, thyme, nutmeg, and pepper flakes, stir, bring to a simmer, adjust to low and cook within 10 minutes.

2. Put one-third of the potatoes in a baking dish, add 1/3 of the cream, repeat the process with the remaining potatoes and the cream, sprinkle the cheddar on top, cover with tin foil, introduce in the oven and cook at 375 degrees F for 45 minutes. Uncover the dish, sprinkle the parmesan, bake everything for 20 minutes, divide between plates, and serve as a side dish.

Nutrition: Calories: 132; Carbs: 21g; Fat: 4g; Protein: 2g; Sodium: 56 mg

471. Italian Roasted Cabbage

Preparation time: 15 minutes
Cooking time: 15 minutes
Servings: 8
Ingredients:
- Cabbage, sliced into 8 wedges – 1
- Black pepper, ground – 1.5 teaspoons
- Extra virgin olive oil - .66 cup
- Italian herb seasoning – 2 teaspoons
- Parmesan cheese, low-sodium, grated - .66 cup

Directions:
1. Warm the oven to Fahrenheit 425 degrees. Prepare a large lined baking sheet with aluminum foil and then spray it with non-stick cooking spray.
2. Slice your cabbage in half, remove the stem, and then cut each half into four wedges so that you are left with eight wedges in total.
3. Arrange the cabbage wedges on the baking sheet and then drizzle half of the extra virgin olive oil over them. Sprinkle half of the seasonings and Parmesan cheese over the top.
4. Place the baking sheet in the hot oven, allow the cabbage to roast for fifteen minutes, and then flip the wedges. Put the rest of the olive oil over the top and then sprinkle the remaining seasonings and cheese over the top as well.
5. Return the cabbage to the oven and allow it to roast for fifteen more minutes, until tender. Serve fresh and hot.

Nutrition: Calories: 17; Carbs: 4g; Fat: 0g; Protein: 1g; Sodium: 27mg; Potassium: 213mg

472. Tex-Mex Cole Slaw

Preparation time: 15 minutes
Cooking time: 0 minutes
Servings: 12
Ingredients:
- Black beans, cooked – 2 cups
- Grape tomatoes, sliced in half – 1.5 cups
- Grilled corn kernels – 1.5 cups
- Jalapeno, seeded and minced – 1
- Cilantro, chopped – .5 cup
- Bell pepper, diced – 1
- Coleslaw cabbage mix – 16 ounces
- Lime juice – 3 tablespoons
- Light sour cream - .66 cup
- Olive oil mayonnaise, reduced-fat – 1 cup
- Chili powder – 1 tablespoon
- Cumin, ground – 1 teaspoon
- Onion powder – 1 teaspoon
- Garlic powder – 1 teaspoon

Directions:

1. Mix the sour cream, mayonnaise, lime juice, garlic powder, onion powder, cumin, and chili powder in a bowl to create the dressing.
2. In a large bowl, toss the vegetables and then add in the prepared dressing and toss again until evenly coated. Chill the mixture in the fridge for thirty minutes to twelve hours before serving.

Nutrition: Calories: 50, Carbs: 10g; Fat: 1g; Protein: 3g; Sodium: 194mg; Potassium: 345mg

473. Roasted Okra

Preparation time: 15 minutes
Cooking time: 20 minutes
Servings: 4
Ingredients:

- Okra, fresh – 1 pound
- Extra virgin olive oil – 2 tablespoons
- Cayenne pepper, ground - .125 teaspoon
- Paprika – 1 teaspoon
- Garlic powder - .25 teaspoon

Directions:

1. Warm the oven to Fahrenheit 450 degrees and prepare a large baking sheet. Cut the okra into pieces appropriate 1/2-inch in size.
2. Place the okra on the baking pan and top it with the olive oil and seasonings, giving it a good toss until evenly coated. Roast the okra in the heated oven until it is tender and lightly browned and seared. Serve immediately while hot.

Nutrition: Calories: 65; Carbs: 6g; Fat: 5g; Protein: 2g; Sodium: 9mg; Potassium: 356mg

474. Brown Sugar Glazed Carrots

Preparation time: 15 minutes
Cooking time: 25 minutes
Servings: 6
Ingredients:

- Carrots, sliced into 1-inch pieces – 2 pounds
- Light olive oil - .33 cup
- Truvia Brown Sugar Blend - .25 cup
- Black pepper, ground - .25 teaspoon

Directions:

1. Warm the oven to Fahrenheit 400 degrees and prepare a large baking sheet. Toss the carrots with the oil, Truvia, and black pepper until evenly coated and then spread them out on the prepared baking sheet.
2. Place the carrots in the oven and allow them to roast until tender, about twenty to twenty-five minutes. Halfway through the cooking time, give the carrots a good serve. Remove the carrots from the oven and serve them alone or topped with fresh parsley.

Nutrition: Calories: 110; Carbs: 16g; Fat: 4g; Protein: 1g; Sodium: 105mg; Potassium: 486mg

475. Oven-Roasted Beets with Honey Ricotta

Preparation time: 15 minutes
Cooking time: 40 minutes
Servings: 6
Ingredients:

- Purple beets – 1 pound
- Golden beets – 1 pound
- Ricotta cheese, low-fat - .5 cup
- Extra virgin olive oil – 3 tablespoons
- Honey – 1 tablespoon
- Rosemary, fresh, chopped – 1 teaspoon
- Black pepper, ground - .25 teaspoon

Directions:

1. Warm the oven to Fahrenheit 375 degrees and prepare a large baking sheet by lining it with kitchen parchment. Slice the beets into 1/2-inch cubes before tossing them with the extra virgin olive oil and black pepper.
2. Put the beets on the prepared baking sheet and allow them to roast until tender, about thirty-five to forty minutes. Halfway through the cooking process, flip the beets over.
3. Meanwhile, in a small bowl, whisk the ricotta with the rosemary and honey. Fridge until ready to serve. Once the beets are done cooking, serve them topped with the ricotta mixture, and enjoy.

Nutrition: Calories: 195; Carbs: 24; Fat: 8g; Protein: 8g; Sodium: 139mg; Potassium: 521mg

476. Creamy Broccoli Cheddar Rice

Preparation time: 15 minutes
Cooking time: 40 minutes
Servings: 6
Ingredients:

- Brown rice – 1 cup
- Chicken broth, low-sodium – 2 cups
- Onion, minced – 1
- Extra virgin olive oil, divided – 3 tablespoons
- Garlic, minced – 2 cloves
- Skim milk - .5 cup
- Black pepper, ground - .25 teaspoon
- Broccoli, chopped – 1.5 cups
- Cheddar cheese, low-sodium, shredded – 1 cup

Directions:

1. Put one tablespoon of the extra virgin olive oil in a large pot and sauté the onion plus garlic over medium heat within two minutes.
2. Put the chicken broth in a pot and wait for it to come to a boil before adding in the rice. Simmer the rice over low heat for twenty-five minutes.
3. Stir the skim milk, black pepper, and remaining two tablespoons of olive oil into the rice. Simmer again within five more minutes. Stir in the broccoli and cook the rice for five more minutes, until the broccoli is tender. Stir in the rice and serve while warm.

Nutrition: Calories: 200, Carbs: 33g, Fat: 3g, Protein: 10g; Sodium: 50mg; Potassium: 344mg

477. Smashed Brussels sprouts

Preparation time: 15 minutes
Cooking time: 40 minutes
Servings: 6
Ingredients:

- Brussels sprouts – 2 pounds
- Garlic, minced – 3 cloves
- Balsamic vinegar – 3 tablespoons
- Extra virgin olive oil - .5 cup
- Black pepper, ground - .5 teaspoon
- Leek washed and thinly sliced – 1
- Parmesan cheese, low-sodium, grated - .5 cup

Directions:

1. Warm the oven to Fahrenheit 450 degrees and prepare two large baking sheets. Trim the yellow leaves and stems off of the Brussels sprouts and then steam them until tender, about twenty to twenty-five minutes.
2. Mix the garlic, black pepper, balsamic vinegar, and extra virgin olive oil in a large bowl. Add the steamed Brussels sprouts and leeks to the bowl and toss until evenly coated.
3. Spread the Brussels sprouts and leaks divided onto the prepared baking sheets.
4. Use a fork or a glass and press down on each of the Brussels sprouts to create flat patties. Put the Parmesan cheese on top and place the smashed sprouts in the oven for fifteen minutes until crispy. Enjoy hot and fresh from the oven.

Nutrition: Calories: 116; Carbs: 11g; Fat: 5g; Protein: 10g; Sodium: 49mg; Potassium: 642mg

478. Cilantro Lime Rice

Preparation time: 15 minutes
Cooking time: 40 minutes
Servings: 6
Ingredients:

- Brown rice – 1.5 cups
- Lime juice – 2 tablespoons
- Lemon juice – 1.5 teaspoons
- Lime zest - .5 teaspoon
- Cilantro, chopped - .25 cup
- Bay leaf – 1
- Extra virgin olive oil – 1 tablespoon
- Water

Directions:

1. Cook rice and bay leaf in a pot with boiling water. Mix the mixture and allow it to boil for thirty minutes, reducing the heat slightly if need be.
2. Once the rice is tender, drain off the water and return the rice to the pot. Let it sit off of the heat within ten minutes. Remove the bay leaf and use a fork to fluff the rice. Stir the rest of the fixing into the rice and then serve immediately.

Nutrition: Calories: 94; Carbs: 15g; Fat: 3g; Protein: 2g; Sodium: 184mg; Potassium: 245mg

479. Corn Salad with Lime Vinaigrette

Preparation time: 15 minutes
Cooking time: 7 minutes
Servings: 6
Ingredients:

- Corn kernels, fresh – 4.5 cups
- Lemon juice – 1 tablespoon
- Red bell pepper, diced – 1
- Grape tomatoes halved – 1 cup
- Cilantro, chopped - .25 cup
- Green onion, chopped - .25 cup
- Jalapeno, diced – 1
- Red onion, thinly sliced - .25
- Feta cheese - .5 cup
- Truvia baking blend – 2 tablespoons
- Extra virgin olive oil – 2 tablespoons
- Honey - .5 tablespoon
- Lime juice – 3 tablespoons
- Black pepper, ground - .125 teaspoon
- Cayenne pepper, ground - .125 teaspoon
- Garlic powder - .125 teaspoon
- Onion powder - .125 teaspoon

Directions:

1. To create your lime vinaigrette, add the lime juice, onion powder, garlic powder, black pepper, cayenne pepper, and honey to a bowl. Mix, then slowly add in the extra virgin olive oil while whisking vigorously.
2. Boil a pot of water and add in the lemon juice, Baking Truvia, and corn kernels. Allow the corn to boil for seven minutes until tender. Strain the boiling water and add the corn kernels to a bowl of ice water to stop the cooking process and cool the kernels. Drain off the ice water and reserve the corn.
3. Add the tomatoes, red pepper, jalapeno, green onion, red onion, cilantro, and cooked corn to a large bowl and toss it until the vegetables are well distributed. Add the feta cheese and vinaigrette to the vegetables and then toss until well combined and evenly coated. Serve immediately.

Nutrition: Calories: 88; Carbs: 23g; Fat: 0g; Protein: 3g; Sodium: 124mg; Potassium: 508mg

480. Mediterranean Chickpea Salad

Preparation time: 15 minutes
Cooking time: 0 minutes
Servings: 6
Ingredients:

- Chickpeas, cooked – 4 cups
- Bell pepper, diced – 2 cups
- Cucumber, chopped – 1 cup
- Tomato, chopped – 1 cup
- Avocado, diced – 1
- Red wine vinegar – 2.5 tablespoons
- Lemon juice – 1 tablespoon
- Extra virgin olive oil – 3 tablespoons

- Parsley, fresh, chopped – 1 teaspoon
- Oregano, dried - .5 teaspoon
- Garlic, minced – 1 teaspoon
- Dill weed, dried - .25 teaspoon
- Black pepper, ground - .25 teaspoon

Directions:

1. Add the diced vegetables except for the avocado and the chickpeas to a large bowl and toss them. In a separate bowl, whisk the seasonings, lemon juice, red wine vinegar, and extra virgin olive oil to create a vinaigrette. Once combined, pour the mixture over the salad and toss to combine.
2. Place the salad in the fridge and allow it to marinate for at least a couple of hours before serving or up to two days. Immediately before serving the salad, dice the avocado and toss it in.

Nutrition: Calories: 120; Carbs: 14g; Fat: 5g; Protein: 4g; Sodium: 15mg; Potassium: 696mg

481. Spanish rice

Preparation time: 15 minutes
Cooking time: 1 hour & 35 minutes
Servings: 8
Ingredients:

- Brown rice – 2 cups
- Extra virgin olive oil – .25 cup
- Garlic, minced – 2 cloves
- Onion, diced – 1
- Tomatoes, diced – 2
- Jalapeno, seeded and diced – 1
- Tomato paste – 1 tablespoon
- Cilantro, chopped - .5 cup
- Chicken broth, low-sodium – 2.5 cups

Directions:

1. Warm the oven to Fahrenheit 375 degrees. Puree the tomatoes, onion, plus garlic using a blender or food processor. Measure out two cups of this vegetable puree to use and discard the excess.
2. Into a large oven-safe Dutch pan, heat the extra virgin olive oil over medium heat until hot and shimmering. Add in the jalapeno and rice to toast, cooking while occasionally stirring for two to three minutes.
3. Slowly stir the chicken broth into the rice, followed by the vegetable puree and tomato paste. Stir until combine and increase the heat to medium-high until the broth reaches a boil.
4. Cover the Dutch pan with an oven-safe lid, transfer the pot to the preheated oven, and bake within 1 hour and 15 minutes. Remove and stir the cilantro into the rice. Serve.

Nutrition: Calories: 265; Sodium: 32mg; Potassium: 322mg; Carbs: 40g; Fat: 3g; Protein: 5g

482. Sweet Potatoes and Apples

Preparation time: 15 minutes
Cooking time: 40 minutes
Servings: 4
Ingredients:

- Sweet potatoes, sliced into 1" cubes – 2
- Apples, cut into 1" cubes – 2
- Extra virgin olive oil, divided – 3 tablespoons
- Black pepper, ground - .25 teaspoon
- Cinnamon, ground – 1 teaspoon
- Maple syrup – 2 tablespoons

Directions:

1. Warm the oven to Fahrenheit 425 degrees and grease a large baking sheet with non-stick cooking spray. Toss the cubed sweet potatoes with two tablespoons of the olive oil and black pepper until coated. Roast the potatoes within twenty minutes, stirring them once halfway through the process.
2. Meanwhile, toss the apples with the remaining tablespoon of olive oil, cinnamon, and maple syrup until evenly coated. After the sweet potatoes have cooked for twenty minutes, add the apples to the baking sheet and toss the sweet potatoes and apples.
3. Return to the oven, then roast it for twenty more minutes, once again giving it a good stir halfway through. Once the potatoes and apples are caramelized from the maple syrup, remove them from the oven and serve hot.

Nutrition: Calories: 100; Carbs: 22g; Fat: 0g; Protein: 2g; Sodium: 38mg; Potassium: 341mg

483. Roasted Turnips

Preparation time: 15 minutes
Cooking time: 30 minutes
Servings: 4
Ingredients:

- Turnips, peels, and cut into ½" cubes – 2 cups
- Black pepper, ground - .25 teaspoon
- Garlic powder - .5 teaspoon
- Onion powder - .5 teaspoon
- Extra virgin olive oil – 1 tablespoon

Directions:

1. Warm the oven to Fahrenheit 400 degrees and prepare a large baking sheet, setting it aside. Begin by trimming the top and bottom edges off of the turnips and peeling them if you wish. Slice them into 1/2-inch cubes.
2. Toss the turnips with the extra virgin olive oil and seasonings and then spread them out on the prepared baking sheet. Roast the turnips until tender, stirring them halfway through, about thirty minutes in total.

Nutrition: Calories: 50; Carbs: 5g; Fat: 4g; Protein: 1g; Sodium: 44mg; Potassium: 134mg

484. No-Mayo Potato Salad

Preparation time: 15 minutes
Cooking time: 20 minutes
Servings: 8
Ingredients:

- Red potatoes – 3 pounds
- Extra virgin olive oil - .5 cup
- White wine vinegar, divided – 5 tablespoons
- Dijon mustard – 2 teaspoons
- Red onion, sliced – 1 cup
- Black pepper, ground - .5 teaspoon
- Basil, fresh, chopped – 2 tablespoons

- Dill weed, fresh, chopped – 2 tablespoons
- Parsley, fresh, chopped – 2 tablespoons

Directions:
1. Add the red potatoes to a large pot and cover them with water until the water level is two inches above the potatoes. Put the pot on high heat, then boil potatoes until they are tender when poked with a fork, about fifteen to twenty minutes. Drain off the water.
2. Let the potatoes to cool until they can easily be handled but are still warm, then cut it in half and put them in a large bowl. Stir in three tablespoons of the white wine vinegar, giving the potatoes a good stir so that they can evenly absorb the vinegar.
3. Mix the rest of two tablespoons of vinegar, extra virgin olive oil, Dijon mustard, and black pepper in a small bowl. Add this mixture to the potatoes and give them a good toss to thoroughly coat the potatoes.
4. Toss in the red onion and minced herbs. Serve at room temperature or chilled. Serve immediately or store in the fridge for up to four days.

Nutrition: Calories: 144; Carbs: 19g; Fat: 7g; Protein: 2g; Sodium: 46m; Potassium: 814mg

485. Zucchini Tomato Bake

Preparation time: 15 minutes
Cooking time: 30 minutes
Servings: 4
Ingredients:
- Grape tomatoes, cut in half – 10 ounces
- Zucchini – 2
- Garlic, minced – 5 cloves
- Italian herb seasoning – 1 teaspoon
- Black pepper, ground - .25 teaspoon
- Parsley, fresh, chopped - .33 cup
- Parmesan cheese, low-sodium, grated - .5 cup

Directions:
1. Warm the oven to Fahrenheit 350 degrees and coat a large baking sheet with non-stick cooking spray. Mix the tomatoes, zucchini, garlic, Italian herb seasoning, Black pepper, and Parmesan cheese in a bowl.
2. Put the mixture out on the baking sheet and roast until the zucchini for thirty minutes. Remove, and garnish with parsley over the top before serving.

Nutrition: Calories: 35; Carbs: 4g; Fat: 2g; Protein: 2g; Sodium: 30mg; Potassium: 649mg

486. Avocado, Tomato, and Olives Salad

Preparation time: 5 minutes
Cooking time: 0 minutes
Servings: 4
Ingredients:
- 2 tablespoons olive oil
- 2 avocados, cut into wedges
- 1 cup Kalamata olives, pitted and halved
- 1 cup tomatoes, cubed
- 1 tablespoon ginger, grated
- A pinch of black pepper

- 2 cups baby arugula
- 1 tablespoon balsamic vinegar

Directions:
1. In a bowl, combine the avocados with the Kalamata and the other ingredients, toss and serve as a side dish.

Nutrition: Calories 320; Protein 3g; Carbohydrates 13.9g; Fat 30.4g; Fiber 8.7g; Sodium 305mg; Potassium 655mg

487. Radish and Olives Salad

Preparation time: 5 minutes
Cooking time: 0 minutes
Servings: 4
Ingredients:
- 2 green onions, sliced
- 1-pound radishes, cubed
- 2 tablespoons balsamic vinegar
- 2 tablespoon olive oil
- 1 teaspoon chili powder
- 1 cup black olives, pitted and halved
- A pinch of black pepper

Directions:
1. Mix radishes with the onions and the other ingredients in a large salad bowl, toss, and serve as a side dish.

Nutrition: Calories 123; Protein 1.3; Carbohydrates 6.9g; Fat 10.8g; Fiber 3.3g; Sodium 345mg; Potassium 306mg

488. Spinach and Endives Salad

Preparation time: 5 minutes
Cooking time: 0 minutes
Servings: 4
Ingredients:
- 2 endives, roughly shredded
- 1 tablespoon dill, chopped
- ¼ cup lemon juice
- ¼ cup olive oil
- 2 cups baby spinach
- 2 tomatoes, cubed
- 1 cucumber, sliced
- ½ cups walnuts, chopped

Directions:
1. In a large bowl, combine the endives with the spinach and the other ingredients, toss and serve as a side dish.

Nutrition: Calories 238; Protein 5.7g; Carbohydrates 8.4g; Fat 22.3g; Fiber 3.1g; Sodium 24mg; Potassium 506mg

489. Basil Olives Mix

Preparation time: 5 minutes
Cooking time: 0 minutes
Servings: 4
Ingredients:
- 2 tablespoons olive oil
- 1 tablespoon balsamic vinegar
- A pinch of black pepper
- 4 cups corn

- 2 cups black olives, pitted and halved
- 1 red onion, chopped
- ½ cup cherry tomatoes halved
- 1 tablespoon basil, chopped
- 1 tablespoon jalapeno, chopped
- 2 cups romaine lettuce, shredded

Directions:
1. Mix the corn with the olives, lettuce, and the other ingredients in a large bowl, toss well, divide between plates and serve as a side dish.

Nutrition: Calories 290; Protein 6.2g; Carbohydrates 37.6g; Fat 16.1g; Fiber 7.4g; Sodium 613mg; Potassium 562mg

490. Arugula Salad

Preparation time: 5 minutes
Cooking time: 0 minutes
Servings: 4
Ingredients:
- ¼ cup pomegranate seeds
- 5 cups baby arugula
- 6 tablespoons green onions, chopped
- 1 tablespoon balsamic vinegar
- 2 tablespoons olive oil
- 3 tablespoons pine nuts
- ½ shallot, chopped

Directions:
1. In a salad bowl, combine the arugula with the pomegranate and the other ingredients, toss and serve.

Nutrition: Calories 120; Protein 1.8g; Carbohydrates 4.2g; Fat 11.6g; Fiber 0.9g; Sodium 9mg; Potassium 163mg

491. Balsamic Cabbage

Preparation time: 10 minutes
Cooking time: 20 minutes
Servings: 4
Ingredients:
- 1-pound green cabbage, roughly shredded
- 2 tablespoons olive oil
- A pinch of black pepper
- 1 shallot, chopped
- 2 garlic cloves, minced
- 2 tablespoons balsamic vinegar
- 2 teaspoons hot paprika
- 1 teaspoon sesame seeds

Directions:
1. Heat-up a pan with the oil over medium heat, add the shallot and the garlic, and sauté for 5 minutes. Add the cabbage and the other ingredients, toss, cook over medium heat for 15 minutes, divide between plates and serve.

Nutrition: Calories 100; Protein 1.8g; Carbohydrates 8.2g; Fat 7.5g; Fiber 3g; Sodium 22mg; Potassium 225mg

492. Chili Broccoli

Preparation time: 10 minutes
Cooking time: 30 minutes

Servings: 4
Ingredients:
- 2 tablespoons olive oil
- 1-pound broccoli florets
- 2 garlic cloves, minced
- 2 tablespoons chili sauce
- 1 tablespoon lemon juice
- A pinch of black pepper
- 2 tablespoons cilantro, chopped

Directions:
1. In a baking pan, combine the broccoli with the oil, garlic, and the other, toss a bit, and bake at 400 degrees F for 30 minutes. Divide the mix between plates and serve as a side dish.

Nutrition: Calories 103; Protein 3.4g; Carbohydrates 8.3gz; 7.4g fat; 3g fiber; Sodium 229mg; Potassium 383mg

493. Hot Brussels sprouts

Preparation time: 10 minutes
Cooking time: 25 minutes
Servings: 4
Ingredients:
- 1 tablespoon olive oil
- 1-pound Brussels sprouts, trimmed and halved
- 2 garlic cloves, minced
- ½ cup low-fat mozzarella, shredded
- A pinch of pepper flakes, crushed

Directions:
1. In a baking dish, combine the sprouts with the oil and the other ingredients except for the cheese and toss. Sprinkle the cheese on top, introduce in the oven and bake at 400 degrees F for 25 minutes. Divide between plates and serve as a side dish.

Nutrition: Calories 111; Protein 10g; Carbohydrates 11.6g; Fat 3.9g; Fiber 5g; Cholesterol 4mg; Sodium 209mg; Potassium 447mg

494. Paprika Brussels sprouts

Preparation time: 10 minutes
Cooking time: 25 minutes
Servings: 4
Ingredients:
- 2 tablespoons olive oil
- 1-pound Brussels sprouts, trimmed and halved
- 3 green onions, chopped
- 2 garlic cloves, minced
- 1 tablespoon balsamic vinegar
- 1 tablespoon sweet paprika
- A pinch of black pepper

Directions:
1. In a baking pan, combine the Brussels sprouts with the oil and the other ingredients, toss and bake at 400 degrees F within 25 minutes. Divide the mix between plates and serve.

Nutrition: Calories 121; Protein 4.4g; Carbohydrates 12.6g; Fat 7.6g; Fiber 5.2g; Sodium 31mg; Potassium 521mg

495. Creamy Cauliflower Mash

Preparation time: 10 minutes
Cooking time: 25 minutes
Servings: 4
Ingredients:
- 2 pounds cauliflower florets
- ½ cup of coconut milk
- A pinch of black pepper
- ½ cup low-fat sour cream
- 1 tablespoon cilantro, chopped
- 1 tablespoon chives, chopped

Directions:
1. Put the cauliflower in a pot, add water to cover, bring to a boil over medium heat, and cook for 25 minutes and drain. Mash the cauliflower, add the milk, black pepper, and the cream, whisk well, divide between plates, sprinkle the rest of the ingredients on top, and serve.

Nutrition: Calories 188; Protein 6.1g; Carbohydrates 15g; Fat 13.4g; Fiber 6.4g; Cholesterol 13mg; Sodium 88mg; Potassium 811mg

496. Turmeric Endives

Preparation time: 10 minutes
Cooking time: 20 minutes
Servings: 4
Ingredients:
- 2 endives, halved lengthwise
- 2 tablespoons olive oil
- 1 teaspoon rosemary, dried
- ½ teaspoon turmeric powder
- A pinch of black pepper

Directions:
1. Mix the endives with the oil and the other ingredients in a baking pan, toss gently, and bake at 400 degrees F within 20 minutes. Serve as a side dish.

Nutrition: Calories 64; Protein 0.2g; Carbohydrates 0.8g; Fat 7.1g; Fiber 0.6g; Sodium 3mg; Potassium 50mg

497. Parmesan Endives

Preparation time: 10 minutes
Cooking time: 20 minutes
Servings: 4
Ingredients:
- 4 endives, halved lengthwise
- 1 tablespoon lemon juice
- 1 tablespoon lemon zest, grated
- 2 tablespoons fat-free parmesan, grated
- 2 tablespoons olive oil
- A pinch of black pepper

Directions:
1. In a baking dish, combine the endives with the lemon juice and the other ingredients except for the parmesan and toss. Sprinkle the parmesan on top, bake the endives at 400 degrees F for 20 minutes, and serve.

Nutrition: Calories 71; Protein 0.9g; Carbohydrates 2.2g; Fat 7.1g; Fiber 0.9g; Sodium 71mg; Potassium 88mg

498. Lemon Asparagus

Preparation time: 10 minutes
Cooking time: 20 minutes
Servings: 4
Ingredients:
- 1-pound asparagus, trimmed
- 2 tablespoons basil pesto
- 1 tablespoon lemon juice
- A pinch of black pepper
- 3 tablespoons olive oil
- 2 tablespoons cilantro, chopped

Directions:
1. Arrange the asparagus n a lined baking sheet, add the pesto and the other ingredients, toss, bake at 400 degrees F within 20 minutes. Serve as a side dish.

Nutrition: Calories 114; Protein 2.6g; Carbohydrates 4.5g; Fat 10.7g; Fiber 2.4g; Sodium 3mg; Potassium 240mg

499. Lime Carrots

Preparation time: 10 minutes
Cooking time: 30 minutes
Servings: 4
Ingredients:
- 1-pound baby carrots, trimmed
- 1 tablespoon sweet paprika
- 1 teaspoon lime juice
- 3 tablespoons olive oil
- A pinch of black pepper
- 1 teaspoon sesame seeds

Directions:
1. Arrange the carrots on a lined baking sheet, add the paprika and the other ingredients except for the sesame seeds, toss, and bake at 400 degrees F within 30 minutes. Divide the carrots between plates, sprinkle sesame seeds on top and serve as a side dish.

Nutrition: Calories 139; Protein 1.1g; Carbohydrates 10.5g; Fat 11.2g; 4g fiber; Sodium 89mg; Potassium 313mg

500. Garlic Potato Pan

Preparation time: 10 minutes
Cooking time: 1 hour
Servings: 8
Ingredients:
- 1-pound gold potatoes, peeled and cut into wedges
- 2 tablespoons olive oil
- 1 red onion, chopped
- 2 garlic cloves, minced
- 2 cups coconut cream
- 1 tablespoon thyme, chopped
- ¼ teaspoon nutmeg, ground
- ½ cup low-fat parmesan, grated

Directions:
1. Warm-up a pan with the oil over medium heat, put the onion plus the garlic, and sauté for 5 minutes. Add the potatoes and brown them for 5 minutes more.
2. Add the cream and the rest of the ingredients, toss gently, bring to a simmer and cook over medium heat within 40

minutes more. Divide the mix between plates and serve as a side dish.

Nutrition: Calories 230; Protein 3.6g; Carbohydrates 14.3g; Fat 19.1g; Fiber 3.3g; Cholesterol 6mg; Sodium 105mg; Potassium 426mg

SEAFOOD

501. Lemon Garlic Shrimp

Preparation time: 15 minutes
Cooking time: 10 minutes
Servings: 4
Ingredients:
1. 2 tablespoons extra-virgin olive oil
2. 3 garlic cloves, sliced
3. ½ teaspoon kosher salt
4. ¼ teaspoon red pepper flakes
5. 1-pound large shrimp, peeled and deveined
6. ½ cup white wine
7. 3 tablespoons fresh parsley, minced
8. Zest of ½ lemon
9. Juice of ½ lemon

Directions:
- Heat-up the olive oil in a wok or large skillet over medium-high heat. Add the garlic, salt, and red pepper flakes and sauté until the garlic starts to brown, 30 seconds to 1 minute.
- Add the shrimp and cook within 2 to 3 minutes on each side. Pour in the wine and deglaze the wok, scraping up any flavorful brown bits, for 1 to 2 minutes. Turn off the heat; mix in the parsley, lemon zest, and lemon juice.

Nutrition: Calories: 200; Fat: 9g; Sodium: 310mg; Carbohydrates: 3g; Protein: 23g

502. Shrimp Fra Diavolo

Preparation time: 15 minutes
Cooking time: 10 minutes
Servings: 4
Ingredients:
1. 2 tablespoons extra-virgin olive oil
2. onion, diced small
3. 1 fennel bulb, cored and diced small, plus ¼ cup fronds for garnish
4. 1 bell pepper, diced small
5. ½ teaspoon dried oregano
6. ½ teaspoon dried thyme
7. ½ teaspoon kosher salt
8. ¼ teaspoon red pepper flakes
9. 1 (14.5-ounce) can no-salt-added diced tomatoes
10. 1-pound shrimp, peeled and deveined
11. Juice of 1 lemon
12. Zest of 1 lemon
13. tablespoons fresh parsley, chopped, for garnish

Directions:
- Heat-up the olive oil in a large skillet or sauté pan over medium heat. Add the onion, fennel, bell pepper, oregano, thyme, salt, and red pepper flakes and sauté until translucent, about 5 minutes.
- Drizzle the pan using the canned tomatoes' juice, scraping up any brown bits, and bringing to a boil. Add the diced

tomatoes and the shrimp. Lower heat to a simmer within 3 minutes.
- Turn off the heat. Add the lemon juice and lemon zest, and toss well to combine. Garnish with the parsley and the fennel fronds.

Nutrition: Calories: 240; Fat: 9g; Sodium: 335mg; Carbohydrates: 13g; Protein: 25g

503. Fish Amandine

Preparation time: 15 minutes
Cooking time: 15 minutes
Servings: 4
Ingredients:
1. 4-ounce skinless tilapia, trout, or halibut fillets, 1/2- to 1-inch thick
2. ¼ cup buttermilk
3. ½ teaspoon dry mustard
4. 1/8 teaspoon crushed red pepper
5. tablespoon butter, melted
6. ¼ teaspoon salt
7. ½ cup panko bread crumbs
8. tbsp. chopped fresh parsley
9. ¼ cup sliced almonds, coarsely chopped
10. tablespoons grated Parmesan cheese

Directions:
1. Defrost fish, if frozen. Preheat oven to 450oF. Grease a shallow baking pan; set aside. Rinse fish; pat dry with paper towels.
2. Pour buttermilk into a shallow dish. In an extra shallow dish, mix bread crumbs, dry mustard, parsley, and salt. Soak fish into buttermilk, then into crumb mixture, turning to coat. Put coated fish in the ready baking pan.
3. Flavor the fish with almonds plus Parmesan cheese; drizzle with melted butter. Sprinkle with crinkled red pepper. Bake for 5 minutes per 1/2-inch thickness of fish or until fish flakes easily when checked with a fork.

Nutrition: Calories 209; Fat 8.7 g; Sodium 302 mg; Carbohydrates 6.7 g; Protein 26.2 g

504. Air-Fryer Fish Cakes

Preparation time: 15 minutes
Cooking time: 10 minutes
Servings: 2
Ingredients:
- Cooking spray
- 10 oz. finely chopped white fish
- 2/3 cup whole-wheat panko breadcrumbs
- 3 tablespoons finely chopped fresh Cilantro
- 2 tablespoons Thai sweet chili sauce
- 2 tablespoons canola mayonnaise
- large egg

- 1/8 teaspoon salt
- ¼ teaspoon ground pepper
- lime wedges

Directions:
3. Oiled the basket of an air fryer with cooking spray. Put fish, cilantro, panko, chili sauce, egg, mayonnaise, pepper, and salt in a medium bowl; stir until well mixed. Shape the mixture into four 3-inch-diameter cakes.
4. Oiled the cakes with cooking spray; place in the basket. Cook at 400oF until the cakes are browned for 9 to 10 minutes. Serve with lime wedges.

Nutrition: Calories 399; Fat 15.5 g; Sodium 537 mg; Carbohydrates 27.9 g; Protein 34.6 g

505. Pesto Shrimp Pasta

Preparation time: 15 minutes
Cooking time: 12 minutes
Servings: 4
Ingredients:
- 1/8 teaspoon freshly cracked pepper
- cup dried orzo
- 4 tsp. packaged pesto sauce mix
- 1 lemon, halved
- 1/8 teaspoon coarse salt
- 1-pound medium shrimp, thawed
- 1 medium zucchini, halved lengthwise and sliced
- tablespoons olive oil, divided
- 1-ounce shaved Parmesan cheese

Directions:
- Prepare orzo pasta concerning package directions. Drain; reserving ¼ cup of the pasta cooking water. Mix 1 teaspoon of the pesto mix into the kept cooking water and set aside.
- Mix 3 teaspoons of the pesto mix plus 1 tablespoon of the olive oil in a large plastic bag. Seal and shake to mix. Put the shrimp in the bag; seal and turn to coat. Set aside.
- Sauté zucchini in a big skillet over moderate heat for 1 to 2 minutes, stirring repeatedly. Put the pesto-marinated shrimp in the skillet and cook for 5 minutes or until shrimp is dense.
- Put the cooked pasta in the skillet with the zucchini and shrimp combination. Stir in the kept pasta water until absorbed, grating up any seasoning in the bottom of the pan. Season with pepper and salt. Squeeze the lemon over the pasta. Top with Parmesan, then serve.

Nutrition: Calories 361; Fat 10.1 g; Sodium 502 mg; Carbohydrates 35.8 g; Protein 31.6 g

506. Monkfish with Sautéed Leeks, Fennel, and Tomatoes

Preparation time: 15 minutes
Cooking time: 35 minutes
Servings: 4
Ingredients:
- to 1½ pounds monkfish
- tablespoons lemon juice, divided

- teaspoon kosher salt, divided
- 1/8 teaspoon freshly ground black pepper
- tablespoons extra-virgin olive oil
- 1 leek, sliced in half lengthwise and thinly sliced
- ½ onion, julienned
- garlic cloves, minced
- bulbs fennel, cored and thinly sliced, plus ¼ cup fronds for garnish
- 1 (14.5-ounce) can no-salt-added diced tomatoes
- tablespoons fresh parsley, chopped
- 2 tablespoons fresh oregano, chopped
- ¼ teaspoon red pepper flakes

Directions:
1. Place the fish in a medium baking dish and add 2 tablespoons of the lemon juice, ¼ teaspoon of the salt, plus the black pepper. Place in the refrigerator.
2. Warm-up olive oil in a large skillet over medium heat, then put the leek and onion and sauté until translucent, about 3 minutes. Add the garlic and sauté within 30 seconds. Add the fennel and sauté 4 to 5 minutes. Add the tomatoes and simmer for 2 to 3 minutes.
3. Stir in the parsley, oregano, red pepper flakes, the remaining ¾ teaspoon salt, and the remaining 1 tablespoon lemon juice. Put the fish over the leek mixture, cover, and simmer for 20 to 25 minutes. Garnish with the fennel fronds.

Nutrition: Calories: 220; Fat: 9g; Sodium: 345mg; Carbohydrates: 11g; Protein: 22g

507. Caramelized Fennel and Sardines with Penne

Preparation time: 15 minutes
Cooking time: 30 minutes
Servings: 4
Ingredients:
- 8 ounces whole-wheat penne
- 2 tablespoons extra-virgin olive oil
- bulb fennel, cored and thinly sliced, plus ¼ cup fronds
- celery stalks, thinly sliced, plus ½ cup leaves
- garlic cloves, sliced
- ¾ teaspoon kosher salt
- ¼ teaspoon freshly ground black pepper
- Zest of 1 lemon
- Juice of 1 lemon
- 2 (4.4-ounce) cans boneless/skinless sardines packed in olive oil, undrained

Directions:
1. Cook the penne, as stated in the package directions. Drain, reserving 1 cup of pasta water. Warm-up olive oil in a large skillet over medium heat, then put the fennel and celery and cook within 10 to 12 minutes. Add the garlic and cook within 1 minute.
2. Add the penne, reserved pasta water, salt, and black pepper. Adjust the heat to medium-high and cook for 1 to 2 minutes.
3. Remove, then stir in the lemon zest, lemon juice, fennel fronds, and celery leaves. Break the sardines into bite-size pieces and gently mix in, along with the oil they were packed in.

Nutrition: Calories: 400; Fat: 15g; Sodium: 530mg; Carbohydrates: 46g; Protein: 22g

508. Coppin

Preparation time: 15 minutes
Cooking time: 35 minutes
Servings: 4
Ingredients:

- 2 tablespoons extra-virgin olive oil
- onion, diced
- bulb fennel, chopped, plus ½ cup fronds for garnish
- 1-quart no-salt-added vegetable stock
- 4 garlic cloves, smashed
- 8 thyme sprigs
- teaspoon kosher salt
- ¼ teaspoon red pepper flakes
- dried bay leaf
- bunch kale, stemmed and chopped
- dozen littleneck clams tightly closed, scrubbed
- 1-pound fish (cod, halibut, and bass are all good choices)
- ¼ cup fresh parsley, chopped

Directions:
1. Heat-up the olive oil in a large stockpot over medium heat. Add the onion and fennel and sauté for about 5 minutes. Add the vegetable stock, garlic, thyme, salt, red pepper flakes, and bay leaf. Adjust the heat to medium-high, and simmer. Add the kale, cover, and simmer within 5 minutes.
2. Carefully add the clams, cover, and simmer about 15 minutes until they open. Remove the clams and set aside. Discard any clams that do not open.
3. Add the fish, cover, and simmer within 5 to 10 minutes, depending on the fish's thickness, until opaque and easily separated. Gently mix in the parsley. Divide the cioppino among 4 bowls. Place 3 clams in each bowl and garnish with the fennel fronds.

Nutrition: Calories: 285; Fat: 9g; Sodium: 570mg; Carbohydrates: 19g; Protein: 32g

509. Green Goddess Crab Salad with Endive

Preparation time: 15 minutes
Cooking time: 10 minutes
Servings: 4
Ingredients:

- 1-pound lump crabmeat
- 2/3 cup plain Greek yogurt
- 3 tablespoons mayonnaise
- 3 tablespoons fresh chives, chopped, plus additional for garnish
- 3 tablespoons fresh parsley, chopped, plus extra for garnish
- 3 tablespoons fresh basil, chopped, plus extra for garnish
- Zest of 1 lemon
- Juice of 1 lemon
- ½ teaspoon kosher salt
- ¼ teaspoon freshly ground black pepper
- 4 endives, ends cut off and leaves separated

Directions:

1. In a medium bowl, combine the crab, yogurt, mayonnaise, chives, parsley, basil, lemon zest, lemon juice, salt, plus black pepper and mix until well combined.
2. Place the endive leaves on 4 salad plates. Divide the crab mixture evenly on top of the endive. Garnish with additional herbs, if desired.

Nutrition: Calories: 200; Fat: 9g; Sodium: 570mg; Carbohydrates: 44g; Protein: 25g

510. Seared Scallops with Blood Orange Glaze

Preparation time: 15 minutes
Cooking time: 20 minutes
Servings: 4
Ingredients:

- 3 tablespoons extra-virgin olive oil, divided
- 3 garlic cloves, minced
- ½ teaspoon kosher salt, divided
- 4 blood oranges, juiced
- teaspoon blood orange zest
- ½ teaspoon red pepper flakes
- 1-pound scallops, small side muscle removed
- ¼ teaspoon freshly ground black pepper
- ¼ cup fresh chives, chopped

Directions:
1. Heat-up 1 tablespoon of the olive oil in a small saucepan over medium-high heat. Add the garlic and ¼ teaspoon of the salt and sauté for 30 seconds.
2. Add the orange juice and zest, bring to a boil, reduce the heat to medium-low, and cook within 20 minutes, or until the liquid reduces by half and becomes a thicker syrup consistency. Remove and mix in the red pepper flakes.
3. Pat the scallops dry with a paper towel and season with the remaining ¼ teaspoon salt and the black pepper. Heat-up the remaining 2 tablespoons of olive oil in a large skillet on medium-high heat. Add the scallops gently and sear.
4. Cook on each side within 2 minutes. If cooking in 2 batches, use 1 tablespoon of oil per batch. Serve the scallops with the blood orange glaze and garnish with the chives.

Nutrition: Calories: 140; Fat: 4g; Sodium: 570mg; Carbohydrates: 12g; Protein: 15g

511. Flounder with Tomatoes and Basil

Preparation time: 15 minutes
Cooking time: 20 minutes
Servings: 4
Ingredients:

- 1-pound cherry tomatoes
- 4 garlic cloves, sliced
- 2 tablespoons extra-virgin olive oil
- 2 tablespoons lemon juice
- 2 tablespoons basil, cut into ribbons
- ½ teaspoon kosher salt
- ¼ teaspoon freshly ground black pepper

- 4 (5- to 6-ounce) flounder fillets

Directions:
1. Preheat the oven to 425°F.
2. Mix the tomatoes, garlic, olive oil, lemon juice, basil, salt, and black pepper in a baking dish. Bake for 5 minutes.
3. Remove, then arrange the flounder on top of the tomato mixture. Bake until the fish is opaque and begins to flake, about 10 to 15 minutes, depending on thickness.

Nutrition: Calories: 215; Fat: 9g; Sodium: 261mg; Carbohydrates: 6g; Protein: 28g

512. Grilled Mahi-Mahi with Artichoke Caponata

Preparation time: 15 minutes
Cooking time: 30 minutes
Servings: 4
Ingredients:
- 2 tablespoons extra-virgin olive oil
- 2 celery stalks, diced
- onion, diced
- garlic cloves, minced
- ½ cup cherry tomatoes, chopped
- ¼ cup white wine
- tablespoons white wine vinegar
- 1 can artichoke hearts, drained and chopped
- ¼ cup green olives, pitted and chopped
- 1 tablespoon capers, chopped
- ¼ teaspoon red pepper flakes
- 2 tablespoons fresh basil, chopped
- (5- to 6-ounces each) skinless mahi-mahi fillets
- ½ teaspoon kosher salt
- ¼ teaspoon freshly ground black pepper
- Olive oil cooking spray

Directions:
1. Warm-up olive oil in a skillet over medium heat, then put the celery and onion, and sauté 4 to 5 minutes. Add the garlic and sauté 30 seconds. Add the tomatoes and cook within 2 to 3 minutes. Add the wine and vinegar to deglaze the pan, increasing the heat to medium-high.
2. Add the artichokes, olives, capers, and red pepper flakes and simmer, reducing the liquid by half, about 10 minutes. Mix in the basil.
3. Season the mahi-mahi with salt and pepper. Heat a grill skillet or grill pan over medium-high heat and coat with olive oil cooking spray. Add the fish and cook within 4 to 5 minutes per side. Serve topped with the artichoke caponata.

Nutrition: Calories: 245; Fat: 9g; Sodium: 570mg; Carbohydrates: 10g; Protein: 28g

513. Cod and Cauliflower Chowder

Preparation time: 15 minutes
Cooking time: 40 minutes
Servings: 4
Ingredients:
- 2 tablespoons extra-virgin olive oil

- leek, sliced thinly
- 4 garlic cloves, sliced
- 1 medium head cauliflower, coarsely chopped
- 1 teaspoon kosher salt
- ¼ teaspoon freshly ground black pepper
- pints cherry tomatoes
- cups no-salt-added vegetable stock
- ¼ cup green olives, pitted and chopped
- 1 to 1½ pounds cod
- ¼ cup fresh parsley, minced

Directions:
1. Heat-up the olive oil in a Dutch oven or large pot over medium heat. Add the leek and sauté until lightly golden brown, about 5 minutes.
2. Add the garlic and sauté within 30 seconds. Add the cauliflower, salt, and black pepper and sauté 2 to 3 minutes.
3. Add the tomatoes and vegetable stock, increase the heat to high and boil, then turn the heat to low and simmer within 10 minutes.
4. Add the olives and mix. Add the fish, cover, and simmer 20 minutes or until fish is opaque and flakes easily. Gently mix in the parsley.

Nutrition: Calories: 270; Fat: 9g; Sodium: 545mg; Potassium: 1475mg; Carbohydrates: 19g; Protein: 30g

514. Sardine Bruschetta with Fennel and Lemon Cream

Preparation time: 15 minutes
Cooking time: 0 minutes
Servings: 4
Ingredients:
- 1/3 cup plain Greek yogurt
- 2 tablespoons mayonnaise
- 2 tablespoons lemon juice, divided
- 2 teaspoons lemon zest
- ¾ teaspoon kosher salt, divided
- fennel bulb, cored and thinly sliced
- ¼ cup parsley, chopped, plus more for garnish
- ¼ cup fresh mint, chopped2 teaspoons extra-virgin olive oil
- 1/8 teaspoon freshly ground black pepper
- 8 slices multigrain bread, toasted
- (4.4-ounce) cans of smoked sardines

Directions:
1. Mix the yogurt, mayonnaise, 1 tablespoon of the lemon juice, the lemon zest, and ¼ teaspoon of the salt in a small bowl.
2. Mix the remaining ½ teaspoon salt, the remaining 1 tablespoon lemon juice, the fennel, parsley, mint, olive oil, and black pepper in a separate small bowl.
3. Spoon 1 tablespoons of the yogurt mixture on each piece of toast. Divide the fennel mixture evenly on top of the yogurt mixture. Divide the sardines among the toasts, placing them on top of the fennel mixture. Garnish with more herbs, if desired.

Nutrition: Calories: 400; Fat: 16g; Sodium: 565mg; Carbohydrates: 51g; Protein: 16g

515. Chopped Tuna Salad

Preparation time: 15 minutes
Cooking time: 0 minutes
Servings: 4
Ingredients:

- 2 tablespoons extra-virgin olive oil
- 2 tablespoons lemon juice
- 2 teaspoons Dijon mustard
- ½ teaspoon kosher salt
- ¼ teaspoon freshly ground black pepper
- 12 olives, pitted and chopped
- ½ cup celery, diced
- ½ cup red onion, diced
- ½ cup red bell pepper, diced
- ½ cup fresh parsley, chopped
- 2 (6-ounce) cans no-salt-added tuna packed in water, drained
- 6 cups baby spinach

Directions:
1. Mix the olive oil, lemon juice, mustard, salt, and black pepper in a medium bowl. Add in the olives, celery, onion, bell pepper, and parsley and mix well. Add the tuna and gently incorporate. Divide the spinach evenly among 4 plates or bowls. Spoon the tuna salad evenly on top of the spinach.

Nutrition: Calories: 220; Fat: 11g; Sodium: 396mg; Carbohydrates: 7g; Protein: 25g

516. Shrimp, Snow Peas and Bamboo Soup

Preparation time: 10 minutes
Cooking time: 10 minutes
Servings: 4
Ingredients:

- 4 scallions, chopped
- and ½ tablespoons olive oil
- 1 teaspoon garlic, minced
- 8 cups low-sodium chicken stock
- ¼ cup coconut aminos
- 5 ounces canned bamboo shoots, no-salt-added sliced
- Black pepper to the taste
- 1 pound shrimp, peeled and deveined
- ½ pound snow peas

Directions:
1. Heat up a pot with the oil over medium heat, add scallions and ginger, stir and cook for 2 minutes.
2. Add coconut aminos, stock and black pepper, stir and bring to a boil.
3. Add shrimp, snow peas and bamboo shoots, stir, cook for 5 minutes, ladle into bowls and serve.
4. Enjoy!

Nutrition: Calories 200, Fat 3, Fiber 2, Carbs 4, Protein 14

517. Lemony Mussels

Preparation time: 5 minutes
Cooking time: 5 minutes

Servings: 4
Ingredients:

- 2 pound mussels, scrubbed
- 2 garlic cloves, minced
- tablespoon olive oil
- Juice of 1 lemon

Directions:
1. Put some water in a pot, add mussels, bring to a boil over medium heat, cook for 5 minutes, discard unopened mussels and transfer them to a bowl.
2. In another bowl, mix the oil with garlic and lemon juice, whisk well, and add over the mussels, toss and serve.
3. Enjoy!

Nutrition: Calories 140, Fat 4, Fiber 4, Carbs 8, Protein 8

518. Citrus-Glazed Salmon with Zucchini Noodles

Preparation time: 15 minutes
Cooking time: 20 minutes
Servings: 4
Ingredients:

- 4 (5- to 6-ounce) pieces salmon
- ½ teaspoon kosher salt
- ¼ teaspoon freshly ground black pepper
- tablespoon extra-virgin olive oil
- cup freshly squeezed orange juice
- 1 teaspoon low-sodium soy sauce
- zucchinis (about 16 ounces), spiralized
- 1 tablespoon fresh chives, chopped
- 1 tablespoon fresh parsley, chopped

Directions:
1. Preheat the oven to 350°F. Flavor the salmon with salt plus black pepper. Heat-up the olive oil in a large oven-safe skillet or sauté pan over medium-high heat. Add the salmon, skin-side down, and sear for 5 minutes, or until the skin is golden brown and crispy.
2. Flip the salmon over, then transfer to the oven until your desired doneness is reached—about 5 minutes. Place the salmon on a cutting board to rest.
3. Place the same pan on the stove over medium-high heat. Add the orange juice and soy sauce to deglaze the pan. Bring to a simmer, scraping up any brown bits, and simmering 5 to 7 minutes.
4. Split or divide the zucchini noodles into 4 plates and place 1 piece of salmon on each. Pour the orange glaze over the salmon and zucchini noodles. Garnish with the chives and parsley.

Nutrition: Calories: 280; Fat: 13g; Sodium: 255mg; Carbohydrates: 11g; Protein: 30g

519. Salmon Cakes with Bell Pepper plus Lemon Yogurt

Preparation time: 15 minutes
Cooking time: 15 minutes
Servings: 4
Ingredients:

- ¼ cup whole-wheat bread crumbs
- ¼ cup mayonnaise

- large egg, beaten
- 1 tablespoon chives, chopped
- 1 tablespoon fresh parsley, chopped
- Zest of 1 lemon
- ¾ teaspoon kosher salt, divided
- ¼ teaspoon freshly ground black pepper
- (5- to 6-ounce) cans no-salt boneless/skinless salmon, drained and finely flaked
- ½ bell pepper, diced small tablespoons extra-virgin olive oil, divided
- 1 cup plain Greek yogurt
- Juice of 1 lemon

Directions:

1. Mix the bread crumbs, mayonnaise, egg, chives, parsley, lemon zest, ½ teaspoon of salt, and black pepper in a large bowl. Add the salmon and the bell pepper and stir gently until well combined. Shape the mixture into 8 patties.
2. Heat-up 1 tablespoon of the olive oil in a large skillet over medium-high heat. Cook half the cakes until the bottoms are golden brown, 4 to 5 minutes. Adjust the heat to medium if the bottoms start to burn.
3. Flip the cakes and cook until golden brown, an additional 4 to 5 minutes. Repeat process with the rest of the 1 tablespoon olive oil and the rest of the cakes.
4. Mix the yogurt, lemon juice, and the remaining ¼ teaspoon salt in a small bowl. Serve with the salmon cakes.

Nutrition: Calories: 330; Fat: 23g; Sodium: 385mg; Carbohydrates: 9g; Protein: 21g

520. Halibut in Parchment with Zucchini, Shallots, and Herbs

Preparation time: 15 minutes
Cooking time: 15 minutes
Servings: 4
Ingredients:

- ½ cup zucchini, diced small
- shallot, minced
- 4 (5-ounce) halibut fillets (about 1 inch thick)
- 4 teaspoons extra-virgin olive oil
- ¼ teaspoon kosher salt
- 1/8 teaspoon freshly ground black pepper
- 1 lemon, sliced into 1/8 -inch-thick rounds
- 8 sprigs of thyme

Directions:

1. Preheat the oven to 450°F. Combine the zucchini and shallots in a medium bowl. Cut 4 (15-by-24-inch) pieces of parchment paper. Fold each sheet in half horizontally.
2. Draw a large half heart on one side of each folded sheet, with the fold along the heart center. Cut out the heart, open the parchment, and lay it flat.
3. Place a fillet near the center of each parchment heart. Drizzle 1 teaspoon olive oil on each fillet. Sprinkle with salt and pepper. Top each fillet with lemon slices and 2 sprigs of thyme. Sprinkle each fillet with one-quarter of the zucchini and shallot mixture. Fold the parchment over.

4. Starting at the top, fold the parchment edges over, and continue all the way around to make a packet. Twist the end tightly to secure. Arrange the 4 packets on a baking sheet. Bake for about 15 minutes. Place on plates; cut open. Serve immediately.

Nutrition: Calories: 190; Fat: 7g; Sodium: 170mg; Carbohydrates: 5g; Protein: 27g

521. Basil Tilapia

Preparation time: 10 minutes
Cooking time: 10 minutes
Servings: 4
Ingredients:

- 4 tilapia fillets, boneless
- Black pepper to the taste
- ½ cup low-fat parmesan, grated
- 4 tablespoons avocado mayonnaise
- 2 teaspoons basil, dried
- 2 tablespoons lemon juice
- ¼ cup olive oil

Directions:

1. Grease a baking dish with the oil, add tilapia fillets, black pepper, spread mayo, basil, drizzle lemon juice and top with the parmesan, introduce in preheated broiler and cook over medium-high heat for 5 minutes on each side.
2. Divide between plates and serve with a side salad.
3. Enjoy!

Nutrition: Calories 215, Fat 10, Fiber 5, Carbs 7, Protein 11

522. Salmon Meatballs with Garlic

Preparation time: 10 minutes
Cooking time: 30 minutes
Servings: 4
Ingredients:

- Cooking spray
- 2 garlic cloves, minced
- yellow onion, chopped
- 1 pound wild salmon, boneless and minced
- ¼ cup chives, chopped
- 1 egg
- tablespoons Dijon mustard
- 1 tablespoon coconut flour
- A pinch of salt and black pepper

Directions:

1. In a bowl, mix onion with garlic, salmon, chives, coconut flour, salt, pepper, mustard and egg, stir well, shape medium meatballs, arrange them on a baking sheet, grease them with cooking spray, introduce in the oven at 350 degrees F and bake for 25 minutes.
2. Divide the meatballs between plates and serve with a side salad.
3. Enjoy!

Nutrition: Calories 211, Fat 4, Fiber 1, Carbs 6, Protein 13

523. Tuna Cakes

Preparation time: 10 minutes

Cooking time: 10 minutes
Servings: 12
Ingredients:

- 15 ounces canned tuna, drain well and flaked
- 3 eggs
- ½ teaspoon dill, dried
- teaspoon parsley, dried
- ½ cup red onion, chopped
- 1 teaspoon garlic powder
- A pinch of salt and black pepper
- Olive oil for frying

Directions:

1. In a bowl, mix tuna with salt, pepper, dill, parsley, onion, garlic powder and eggs, stir and shape medium cakes out of this mix.
2. Heat up a pan with oil over medium-high heat, add tuna cakes, cook for 5 minutes on each side, divide between plates and serve with a side salad.
3. Enjoy!

Nutrition: Calories 210, Fat 2, Fiber 2, Carbs 6, Protein 6

524. Spiced Cod Mix

Preparation time: 10 minutes
Cooking time: 25 minutes
Servings: 4
Ingredients:

- 4 cod fillets, skinless and boneless
- ½ teaspoon mustard seeds
- A pinch of black pepper
- 2 green chilies, chopped
- teaspoon ginger, grated
- 1 teaspoon curry powder
- ¼ teaspoon cumin, ground
- 4 tablespoons olive oil
- 1 teaspoon turmeric powder
- 1 red onion, chopped
- ¼ cup cilantro, chopped
- 1 and ½ cups coconut cream
- garlic cloves, minced

Directions:

1. Heat up a pot with half of the oil over medium heat, add mustard seeds, ginger, onion and garlic, stir and cook for 5 minutes.
2. Add turmeric, curry powder, chilies and cumin, stir and cook for 5 minutes more.
3. Add coconut milk, salt and pepper, stir, bring to a boil and cook for 15 minutes.
4. Heat up another pan with the rest of the oil over medium heat, add fish, stir, cook for 3 minutes, add over the curry mix, also add cilantro, toss, cook for 5 minutes more, divide into bowls and serve.
5. Enjoy!

Nutrition: Calories 200, Fat 14, Fiber 7, Carbs 6, Protein 9

525. Italian Shrimp

Preparation time: 10 minutes
Cooking time: 22 minutes
Servings: 4

Ingredients:

- 8 ounces mushrooms, chopped
- asparagus bunch, cut into medium pieces
- pound shrimp, peeled and deveined
- Black pepper to the taste
- tablespoons olive oil
- teaspoons Italian seasoning
- 1 yellow onion, chopped
- 1 teaspoon red pepper flakes, crushed
- 1 cup low-fat parmesan cheese, grated
- garlic cloves, minced
- 1 cup coconut cream

Directions:

1. Put water in a pot, bring to a boil over medium heat, add asparagus, steam for 2 minutes, transfer to a bowl with ice water, drain and put in a bowl.
2. Heat up a pan with the oil over medium heat, add onions and mushrooms, stir and cook for 7 minutes.
3. Add pepper flakes, Italian seasoning, black pepper and asparagus, stir and cook for 5 minutes more.
4. Add cream, shrimp, garlic and parmesan, toss, cook for 7 minutes, divide into bowls and serve.
5. Enjoy!

Nutrition: Calories 225, Fat 6, Fiber 5, Carbs 6, Protein 8

526. Salmon with Mushroom

Preparation time: 30 minutes
Cooking time: 10 minutes
Servings: 4
Ingredients:

- 8 ounces salmon fillets, boneless
- 2 tablespoons olive oil
- Black pepper to the taste
- 2 ounces white mushrooms, sliced
- ½ shallot, chopped
- 2 tablespoons balsamic vinegar
- 2 teaspoons mustard
- 3 tablespoons parsley, chopped

Directions:

1. Brush salmon fillets with 1 tablespoon olive oil, season with black pepper, place on preheated grill over medium heat, cook for 4 minutes on each side and divide between plates.
2. Heat up a pan with the rest of the oil over medium-high heat, add mushrooms, shallot and some black pepper, stir and cook for 5 minutes.
3. Add the mustard, the vinegar and the parsley, stir, cook for 2-3 minutes more, add over the salmon and serve.
4. Enjoy!

Nutrition: Calories 220, Fat 4, Fiber 8, Carbs 6, Protein 12

527. Cod Sweet Potato Chowder

Preparation time: 10 minutes
Cooking time: 20 minutes
Servings: 4
Ingredients:

- 3 cups sweet potatoes, cubed

- 4 cod fillets, skinless and boneless
- cup celery, chopped
- 1 cup onion, chopped
- Black pepper to the taste
- tablespoons garlic, minced
- tablespoons olive oil
- 2 tablespoons tomato paste, no-salt-added
- cups veggie stock
- 1 and ½ cups tomatoes, chopped
- 1 and ½ teaspoons thyme

Directions:
1. Heat up a pot with the oil over medium heat, add tomato paste, celery, onion and garlic, stir and cook for 5 minutes.
2. Add tomatoes, tomato paste, potatoes and pepper, stir, bring to a boil, reduce heat and cook for 10 minutes.
3. Add thyme and cod, stir, cook for 5 minutes more, ladle into bowls and serve.
4. Enjoy!

Nutrition: Calories 250, Fat 6, Fiber 5, Carbs 7, Protein 12

528. Salmon with Cinnamon

Preparation time: 10 minutes
Cooking time: 10 minutes
Servings: 2
Ingredients:
- 2 salmon fillets, boneless and skin-on
- Black pepper to the taste
- tablespoon cinnamon powder
- 1 tablespoon olive oil

Directions:
1. Heat up a pan with the oil over medium heat, add pepper and cinnamon and stir well.
2. Add salmon, skin side up, cook for 5 minutes on each side, divide between plates and serve with a side salad.
3. Enjoy!

Nutrition: Calories 220, Fat 8, Fiber 4, Carbs 11, Protein 8

529. Scallops and Strawberry Mix

Preparation time: 10 minutes
Cooking time: 6 minutes
Servings: 2
Ingredients:
- 4 ounces scallops
- ½ cup Pico de Gallo
- ½ cup strawberries, chopped
- tablespoon lime juice
- Black pepper to the taste

Directions:
1. Heat up a pan over medium heat, add scallops, cook for 3 minutes on each side and take off heat,
2. In a bowl, mix strawberries with lime juice, Pico de Gallo, scallops and pepper, toss and serve cold.
3. Enjoy!

Nutrition: Calories 169, Fat 2, Fiber 2, Carbs 8, Protein 13

530. Baked Haddock with Avocado Mayonnaise

Preparation time: 10 minutes
Cooking time: 30 minutes
Servings: 4
Ingredients:
- pound haddock, boneless
- teaspoons water
- tablespoons lemon juice
- A pinch of salt and black pepper
- 2 tablespoons avocado mayonnaise
- teaspoon dill, chopped
- Cooking spray

Directions:
1. Spray a baking dish with some cooking oil, add fish, water, lemon juice, salt, black pepper, mayo and dill, toss, introduce in the oven and bake at 350 degrees F for 30 minutes.
2. Divide between plates and serve.
3. Enjoy!

Nutrition: Calories 264, Fat 4, Fiber 5, Carbs 7, Protein 12

531. Salmon Casserole

Preparation time: 10 minutes
Cooking time: 1 hour
Servings: 4
Ingredients:
- 8 sweet potatoes, sliced
- 4 cups salmon, cooked and flaked
- red onion, chopped
- carrots, chopped
- Black pepper to the taste
- celery stalk, chopped
- cups coconut milk
- tablespoons olive oil
- tablespoons chives, chopped
- garlic cloves, minced

Directions:
1. Heat up a pan with the oil over medium heat, add garlic, stir and cook for 1 minute.
2. Add coconut milk, black pepper, carrots, celery, chives, onion and salmon, stir and take off heat.
3. Arrange a layer of potatoes in a baking dish, add the salmon mix, top with the rest of the potatoes, introduce in the oven and bake at 375 degrees F for 1 hour.
4. Slice, divide between plates and serve.
5. Enjoy!

Nutrition: Calories 220, Fat 9, Fiber 6, Carbs 8, Protein 12

532. Scallops, Sweet Potatoes and Cauliflower Mix

Preparation time: 10 minutes
Cooking time: 10 minutes
Servings: 4
Ingredients:

- 12 sea scallops
- 3 garlic cloves, minced
- Black pepper to the taste
- 2 cups cauliflower florets, chopped
- 2 tablespoons olive oil
- 2 cups sweet potatoes, chopped
- tablespoon thyme, chopped
- ¼ cup pine nuts, toasted
- 1 cup low-sodium veggie stock
- tablespoons chives, finely chopped

Directions:
1. Heat up a pan with the oil over medium-high heat, add thyme and garlic, stir and cook for 2 minutes.
2. Add scallops, cook them for 2 minutes, season them black pepper, add cauliflower, sweet potatoes and the stock, toss and cook for 5 minutes more.
3. Divide the scallops mix between plates, sprinkle chives and pine nuts on top and serve.
4. Enjoy!

Nutrition: Calories 200, Fat 10, Fiber 4, Carbs 9, Protein 10

533. Spiced Salmon

Preparation time: 10 minutes
Cooking time: 10 minutes
Servings: 4
Ingredients:
- 4 salmon fillets
- 2 tablespoons olive oil
- teaspoon cumin, ground
- teaspoon sweet paprika
- teaspoon onion powder
- teaspoon chili powder
- ½ teaspoon garlic powder
- A pinch of salt and black pepper

Directions:
1. In a bowl, combine the cumin with paprika, onion powder, chili powder, garlic powder, salt and black pepper, toss and rub the salmon with this mix.
2. Heat up a pan with the oil over medium-high heat, add the salmon, cook for 5 minutes on each side, divide between plates and serve with a side salad.
3. Enjoy!

Nutrition: Calories 220, Fat 10, Carbs 8, Fiber 12, Protein 10

534. Salmon and Tomatoes Salad

Preparation time: 10 minutes
Cooking time: 0 minutes
Servings: 2
Ingredients:
- 4 cups cherry tomatoes, halved
- red onion, sliced
- 8 ounces smoked salmon, thinly sliced
- 4 tablespoons olive oil
- ½ teaspoon garlic, minced
- tablespoons lemon juice
- tablespoon oregano, chopped

- Black pepper to the taste
- 1 teaspoon balsamic vinegar

Directions:
1. In a salad bowl, combine the tomatoes with the onion, salmon, oil, garlic, lemon juice, oregano, black pepper and vinegar, toss and serve cold.
2. Enjoy!

Nutrition: Calories 159, Fat 8, Fiber 3, Carbs 7, Protein 7

535. Coconut Cream Shrimp

Preparation time: 10 minutes
Cooking time: 0 minutes
Servings: 2
Ingredients:
- pound shrimp, cooked, peeled and deveined
- 1 tablespoon coconut cream
- ¼ teaspoon jalapeno, chopped
- ½ teaspoon lime juice
- 1 tablespoon parsley, chopped
- A pinch of black pepper

Directions:
1. In a bowl, mix the shrimp with the cream, jalapeno, lime juice, parsley and black pepper, toss, divide into small bowls and serve.
2. Enjoy!

Nutrition: Calories 183, Fat 5, Fiber 3, Carbs 12, Protein 8

536. Tuna Pate

Preparation time: 10 minutes
Cooking time: 0 minutes
Servings: 10
Ingredients:
- 6 ounces canned tuna, drained and flaked
- 3 teaspoons lemon juice
- teaspoon onion, minced
- 8 ounces low-fat cream cheese
- ¼ cup parsley, chopped

Directions:
1. In a bowl, mix tuna with cream cheese, lemon juice, parsley and onion, stir really well and serve cold.
2. Enjoy!

Nutrition: Calories 172, Fat 2, Fiber 3, Carbs 8, Protein 4

537. Shrimp and Avocado Salad

Preparation time: 10 minutes
Cooking time: 0 minutes
Servings: 2
Ingredients:
- 2 green onions, chopped
- 2 avocados, pitted, peeled and cut into medium chunks
- 2 tablespoons cilantro, chopped
- cup shrimp, already cooked, peeled and deveined
- A pinch of salt and black pepper

Directions:

1. In a salad bowl, mix shrimp with avocado, green onions, cilantro, salt and pepper, toss and serve cold.
2. Enjoy!

Nutrition: Calories 160, Fat 2, Fiber 3, Carbs 10, Protein 6

538. Shrimp with Cilantro Sauce

Preparation time: 10 minutes
Cooking time: 4 minutes
Servings: 2
Ingredients:
- pound shrimp, peeled and deveined
- tablespoons cilantro, chopped
- tablespoons olive oil
- tablespoon pine nuts
- Zest of 1 lemon, grated
- Juice of ½ lemon

Directions:
1. In your blender, combine the cilantro with 2 tablespoons oil, pine nuts, lemon zest and lemon juice and pulse well.
2. Heat up a pan with the rest of the oil over medium-high heat, add the shrimp and cook for 3 minutes.
3. Add the cilantro mix, toss, cook for 1 minute, divide between plates and serve with a side salad
4. Enjoy!

Nutrition: Calories 210, Fat 5, Fiber 1, Carbs 8, Protein 12

539. Citrus Calamari

Preparation time: 10 minutes
Cooking time: 5 minutes
Servings: 4
Ingredients:
- lime, sliced
- lemon, sliced
- pounds calamari tubes and tentacles, sliced
- Black pepper to the taste
- ¼ cup olive oil
- garlic cloves, minced
- tablespoons lemon juice
- 1 orange, peeled and cut into segments
- tablespoons cilantro, chopped

Directions:
1. In a bowl, mix calamari with black pepper, lime slices, lemon slices, orange slices, garlic, oil, cilantro and lemon juice and toss.
2. Heat up a pan over medium-high heat, add calamari mix, cook for 5 minutes, divide into bowls and serve.
3. Enjoy!

Nutrition: Calories 190, Fat 2, Fiber 1, Carbs 11, Protein 14

540. Mussels Curry with Lime

Preparation time: 10 minutes
Cooking time: 10 minutes
Servings: 4
Ingredients:
- 2 and ½ pounds mussels, scrubbed

- 14 ounces canned coconut milk
- 3 tablespoons red curry paste
- tablespoon olive oil
- Black pepper to the taste
- ½ cup low-sodium chicken stock
- Juice of 1 lime
- Zest of 1 lime, grated
- ¼ cup cilantro, chopped
- tablespoons basil, chopped

Directions:
1. Heat up a pan with the oil over medium-high heat, add curry paste, stir and cook for 2 minutes.
2. Add stock, black pepper, coconut milk, lime juice, lime zest and mussels, toss, cover the pan and cook for 10 minutes.
3. Divide this into bowls, sprinkle cilantro and basil on top and serve.
4. Enjoy!

Nutrition: Calories 260, Fat 12, Fiber 2, Carbs 10, Protein 12

541. Spanish Mussels Mix

Preparation time: 10 minutes
Cooking time: 23 minutes
Servings: 4
Ingredients:
- 3 tablespoons olive oil
- 2 pounds mussels, scrubbed
- Black pepper to the taste
- 3 cups canned tomatoes, crushed
- shallot, chopped
- garlic cloves, minced
- cups low-sodium veggie stock
- 1/3 cup cilantro, chopped

Directions:
1. Heat up a pan with the oil over medium-high heat, add shallot, stir and cook for 3 minutes.
2. Add garlic, stock, tomatoes and black pepper, stir, bring to a simmer and cook for 10 minutes.
3. Add mussels and cilantro, toss, cover the pan, cook for another 10 minutes, divide into bowls and serve.
4. Enjoy!

Nutrition: Calories 210, Fat 2, Fiber 6, Carbs 5, Protein 8

542. Quinoa and Scallops Salad

Preparation time: 10 minutes
Cooking time: 20 minutes
Servings: 6
Ingredients:
- 12 ounces sea scallops
- 4 tablespoons olive oil+ 2 teaspoons
- 4 teaspoons coconut aminos
- and ½ cup quinoa, already cooked
- teaspoons garlic, minced
- 1 cup snow peas, sliced
- 1/3 cup balsamic vinegar
- 1 cup scallions, sliced

- 1/3 cup red bell pepper, chopped
- ¼ cup cilantro, chopped

Directions:
1. In a bowl, mix scallops with half of the aminos and toss.
2. Heat up a pan with 1 tablespoon olive oil over medium heat, add quinoa, stir and cook for 8 minutes.
3. Add garlic and snow peas, stir, cook for 5 more minutes and take off heat.
4. Meanwhile, in a bowl, mix 3 tablespoons olive oil with the rest of the coconut aminos and vinegar, whisk well, add the quinoa mix, scallions and bell pepper and toss.
5. Heat up another pan with 2 teaspoons olive oil over medium-high heat, add scallops, cook for 1 minute on each side, add over the quinoa mix, toss a bit, sprinkle cilantro on top and serve.
6. Enjoy!

Nutrition: Calories 221, Fat 5, Fiber 2, Carbs 7, Protein 8

543. Salmon and Veggies Soup

Preparation time: 10 minutes
Cooking time: 22 minutes
Servings: 6
Ingredients:
- 2 tablespoon olive oil
- leek, chopped
- red onion, chopped
- Black pepper to the taste
- carrots, chopped
- cups low-stock veggie stock
- ounces salmon, skinless, boneless and cubed
- ½ cup coconut cream
- 1 tablespoon dill, chopped

Directions:
1. Heat up a pan with the oil over medium heat, add leek and onion, stir and cook for 7 minutes.
2. Add black pepper, add carrots and stock, stir, bring to a boil and cook for 10 minutes.
3. Add salmon, cream and dill, stir, boil everything for 5-6 minutes more, ladle into bowls and serve.
4. Enjoy!

Nutrition: Calories 232, Fat 3, Fiber 4, Carbs 7, Protein 12

544. Salmon Salsa

Preparation time: 10 minutes
Cooking time: 0 minutes
Servings: 12
Ingredients:
- 3 yellow tomatoes, seedless and chopped
- 1-pound smoked salmon, boneless, skinless and flaked
- red tomato, seedless and chopped
- Black pepper to the taste
- 1 cup watermelon, seedless and chopped
- 1 red onion, chopped
- 1 mango, peeled, seedless and chopped
- jalapeno peppers, chopped
- ¼ cup parsley, chopped
- tablespoons lime juice

Directions:
1. In a bowl, mix all the tomatoes with mango, watermelon, onion, salmon, black pepper, jalapeno, parsley and lime juice, toss and serve cold.
2. Enjoy!

Nutrition: Calories 123, Fat 2, Fiber 4, Carbs 5, Protein 5

545. Salmon and Easy Cucumber Salad

Preparation time: 10 minutes
Cooking time: 0 minutes
Servings: 4
Ingredients:
- 2 cucumbers, cubed
- 2 teaspoons lemon juice
- 4 ounces non-fat yogurt
- teaspoon lemon zest, grated
- Black pepper to the taste
- teaspoons dill, chopped
- 8 ounces smoked salmon, flaked

Directions:
1. In a bowl, the cucumbers with the lemon juice, lemon zest, black pepper, dill, salmon and yogurt, toss and serve cold.
2. Enjoy!

Nutrition: Calories 242, Fat 3, Fiber 4, Carbs 8, Protein 3

546. Inspiring Cajun Snow Crab

Preparation time: 10 minutes
Cooking Time: 10 minutes
Serving: 2
Ingredients:
- lemon, fresh and quartered
- tablespoons Cajun seasoning
- bay leaves
- snow crab legs, precooked and defrosted
- Golden ghee

Directions:
1. Take a large pot and fill it about halfway with sunflower seeds and water.
2. Bring the water to a boil.
3. Squeeze lemon juice into the pot and toss in remaining lemon quarters.
4. Add bay leaves and Cajun seasoning.
5. Season for 1 minute.
6. Add crab legs and boil for 8 minutes (make sure to keep them submerged the whole time).
7. Melt ghee in microwave and use as dipping sauce, enjoy!

Nutrition: Calories: 643; Fat: 51g; Carbohydrates: 3g; Protein: 41g

547. Grilled Lime Shrimp

Preparation time: 25 minutes
Cooking Time: 5 minutes
Serving: 8
Ingredients:

- pound medium shrimp, peeled and deveined
- lime, juiced
- ½ cup olive oil
- tablespoons Cajun seasoning

Directions:
1. Take a re-sealable zip bag and add lime juice, Cajun seasoning, and olive oil.
2. Add shrimp and shake it well, let it marinate for 20 minutes.
3. Preheat your outdoor grill to medium heat.
4. Lightly grease the grate.
5. Remove shrimp from marinade and cook for 2 minutes per side.
6. Serve and enjoy!

Nutrition: Calories: 188; Fat: 3g; Net Carbohydrates: 1.2g; Protein: 13g

548. Calamari Citrus

Preparation time: 10 minutes
Cooking Time: 5 minutes
Serving: 4
Ingredients:
- lime, sliced
- lemon, sliced
- pounds calamari tubes and tentacles, sliced
- Pepper to taste
- ¼ cup olive oil
- garlic cloves, minced
- tablespoons lemon juice
- 1 orange, peeled and cut into segments
- tablespoons cilantro, chopped

Directions:
1. Take a bowl and add calamari, pepper, lime slices, lemon slices, orange slices, garlic, oil, cilantro, lemon juice and toss well.
2. Take a pan and place it over medium-high heat.
3. Add calamari mix and cook for 5 minutes.
4. Divide into bowls and serve.
5. Enjoy!

Nutrition: Calories: 190; Fat: 2g; Net Carbohydrates: 11g; Protein: 14g

549. Spiced Up Salmon

Preparation time: 10 minutes
Cooking Time: 10 minutes
Serving: 4
Ingredients:
- 4 salmon fillets
- 2 tablespoons olive oil
- cumin, ground
- 1 teaspoon sweet paprika
- 1 teaspoon chili powder
- ½ teaspoon garlic powder
- Pinch of pepper

Directions:
1. Take a bowl and add cumin, paprika, onion, chili powder, garlic powder, pepper and toss well.
2. Rub the salmon in the mixture.

3. Take a pan and place it over medium heat, add oil and let it heat up.
4. Add salmon and cook for 5 minutes, both sides.
5. Divide between plates and serve.
6. Enjoy!

Nutrition: Calories: 220; Fat: 10g; Net Carbohydrates: 8g; Protein: 10g

550. Coconut Cream Shrimp

Preparation time: 10 minutes
Cooking Time: Nil
Serving: 4
Ingredients:
- pound shrimp, cooked , peeled and deveined
- tablespoon coconut cream
- ¼ teaspoon jalapeno, chopped
- ½ teaspoon lime juice
- 1 tablespoon parsley, chopped
- Pinch of pepper

Directions:
1. Take a bowl and add shrimp, cream, jalapeno, lime juice, parsley, and pepper.
2. Toss well and divide into small bowls.
3. Serve and enjoy!

Nutrition: Calories: 183; Fat: 5g; Net Carbohydrates: 12g; Protein: 8g

551. Salmon and Orange Dish

Preparation time: 10 minutes
Cooking Time: 15 minutes
Serving: 4
Ingredients:
- 4 salmon fillets
- cup orange juice
- tablespoons arrowroot and water mixture
- 1 teaspoon orange peel, grated
- 1 teaspoon black pepper

Directions:
1. Add the listed ingredients to your pot.
2. Lock the lid and cook on HIGH pressure for 12 minutes.
3. Release the pressure naturally.
4. Serve and enjoy!

Nutrition: Calories: 583; Fat: 20g; Carbohydrates: 71g; Protein: 33g

552. Mesmerizing Coconut Haddock

Preparation time: 10 minutes
Cooking Time: 12 minutes
Serving: 3
Ingredients:
- 4 haddock fillets, 5 ounces each, boneless
- 2 tablespoons coconut oil, melted
- cup coconut, shredded and unsweetened
- ¼ cup hazelnuts, ground
- Sunflower seeds to taste

Directions:

1. Preheat your oven to 400 degrees F.
2. Line a baking sheet with parchment paper.
3. Keep it on the side.
4. Pat fish fillets with paper towel and season with sunflower seeds.
5. Take a bowl and stir in hazelnuts and shredded coconut.
6. Drag fish fillets through the coconut mix until both sides are coated well.
7. Transfer to baking dish.
8. Brush with coconut oil.
9. Bake for about 12 minutes until flaky.
10. Serve and enjoy!

Nutrition: Calories: 299; Fat: 24g; Carbohydrates: 1g; Protein: 20g

553. Asparagus and Lemon Salmon Dish

Preparation time: 5 minutes
Cooking Time: 15 minutes
Serving: 3
Ingredients:
- 2 salmon fillets, 6 ounces each, skin on
- Sunflower seeds to taste
- pound asparagus, trimmed
- cloves garlic, minced
- tablespoons almond butter
- ¼ cup cashew cheese

Directions:
1. Preheat your oven to 400 degrees F.
2. Line a baking sheet with oil.
3. Take a kitchen towel and pat your salmon dry, season as needed.
4. Put salmon onto the baking sheet and arrange asparagus around it.
5. Place a pan over medium heat and melt almond butter.
6. Add garlic and cook for 3 minutes until garlic browns slightly.
7. Drizzle sauce over salmon.
8. Sprinkle salmon with cheese and bake for 12 minutes until salmon looks cooked all the way and is flaky.
9. Serve and enjoy!

Nutrition: Calories: 434; Fat: 26g; Carbohydrates: 6g; Protein: 42g

554. Ecstatic "Foiled" Fish

Preparation time: 20 minutes
Cooking Time: 40 minutes
Serving: 4
Ingredients:
- 2 rainbow trout fillets
- tablespoon olive oil
- teaspoon garlic salt
- teaspoon ground black pepper
- fresh jalapeno pepper, sliced
- 1 lemon, sliced

Directions:
1. Preheat your oven to 400 degrees F.
2. Rinse your fish and pat them dry.
3. Rub the fillets with olive oil, season with some garlic salt and black pepper.

4. Place each of your seasoned fillets on a large sized sheet of aluminum foil.
5. Top it with some jalapeno slices and squeeze the juice from your lemons over your fish.
6. Arrange the lemon slices on top of your fillets.
7. Carefully seal up the edges of your foil and form a nice, enclosed packet.
8. Place your packets on your baking sheet.
9. Bake them for about 20 minutes.
10. Once the flakes start to flake off with a fork, the fish is ready!

Nutrition: Calories: 213; Fat: 10g; Carbohydrates: 8g; Protein: 24g

555. Brazilian Shrimp Stew

Preparation time: 20 minutes
Cooking Time: 25 minutes
Serving: 4
Ingredients:
- 4 tablespoons lime juice
- ½ tablespoons cumin, ground
- ½ tablespoons paprika
- ½ teaspoons garlic, minced
- 1 ½ teaspoons pepper
- pounds tilapia fillets, cut into bits
- 1 large onion, chopped
- large bell peppers, cut into strips
- 1 can (14 ounces) tomato, drained
- 1 can (14 ounces) coconut milk
- Handful of cilantro, chopped

Directions:
1. Take a large sized bowl and add lime juice, cumin, paprika, garlic, pepper and mix well.
2. Add tilapia and coat it up.
3. Cover and allow to marinate for 20 minutes.
4. Set your Instant Pot to Sauté mode (HIGH) [MOU10] [F11] and add olive oil.
5. Add onions and cook for 3 minutes until tender.
6. Add pepper strips, tilapia, and tomatoes to a skillet.
7. Pour coconut milk and cover, simmer for 20 minutes.
8. Add cilantro during the final few minutes.
9. Serve and enjoy!

Nutrition: Calories: 471; Fat: 44g; Carbohydrates: 13g; Protein: 12g

556. Simple Sautéed Garlic and Parsley Scallops

Preparation time: 5 minutes
Cooking Time: 25 minutes
Serving: 4
Ingredients:
- 8 tablespoons almond butter
- 2 garlic cloves, minced
- 16 large sea scallops
- Sunflower seeds and pepper to taste
- ½ tablespoons olive oil

Directions:
1. Seasons scallops with sunflower seeds and pepper.
2. Take a skillet, place it over medium heat, add oil and let it heat up.

3. Sauté scallops for 2 minutes per side, repeat until all scallops are cooked.
4. Add almond butter to the skillet and let it melt.
5. Stir in garlic and cook for 15 minutes.
6. Return scallops to skillet and stir to coat.
7. Serve and enjoy!

Nutrition: Calories: 417; Fat: 31g; Net Carbohydrates: 5g; Protein: 29g

557. Salmon and Cucumber Platter

Preparation time: 10 minutes
Cooking Time: Nil
Serving: 4
Ingredients:
- 2 cucumbers, cubed
- 2 teaspoons fresh squeezed lemon juice
- 4 ounces non-fat yogurt
- teaspoon lemon zest, grated
- Pepper to taste
- teaspoons dill, chopped
- 8 ounces smoked salmon, flaked

Directions:
1. Take a bowl and add cucumbers, lemon juice, lemon zest, pepper, dill, salmon, and yogurt and toss well.
2. Serve cold.
3. Enjoy!

Nutrition: Calories: 242; Fat: 3g; Carbohydrates: 3g; Protein: 3g

558. Tuna Pate

Preparation time: 10 minutes
Cooking Time: Nil
Serving: 4
Ingredients:
- 6 ounces canned tuna, drained and flaked
- 3 teaspoons fresh lemon juice
- teaspoon onion, minced
- 8 ounces low-fat cream cheese
- ¼ cup parsley, chopped

Directions:
1. Take a bowl and mix in tuna, cream cheese, lemon juice, parsley, onion and stir well.
2. Serve cold and enjoy!

Nutrition: Calories: 172; Fat: 2g; Carbohydrates: 8g; Protein: 4g

559. Cinnamon Salmon

Preparation time: 10 minutes
Cooking Time: 10 minutes
Serving: 4
Ingredients:
- 2 salmon fillets, boneless and skin on
- Pepper to taste
- tablespoon cinnamon powder
- tablespoon organic olive oil

Directions:

1. Take a pan and place it over medium heat, add oil and let it heat up.
2. Add pepper, cinnamon and stir.
3. Add salmon, skin side up and cook for 5 minutes on both sides.
4. Divide between plates and serve.
5. Enjoy!

Nutrition: Calories: 220; Fat: 8g; Carbohydrates: 11g; Protein: 8g

560. Scallop and Strawberry Mix

Preparation time: 10 minutes
Cooking Time: 6 minutes
Serving: 4
Ingredients:
- 4 ounces scallops
- ½ cup Pico De Gallo
- ½ cup strawberries, chopped
- tablespoon lime juice
- Pepper to taste

Directions:
1. Take a pan and place it over medium heat, add scallops and cook for 3 minutes on both sides.
2. Remove heat.
3. Take a bowl and add strawberries, lime juice, Pico De Gallo, scallops, pepper and toss well.
4. Serve and enjoy!

Nutrition: Calories: 169; Fat: 2g; Carbohydrates: 8g; Protein: 13g

561. Salmon with Peas and Parsley Dressing

Preparation time: 15 minutes
Cooking Time: 15 minutes
Serving: 4
Ingredients:
- 16 ounces salmon fillets, boneless and skin-on
- tablespoon parsley, chopped
- 10 ounces peas
- 9 ounces vegetable stock, low sodium
- cups water
- ½ teaspoon oregano, dried
- ½ teaspoon sweet paprika
- garlic cloves, minced
- A pinch of black pepper

Directions:
1. Add garlic, parsley, paprika, oregano and stock to a food processor and blend.
2. Add water to your Instant Pot.
3. Add steam basket.
4. Add fish fillets inside the steamer basket.
5. Season with pepper.
6. Lock the lid and cook on HIGH pressure for 10 minutes.
7. Release the pressure naturally over 10 minutes.
8. Divide the fish amongst plates.
9. Add peas to the steamer basket and lock the lid again, cook on HIGH pressure for 5 minutes.
10. Quick release the pressure.

11. Divide the peas next to your fillets and serve with the parsley dressing drizzled on top
12. Enjoy!

Nutrition: Calories: 315; Fat: 5g; Carbohydrates: 14g; Protein: 16g

562. Mackerel and Orange Medley

Preparation time: 10 minutes
Cooking Time: 10 minutes
Serving: 4
Ingredients:

- 4 mackerel fillets, skinless and boneless
- 4 spring onion, chopped
- teaspoon olive oil
- 1-inch ginger piece, grated
- Black pepper as needed
- Juice and zest of 1 whole orange
- 1 cup low sodium fish stock

Directions:
1. Season the fillets with black pepper and rub olive oil.
2. Add stock, orange juice, ginger, orange zest and onion to Instant Pot.
3. Place a steamer basket and add the fillets.
4. Lock the lid and cook on HIGH pressure for 10 minutes.
5. Release the pressure naturally over 10 minutes.
6. Divide the fillets amongst plates and drizzle the orange sauce from the pot over the fish.
7. Enjoy!

Nutrition: Calories: 200; Fat: 4g; Carbohydrates: 19g; Protein: 14g

563. Spicy Chili Salmon

Preparation time: 10 minutes
Cooking Time: 7 minutes
Serving: 4
Ingredients:

- 4 salmon fillets, boneless and skin-on
- 2 tablespoons assorted chili peppers, chopped
- Juice of 1 lemon
- lemon, sliced
- 1 cup water
- Black pepper

Directions:
1. Add water to the Instant Pot.
2. Add steamer basket and add salmon fillets, season the fillets with salt and pepper.
3. Drizzle lemon juice on top.
4. Top with lemon slices.
5. Lock the lid and cook on HIGH pressure for 7 minutes.
6. Release the pressure naturally over 10 minutes.
7. Divide the salmon and lemon slices between serving plates.
8. Enjoy!

Nutrition: Calories: 281; Fats: 8g; Carbs: 19g; Protein: 7g

564. Simple One Pot Mussels

Preparation time: 10 minutes

Cooking Time: 5 minutes
Serving: 4
Ingredients:

- 2 tablespoons butter
- 2 chopped shallots
- 4 minced garlic cloves
- ½ cup broth
- ½ cup white wine
- 2 pounds cleaned mussels
- Lemon and parsley for serving

Directions:
1. Clean the mussels and remove the beard.
2. Discard any mussels that do not close when tapped against a hard surface.
3. Set your pot to Sauté mode and add chopped onion and butter.
4. Stir and sauté onions.
5. Add garlic and cook for 1 minute.
6. Add broth and wine.
7. Lock the lid and cook for 5 minutes on HIGH pressure.
8. Release the pressure naturally over 10 minutes.
9. Serve with a sprinkle of parsley and enjoy!

Nutrition: Calories: 286; Fats: 14g; Carbs: 12g; Protein: 28g

565. Lemon Pepper and Salmon

Preparation time: 5 minutes
Cooking Time: 6 minutes
Serving: 3
Ingredients:

- ¾ cup water
- Few sprigs of parsley, basil, tarragon, basil
- pound of salmon, skin on
- teaspoons ghee
- ¼ teaspoon salt
- ½ teaspoon pepper
- ½ lemon, thinly sliced
- 1 whole carrot, julienned

Directions:
1. Set your pot to Sauté mode and water and herbs.
2. Place a steamer rack inside your pot and place salmon.
3. Drizzle the ghee on top of the salmon and season with salt and pepper.
4. Cover lemon slices.
5. Lock the lid and cook on HIGH pressure for 3 minutes.
6. Release the pressure naturally over 10 minutes.
7. Transfer the salmon to a serving platter.
8. Set your pot to Sauté mode and add vegetables.
9. Cook for 1-2 minutes.
10. Serve with vegetables and salmon.
11. Enjoy!

Nutrition: Calories: 464; Fat: 34g; Carbohydrates: 3g; Protein: 34g

566. Roasted Lemon Swordfish

Preparation time: 10 minutes
Cooking Time: 70-80 minutes
Servings: 4

Ingredients:
- ¼ cup parsley, chopped
- ½ teaspoon garlic, chopped
- ½ teaspoon canola oil
- 4 swordfish fillets, 6 ounces each
- ¼ teaspoon sunflower seeds
- tablespoon sugar
- lemons, quartered and seeds removed

Directions:
1. Preheat your oven to 375 degrees F.
2. Take a small-sized bowl and add sugar, sunflower seeds, lemon wedges.
3. Toss well to coat them.
4. Take a shallow baking dish and add lemons, cover with aluminum foil.
5. Roast for about 60 minutes until lemons are tender and browned (Slightly).
6. Heat your grill and place the rack about 4 inches away from the source of heat.
7. Take a baking pan and coat it with cooking spray.
8. Transfer fish fillets to the pan and brush with oil on top spread garlic on top.
9. Grill for about 5 minutes each side until fillet turns opaque.
10. Transfer fish to a serving platter, squeeze roasted lemon on top.
11. Sprinkle parsley serve with a lemon wedge on the side.
12. Enjoy!

Nutrition: Calories: 280; Fat: 12g; Net Carbohydrates: 4g; Protein: 34g

567. Especial Glazed Salmon

Preparation time: 45 minutes
Cooking Time: 10 minutes
Serving: 4
Ingredients:
- 4 pieces salmon fillets, 5 ounces each
- 4 tablespoons coconut aminos
- 4 teaspoon olive oil
- 2 teaspoons ginger, minced
- 4 teaspoons garlic, minced
- 2 tablespoons sugar-free ketchup
- 4 tablespoons dry white wine
- 2 tablespoons red boat fish sauce, low sodium

Directions:
1. Take a bowl and mix in coconut aminos, garlic, ginger, fish sauce and mix.
2. Add salmon and let it marinate for 15-20 minutes.
3. Take a skillet/pan and place it over medium heat.
4. Add oil and let it heat up.
5. Add salmon fillets and cook on high heat for 3-4 minutes per side.
6. Remove dish once crispy.
7. Add sauce and wine.
8. Simmer for 5 minutes on low heat.
9. Return salmon to the glaze and flip until both sides are glazed.
10. Serve and enjoy!

Nutrition: Calories: 372; Fat: 24g; Carbohydrates: 3g; Protein: 35g

568. Generous Stuffed Salmon Avocado

Preparation time: 10 minutes
Cooking Time: 30 minutes
Serving: 2
Ingredients:
- ripe organic avocado
- ounces wild caught smoked salmon
- ounce cashew cheese
- tablespoons extra virgin olive oil
- Sunflower seeds as needed

Directions:
1. Cut avocado in half and deseed.
2. Add the rest of the ingredients to a food processor and process until coarsely chopped.
3. Place mixture into avocado.
4. Serve and enjoy!

Nutrition: Calories: 525; Fat: 48g; Carbohydrates: 4g; Protein: 19g

569. Spanish Mussels

Preparation time: 10 minutes
Cooking Time: 23 minutes
Serving: 4
Ingredients:
- 3 tablespoons olive oil
- 2 pounds mussels, scrubbed
- Pepper to taste
- 3 cups canned tomatoes, crushed
- shallot, chopped
- garlic cloves, minced
- cups low sodium vegetable stock
- 1/3 cup cilantro, chopped

Directions:
1. Take a pan and place it over medium-high heat, add shallot and stir-cook for 3 minutes.
2. Add garlic, stock, tomatoes, pepper, stir and reduce heat, simmer for 10 minutes.
3. Add mussels, cilantro, and toss.
4. Cover and cook for 10 minutes more.
5. Serve and enjoy!

Nutrition: Calories: 210; Fat: 2g; Carbohydrates: 5g; Protein: 8g

570. Tilapia Broccoli Platter

Preparation time: 4 minutes
Cooking Time: 14 minutes
Serving: 2
Ingredients:
- 6 ounce tilapia, frozen
- tablespoon almond butter
- tablespoon garlic, minced
- 1 teaspoon lemon pepper seasoning
- 1 cup broccoli florets, fresh

Directions:
1. Preheat your oven to 350 degrees F.
2. Add fish in aluminum foil packets.
3. Arrange broccoli around fish.
4. Sprinkle lemon pepper on top.

5. Close the packets and seal.
6. Bake for 14 minutes.
7. Take a bowl and add garlic and almond butter, mix well and keep the mixture on the side.
8. Remove the packet from oven and transfer to platter.
9. Place almond butter on top of the fish and broccoli, serve and enjoy!

Nutrition: Calories: 362; Fat: 25g; Carbohydrates: 2g; Protein: 29g

571. Saffron Shrimp

Preparation time: 10 minutes
Cooking time: 30 minutes
Servings: 4
Ingredients:
- teaspoon lemon juice
- Black pepper to the taste
- ½ cup avocado mayo
- ½ teaspoon sweet paprika
- tablespoons olive oil
- fennel bulb, chopped
- 1 yellow onion, chopped
- garlic cloves, minced
- 1 cup canned tomatoes, no-salt-added and chopped
- 1 and ½ pounds big shrimp, peeled and deveined
- ¼ teaspoon saffron powder

Directions:
1. In a bowl, combine the garlic with lemon juice, black pepper, mayo and paprika and whisk.
2. Add the shrimp and toss.
3. Heat up a pan with the oil over medium-high heat, add the shrimp, fennel, onion and garlic mix, toss and cook for 4 minutes.
4. Add tomatoes and saffron, toss, divide into bowls and serve.
5. Enjoy!

Nutrition: Calories 210, Fat 2, Fiber 5, Carbs 8, Protein 4

572. Crab, Zucchini and Watermelon Soup

Preparation time: 4 hours
Cooking time: 0 minutes
Servings: 4
Ingredients:
- ¼ cup basil, chopped
- 2 pounds tomatoes
- 5 cups watermelon, cubed
- ¼ cup red wine vinegar
- 1/3 cup olive oil
- 2 garlic cloves, minced
- zucchini, chopped
- Black pepper to the taste
- 1 cup crabmeat

Directions:
1. In your food processor, mix tomatoes with basil, vinegar, 4 cups watermelon, garlic, 1/3 cup oil and black pepper to the taste, pulse, pour into a bowl and keep in the fridge for 1 hour.

2. Divide this into bowls, add zucchini, crab and the rest of the watermelon and serve.
3. Enjoy!

Nutrition: Calories 231, Fat 3, Fiber 3, Carbs 6, Protein 8

573. Shrimp and Orzo

Preparation time: 10 minutes
Cooking time: 30 minutes
Servings: 4
Ingredients:
- pound shrimp, peeled and deveined
- Black pepper to the taste
- garlic cloves, minced
- tablespoon olive oil
- ½ teaspoon oregano, dried
- 1 yellow onion, chopped
- cups low-sodium chicken stock
- ounces orzo
- ½ cup water
- ounces canned tomatoes, no-salt-added and chopped
- Juice of 1 lemon

Directions:
1. Heat up a pan with the oil over medium-high heat, add onion, garlic and oregano, stir and cook for 4 minutes.
2. Add orzo, stir and cook for 2 more minutes.
3. Add stock and the water, bring to a boil, cover, reduce heat to low and cook for 12 minutes.
4. Add lemon juice, tomatoes, black pepper and shrimp, introduce in the oven and bake at 400 degrees F for 15 minutes.
5. Divide between plates and serve.
6. Enjoy!

Nutrition: Calories 228, Fat 4, Fiber 3, Carbs 7, Protein 8

574. Lemon and Garlic Scallops

Preparation time: 10 minutes
Cooking Time: 5 minutes
Serving: 4
Ingredients:
- tablespoon olive oil
- ¼ pounds dried scallops
- tablespoons all-purpose flour
- ¼ teaspoon sunflower seeds
- 4-5 garlic cloves, minced
- 1 scallion, chopped
- 1 pinch of ground sage
- 1 lemon juice
- tablespoons parsley, chopped

Direction
1. Take a nonstick skillet and place over medium-high heat.
2. Add oil and allow the oil to heat up.
3. Take a medium sized bowl and add scallops alongside sunflower seeds and flour.
4. Place the scallops in the skillet and add scallions, garlic, and sage.
5. Sauté for 3-4 minutes until they show an opaque texture.
6. Stir in lemon juice and parsley.
7. Remove heat and serve hot!

Nutrition: Calories: 151; Fat: 4g; Carbohydrates: 10g; Protein: 18g

575. Walnut Encrusted Salmon

Preparation time: 10 minutes
Cooking Time: 14 minutes
Serving: 34
Ingredients:
- ½ cup walnuts
- 2 tablespoons stevia
- ½ tablespoon Dijon mustard
- ¼ teaspoon dill
- 2 salmon fillets (3 ounces each)
- tablespoon olive oil
- Sunflower seeds and pepper to taste

Directions:
1. Preheat your oven to 350 degrees F.
2. Add walnuts, mustard, stevia to food processor and process until your desired consistency is achieved.
3. Take a frying pan and place it over medium heat.
4. Add oil and let it heat up.
5. Add salmon and sear for 3 minutes.
6. Add walnut mix and coat well.
7. Transfer coated salmon to baking sheet, bake in oven for 8 minutes.
8. Serve and enjoy!

Nutrition: Calories: 373; Fat: 43g; Carbohydrates: 4g; Protein: 20g

576. Smoked Salmon with Capers and Radishes

Preparation time: 10 minutes
Cooking time: 0 minutes
Servings: 8
Ingredients:
- 3 tablespoons beet horseradish, prepared
- 1-pound smoked salmon, skinless, boneless and flaked
- 2 teaspoons lemon zest, grated
- 4 radishes, chopped
- ½ cup capers, drained and chopped
- 1/3 cup red onion, roughly chopped
- 3 tablespoons chives, chopped

Directions:
1. In a bowl, combine the salmon with the beet horseradish, lemon zest, radish, capers, onions and chives, toss and serve cold.
2. Enjoy!

Nutrition: Calories 254, Fat 2, Fiber 1, Carbs 7, Protein 7

577. Trout Spread

Preparation time: 10 minutes
Cooking time: 0 minutes
Servings: 8
Ingredients:
- 4 ounces smoked trout, skinless, boneless and flaked
- ¼ cup coconut cream

- tablespoon lemon juice
- 1/3 cup non-fat yogurt
- 1 and ½ tablespoon parsley, chopped
- tablespoons chives, chopped
- Black pepper to the taste
- A drizzle of olive oil

Directions:
1. In a bowl mix trout with yogurt, cream, black pepper, chives, lemon juice and the dill and stir.
2. Drizzle the olive oil at the end and serve.
3. Enjoy!

Nutrition: Calories 204, Fat 2, Fiber 2, Carbs 8, Protein 15

578. Easy Shrimp and Mango

Preparation time: 10 minutes
Cooking time: 0 minutes
Servings: 4
Ingredients:
- 3 tablespoons balsamic vinegar
- 3 tablespoons coconut sugar
- 6 tablespoons avocado mayonnaise
- 3 mangos, peeled and cubed
- 3 tablespoons parsley, finely chopped
- pound shrimp, peeled, deveined and cooked

Directions:
1. In a bowl, mix vinegar with sugar and mayo and whisk.
2. In another bowl, combine the mango with the parsley and shrimp, add the mayo mix, toss and serve.
3. Enjoy!

Nutrition: Calories 204, Fat 3, Fiber 2, Carbs 8, Protein 8

579. Spring Salmon Mix

Preparation time: 10 minutes
Cooking time: 0 minutes
Servings: 4
Ingredients:
- 2 tablespoons scallions, chopped
- 2 tablespoons sweet onion, chopped
- and ½ teaspoons lime juice
- tablespoon chives, minced
- tablespoon olive oil
- 1 pound smoked salmon, flaked
- 1 cup cherry tomatoes, halved
- Black pepper to the taste
- 1 tablespoon parsley, chopped

Directions:
1. In a bowl, mix the scallions with sweet onion, lime juice, chives, oil, salmon, tomatoes, black pepper and parsley, toss and serve.
2. Enjoy!

Nutrition: Calories 200, Fat 8, Fiber 3, Carbs 8, Protein 6

580. Smoked Salmon and Green Beans

Preparation time: 10 minutes

Cooking time: 0 minutes

Servings: 4

Ingredients:

- 3 tablespoons balsamic vinegar
- 2 tablespoons olive oil
- 1/3 cup Kalamata olives, pitted and minced
- garlic clove, minced
- Black pepper to the taste
- ½ teaspoon lemon zest, grated
- pound green beans, blanched and halved
- ½ pound cherry tomatoes, halved
- ½ fennel bulb, sliced
- ½ red onion, sliced
- cups baby arugula
- ¾ pound smoked salmon, flaked

Directions:

1. In a bowl, combine the green beans with cherry tomatoes, fennel, onion, arugula and salmon and toss.
2. Add vinegar, oil, olives, garlic, black pepper and lemon zest, toss and serve.
3. Enjoy!

Nutrition: Calories 212, Fat 3, Fiber 3, Carbs 6, Protein 4

581. Aromatic Salmon with Fennel Seeds

Preparation Time: 8 minutes

Cooking Time: 10 minutes

Servings: 2

Ingredients:

- 4 medium salmon fillets, skinless and boneless
- tablespoon fennel seeds
- tablespoons olive oil
- 1 tablespoon lemon juice
- 1 tablespoon water

Directions:

1. Heat up olive oil in the skillet.
2. Add fennel seeds and roast them for 1 minute.
3. Add salmon fillets and sprinkle with lemon juice.
4. Add water and roast the fish for 4 minutes per side over the medium heat.

Nutrition: 301 calories, 4.8g protein, 0.8g carbohydrates, 18.2g fat, 0.6g fiber, 78mg cholesterol, 81mg sodium, 713mg potassium

582. Shrimp Quesadillas

Preparation Time: 16 minutes

Cooking Time: 5 minutes

Servings: 2

Ingredients:

- Two whole wheat tortillas
- ½ tsp. ground cumin
- 4 cilantro leaves
- 3 oz. diced cooked shrimp
- de-seeded plump tomato
- ¾ c. grated non-fat mozzarella cheese
- ¼ c. diced red onion

Directions:

1. In medium bowl, combine the grated mozzarella cheese and the warm, cooked shrimp. Add the ground cumin, red onion, and tomato. Mix together. Spread the mixture evenly on the tortillas.
2. Heat a non-stick frying pan. Place the tortillas in the pan, then heat until they crisp.
3. Add the cilantro leaves. Fold over the tortillas.
4. Press down for 1 – 2 minutes. Slice the tortillas into wedges.
5. Serve immediately.

Nutrition: Calories: 99; Fat: 9 g; Carbs: 7.2 g; Protein: 59 g; Sugars: 4 g; Sodium: 500 mg

583. The OG Tuna Sandwich

Preparation Time: 15 minutes

Cooking Time: 5 minutes

Servings: 2

Ingredients:

- 30 g olive oil
- peeled and diced medium cucumber
- ½ g pepper
- whole wheat bread slices
- 85 g diced onion
- 2 ½ g salt
- 1 can flavored tuna
- 85 g shredded spinach

Directions:

1. Grab your blender and add the spinach, tuna, onion, oil, salt and pepper in, and pulse for about 10 to 20 seconds.
2. In the meantime, toast your bread and add your diced cucumber to a bowl, which you can pour your tuna mixture in. Carefully mix and add the mixture to the bread once toasted.
3. Slice in half and serve, while storing the remaining mixture in the fridge.

Nutrition: Calories: 302; Fat: 5.8 g; Carbs: 36.62 g; Protein: 28 g; Sugars: 3.22 g; Sodium: 445 mg

584. Easy to Understand Mussels

Preparation Time: 10 minutes

Cooking Time: 10 minutes

Servings: 2

Ingredients:

- 2 lbs. cleaned mussels
- 4 minced garlic cloves
- 2 chopped shallots
- Lemon and parsley
- 2 tbsps. Butter
- ½ c. broth
- ½ c. white wine

Directions:

1. Clean the mussels and remove the beard
2. Discard any mussels that do not close when tapped against a hard surface
3. Set your pot to Sauté mode and add chopped onion and butter
4. Stir and sauté onions

5. Add garlic and cook for 1 minute
6. Add broth and wine
7. Lock up the lid and cook for 5 minutes on HIGH pressure
8. Release the pressure naturally over 10 minutes
9. Serve with a sprinkle of parsley and enjoy!

Nutrition: Calories: 286; Fat: 14 g; Carbs: 12 g; Protein: 28 g; Sugars: 0 g; Sodium: 314 mg

585. Cheesy Shrimp Mix

Preparation time: 10 minutes
Cooking time: 30 minutes
Servings: 10
Ingredients:
- ½ pound shrimp, already peeled and deveined
- cup avocado mayonnaise
- ½ cup low-fat mozzarella cheese, shredded
- garlic cloves, minced
- ¼ teaspoon hot sauce
- tablespoon lemon juice
- A drizzle of olive oil
- ½ cup scallions, sliced

Directions:
1. In a bowl, mix mozzarella with mayo, hot sauce, and garlic and lemon juice and whisk well.
2. Add scallions and shrimp, toss, pour into a baking dish greased with the olive oil, introduce in the oven at 350 degrees F and bake for 30 minutes.
3. Divide into bowls and serve.
4. Enjoy!

Nutrition: Calories 275, Fat 3, Fiber 5, Carbs 10, Protein 12

586. Cod Salad with Mustard

Preparation time: 12 minutes
Cooking time: 12 minutes
Servings: 4
Ingredients:
- 4 medium cod fillets, skinless and boneless
- 2 tablespoons mustard
- tablespoon tarragon, chopped
- tablespoon capers, drained
- 4 tablespoons olive oil+ 1 teaspoon
- Black pepper to the taste
- cups baby arugula
- small red onion, sliced
- 1 small cucumber, sliced
- tablespoons lemon juice

Directions:
1. In a bowl, mix mustard with 2 tablespoons olive oil, tarragon and capers and whisk.
2. Heat up a pan with 1 teaspoon oil over medium-high heat, add fish, season with black pepper to the taste, and cook for 6 minutes on each side and cut into medium cubes.
3. In a salad bowl, combine the arugula with onion, cucumber, lemon juice, cod and mustard mix, toss and serve.
4. Enjoy!

Nutrition: Calories 258, Fat 12, Fiber 6, Carbs 12, Protein 18

587. Broccoli and Cod Mash

Preparation Time: 10 minutes
Cooking Time: 20 minutes
Servings: 1
Ingredients:
- 2 cups broccoli, chopped
- 4 cod fillets, boneless, chopped
- white onion, chopped
- tablespoons olive oil
- cup of water
- tablespoon low-fat cream cheese
- ½ teaspoon ground black pepper

Directions:
1. Roast the cod in the saucepan with olive oil for 1 minute per side.
2. Then add all remaining ingredients except cream cheese and boil the meal for 18 minutes.
3. After this, drain water, add cream cheese, and stir the meal well.

Nutrition: 186 calories, 21.8g protein, 5.8g carbohydrates, 9.1g fat, 1.8g fiber, 43mg cholesterol, 105mg sodium, 191mg potassium

588. Greek Style Salmon

Preparation Time: 10 minutes
Cooking Time: 10 minutes
Servings: 2
Ingredients:
- 4 medium salmon fillets, skinless and boneless
- tablespoon lemon juice
- 1 tablespoon dried oregano
- 1 teaspoon dried thyme
- ¼ teaspoon onion powder
- 1 tablespoon olive oil

Directions:
1. Heat up olive oil in the skillet.
2. Sprinkle the salmon with dried oregano, thyme, onion powder, and lemon juice.
3. Put the fish in the skillet and cook for 4 minutes per side.

Nutrition: 271 calories, 34.7g protein, 1.1g carbohydrates, 14.7g fat, 0.6g fiber, 78mg cholesterol, 80mg sodium, 711mg potassium

589. Spicy Ginger Sea bass

Preparation Time: 5 minutes
Cooking Time: 10 minutes
Servings: 2
Ingredients:
- tablespoon ginger, grated
- tablespoons sesame oil
- ¼ teaspoon chili powder
- sea bass fillets, boneless
- tablespoon margarine

Directions:
1. Heat up sesame oil and margarine in the skillet.
2. Add chili powder and ginger.
3. Then add sea bass and cook the fish for 3 minutes per side.

4. Then close the lid and simmer the fish for 3 minutes over low heat.

Nutrition: 216 calories, 24g protein, 1.1g carbohydrates, 12.3g fat, 0.2g fiber, 54mg cholesterol, 123mg sodium, 354mg potassium

590. Yogurt Shrimps

Preparation Time: 5 minutes
Cooking Time: 10 minutes
Servings: 2
Ingredients:
- pound shrimp, peeled
- 1 tablespoon margarine
- ¼ cup low-fat yogurt
- 1 teaspoon lemon zest, grated
- 1 chili pepper, chopped

Directions:
1. Melt the margarine in the skillet, add chili pepper, and roast it for 1 minute.
2. Then add shrimps and lemon zest.
3. Roast the shrimps for 2 minutes per side.
4. After this, add yogurt, stir the shrimps well and cook for 5 minutes.

Nutrition: 137 calories, 21.4g protein, 2.4g carbohydrates, 4g fat, 0.1g fiber, 192mg cholesterol, 257mg sodium, 187mg potassium

591. Creamy Salmon and Asparagus Mix

Preparation time: 10 minutes
Cooking time: 10 minutes
Servings: 6
Ingredients:
- tablespoon lemon zest, grated
- tablespoon lemon juice
- Black pepper to the taste
- cup coconut cream
- pound asparagus, trimmed
- 20 ounces salmon, skinless and boneless
- 1-ounce parmesan cheese, grated

Directions:
1. Put some water in a pot, add a pinch of salt, bring to a boil over medium heat, add asparagus, cook for 1 minute, transfer to a bowl filled with ice water, drain and put in a bowl.
2. Heat up the pot with the water again over medium heat, add salmon, cook for 5 minutes and also drain.
3. In a bowl, mix lemon peel with cream and lemon juice and whisk
4. Heat up a pan over medium-high heat, asparagus, cream and pepper, cook for 1 more minute, divide between plates, add salmon and serve with grated parmesan.
5. Enjoy!

Nutrition: Calories 354, Fat 2, Fiber 2, Carbs 2, Protein 4

592. Salmon and Brussels sprouts

Preparation time: 10 minutes
Cooking time: 20 minutes
Servings: 6
Ingredients:
- 2 tablespoons brown sugar
- teaspoon onion powder
- teaspoon garlic powder
- teaspoon smoked paprika
- tablespoons olive oil
- and ¼ pounds Brussels sprouts, halved
- 6 medium salmon fillets, boneless

Directions:
1. In a bowl, mix sugar with onion powder, garlic powder, smoked paprika and 2 tablespoon olive oil and whisk well.
2. Spread Brussels sprouts on a lined baking sheet, drizzle the rest of the olive oil, toss to coat, introduce in the oven at 450 degrees F and bake for 5 minutes.
3. Add salmon fillets brush with sugar mix you've prepared, introduce in the oven and bake for 15 minutes more.
4. Divide everything between plates and serve.
5. Enjoy!

Nutrition: Calories 212, Fat 5, Fiber 3, Carbs 12, Protein 8

593. Salmon and Beets Mix

Preparation time: 10 minutes
Cooking time: 35 minutes
Servings: 4
Ingredients:
- 1-pound medium beets, sliced
- 6 tablespoons olive oil
- and ½ pounds salmon fillets, skinless and boneless
- Black pepper to the taste
- tablespoon chives, chopped
- tablespoon parsley, chopped
- tablespoon shallots, chopped
- tablespoon lemon zest, grated
- ¼ cup lemon juice

Directions:
1. In a bowl, mix beets with ½ tablespoon oil and toss to coat, season with black pepper, spread on a lined baking sheet and bake in the oven at 450 degrees F for 20 minutes.
2. Add salmon, brush it with the rest of the oil, introduce in the oven and bake for 15 minutes more.
3. In a bowl, combine the chives with the parsley, shallots, lemon zest and lemon juice and toss.
4. Divide the salmon and the beets between plates, drizzle the chives mix on top and serve.
5. Enjoy!

Nutrition: Calories 272, Fat 6, Fiber 2, Carbs 12, Protein 9

594. Garlic Shrimp Mix

Preparation time: 10 minutes

Cooking time: 10 minutes
Servings: 4
Ingredients:
- pound shrimp, deveined and peeled
- teaspoons olive oil
- 6 tablespoons lemon juice
- tablespoons dill, chopped
- tablespoon oregano, chopped
- garlic cloves, chopped
- Black pepper to the taste
- ¾ cup non-fat yogurt
- ½ pounds cherry tomatoes, halved

Directions:
1. Heat up a pan with the oil over medium-high heat, add the shrimp and cook for 3 minutes.
2. Add lemon juice, dill, oregano, garlic, black pepper, yogurt and tomatoes, toss, cook for 5 minutes more, divide into bowls and serve.
3. Enjoy!

Nutrition: Calories 253, Fat 6, Fiber 6, Carbs 10, Protein 17

595. Salmon and Potatoes Mix

Preparation time: 10 minutes
Cooking time: 10 minutes
Servings: 4
Ingredients:
- and ½ pounds potatoes, chopped
- tablespoon olive oil
- 4 ounces smoked salmon, chopped
- tablespoon chives, chopped
- teaspoons prepared horseradish
- ¼ cup coconut cream
- Black pepper to the taste

Directions:
1. 4 Heat up a pan with the oil over medium heat, add potatoes and cook for 10 minutes.
2. 5 Add salmon, chives, horseradish, cream and black pepper, toss, cook for 1 minute more, divide between plates and serve.
3. Enjoy!

Nutrition: Calories 233, Fat 6, Fiber 5, Carbs 9, Protein 11

596. Balsamic Salmon and Peaches Mix

Preparation time: 10 minutes
Cooking time: 10 minutes
Servings: 4
Ingredients:
- tablespoon balsamic vinegar
- teaspoon thyme, chopped
- 1 tablespoon ginger, grated
- 4 tablespoons olive oil
- Black pepper to the taste
- red onions, cut into wedges
- peaches cut into wedges
- salmon steaks

Directions:
1. In a small bowl, combine vinegar with ginger, thyme, 3 tablespoons olive oil and black pepper and whisk
2. In another bowl, mix onion with peaches, 1 tablespoon oil and pepper and toss.
3. Season salmon with black pepper, place on preheated grill over medium heat, cook for 5 minutes on each side and divide between plates.
4. Put the peaches and onions on the same grill, cook for 4 minutes on each side, divide next to the salmon, drizzle the vinegar mix and serve.
5. Enjoy!

Nutrition: Calories 200, Fat 2, Fiber 2, Carbs 3, Protein 2

597. Salmon and Bean s Mix

Preparation time: 10 minutes
Cooking time: 20 minutes
Servings: 4
Ingredients:
- 2 tablespoons coconut aminos
- ½ cup olive oil
- and ½ cup low-sodium chicken stock
- 6 ounces salmon fillets
- garlic cloves, minced
- tablespoon ginger, grated
- 1 cup canned black beans, no-salt-added, drained and rinsed
- teaspoons balsamic vinegar
- ¼ cup radishes, grated
- ¼ cup carrots, grated
- ¼ cup scallions, chopped

Directions:
1. In a bowl, combine the aminos with half of the oil and whisk.
2. Put the salmon in a baking dish, pour add coconut aminos and the stock, toss a bit, leave aside in the fridge for 10 minutes, introduce in preheated broiler and cook over medium-high heat for 4 minutes on each side.
3. Heat up a pan with the rest of the oil over medium heat, add garlic, ginger and black beans, stir and cook for 3 minutes.
4. Add vinegar, radishes, carrots and scallions, toss and cook for 5 minutes more.
5. Divide fish and the black beans mix between plates and serve.
6. Enjoy!

Nutrition: Calories 220, Fat 4, Fiber 2, Carbs 12, Protein 7

598. Lemony Salmon and Pomegranate Mix

Preparation time: 20 minutes
Cooking time: 10 minutes
Servings: 4
Ingredients:
- tablespoon olive oil
- 4 salmon fillets, skinless and boneless
- 4 tablespoons sesame paste
- Juice of 1 lemon

- lemon, cut into wedges
- ½ cucumber, chopped
- Seeds from 1 pomegranate
- A bunch of parsley, chopped

Directions:
1. Heat up a pan with the oil over medium heat, add salmon, cook for 5 minutes on each side and divide between plates
2. In a bowl, mix sesame paste and lemon juice and whisk.
3. Add cucumber, parsley and pomegranate seeds and toss
4. Divide this over the salmon and serve.
5. Enjoy!

Nutrition: Calories 254, Fat 3, Fiber 6, Carbs 9, Protein 14

599. Salmon and Veggie Mix

Preparation time: 10 minutes
Cooking time: 30 minutes
Servings: 6
Ingredients:
- 3 red onions, cut into wedges
- ¾ cup green olives, pitted
- 3 red bell peppers, cut into strips
- ½ teaspoon smoked paprika
- Black pepper to the taste
- 5 tablespoons olive oil
- 6 salmon fillets, skinless and boneless
- 2 tablespoons parsley, chopped

Directions:
1. Spread bell peppers, onions and olives on a lined baking sheet, add smoked paprika, black pepper and 3 tablespoons olive oil, toss to coat, bake in the oven at 375 degrees F for 15 minutes and divide between plates.

2. Heat up a pan with the rest of the oil over medium-high heat, add the salmon, season with black pepper, cook for 5 minutes on each side, divide next to the bell peppers and olives mix, sprinkle parsley on top and serve.
3. Enjoy!

Nutrition: Calories 221, Fat 2, Fiber 3, Carbs 8, Protein 10

600. Greek Salmon with Yogurt

Preparation time: 10 minutes
Cooking time: 15 minutes
Servings: 4
Ingredients:
- 4 medium salmon fillets, skinless and boneless
- fennel bulb, chopped
- Black pepper to the taste
- ¼ cup low-sodium veggie stock
- cup non-fat yogurt
- ¼ cup green olives pitted and chopped
- ¼ cup chives, chopped
- tablespoon olive oil
- tablespoon lemon juice

Directions:
1. Arrange the fennel in a baking dish, add salmon fillets, season with black pepper, add stock, bake in the oven at 390 degrees F for 10 minutes and divide everything between plates.
2. In a bowl, mix yogurt with chives, olives, lemon juice, olive oil and black pepper and whisk well.
3. Top the salmon with this mix and serve.
4. Enjoy!

Nutrition: Calories 252, Fat 2, Fiber 4, Carbs 12, Protein 9

POULTRY

601. Chicken Sliders

Preparation time: 10 minutes
Cooking time: 10 minutes
Servings: 4
Ingredients:
- 10 ounces ground chicken breast
- 1 tablespoon black pepper
- 1 tablespoon minced garlic
- 1 tablespoon balsamic vinegar
- 1/2 cup minced onion
- 1 fresh chili pepper, minced
- 1 tablespoon fennel seed, crushed
- 4 whole-wheat mini buns
- 4 lettuce leaves
- 4 tomato slices

Directions:
1. Combine all the ingredients except the wheat buns, tomato, and lettuce. Mix well and refrigerate the mixture for 1 hour. Divide the mixture into 4 patties.
2. Broil these patties in a greased baking tray until golden brown. Place the chicken patties in the wheat buns along with lettuce and tomato. Serve.

Nutrition: Calories 224; Fat 4.5 g; Sodium 212 mg; Carbs 10.2 g; Protein 67.4 g

602. White Chicken Chili

Preparation time: 20 minutes
Cooking time: 15 minutes
Servings: 4
Ingredients:
- 1 can white chunk chicken
- 2 cans low-sodium white beans, drained
- 1 can low-sodium diced tomatoes
- 4 cups of low-sodium chicken broth
- 1 medium onion, chopped
- 1/2 medium green pepper, chopped
- 1 medium red pepper, chopped
- 2 garlic cloves, minced
- 2 teaspoons chili powder
- 1 teaspoon ground cumin
- 1 teaspoon dried oregano
- Cayenne pepper, to taste

- 8 tablespoons shredded reduced-fat Monterey Jack cheese
- 3 tablespoons chopped fresh cilantro

Directions:
1. In a soup pot, add beans, tomatoes, chicken, and chicken broth. Cover this soup pot and let it simmer over medium heat. Meanwhile, grease a nonstick pan with cooking spray. Add peppers, garlic, and onions. Sauté for 5 minutes until soft.
2. Transfer the mixture to the soup pot. Add cumin, chili powder, cayenne pepper, and oregano. Cook for 10 minutes, then garnish the chili with cilantro and 1 tablespoon cheese. Serve.

Nutrition: Calories 225; Fat 12.9 g; Sodium 480 mg; Carbs 24.7 g; Protein 25.3g

603. Sweet Potato-Turkey Meatloaf

Preparation time: 15 minutes
Cooking time: 25 minutes
Servings: 4
Ingredients:
- 1 large sweet potato, peeled and cubed
- 1-pound ground turkey (breast)
- 1 large egg
- 1 small sweet onion, finely chopped
- 2 cloves garlic, minced
- 2 slices whole-wheat bread, crumbs
- ¼ cup honey barbecue sauce
- ¼ cup ketchup
- 2 Tablespoons Dijon Mustard
- 1 Tablespoon fresh ground pepper
- ½ Tablespoon salt

Directions:
1. Warm oven to 350 F. Grease a baking dish. In a large pot, boil a cup of lightly salted water, add the sweet potato. Cook until tender. Drain the water. Mash the potato.
2. Mix the honey barbecue sauce, ketchup, and Dijon mustard in a small bowl. Mix thoroughly. In a large bowl, mix the turkey and the egg. Add the sweet onion, garlic. Pour in the combined sauces. Add the bread crumbs. Season the mixture with salt and pepper.
3. Add the sweet potato. Combine thoroughly with your hands. If the mixture feels wet, add more bread crumbs. Shape the mixture into a loaf. Place in the loaf pan. Bake for 25 – 35 minutes until the meat is cooked through. Broil for 5 minutes. Slice and serve.

Nutrition: Calories – 133; Protein - 85g; Carbohydrates - 50g; Fat - 34g; Sodium - 202mg

604. Oaxacan Chicken

Preparation time: 15 minutes
Cooking time: 28 minutes
Servings: 2
Ingredients:
- 1 4-ounce chicken breast, skinned and halved
- ½ cup uncooked long-grain rice
- 1 teaspoon of extra-virgin olive oil
- ½ cup low-sodium salsa

- ½ cup chicken stock, mixed with 2 Tablespoons water
- ¾ cup baby carrots
- 2 tablespoons green olives, pitted and chopped
- 2 Tablespoons dark raisins
- ½ teaspoon ground Cinnamon
- 2 Tablespoons fresh cilantro or parsley, coarsely chopped

Directions:
1. Warm oven to 350 F. In a large saucepan that can go in the oven, heat the olive oil. Add the rice. Sauté the rice until it begins to pop, approximately 2 minutes.
2. Add the salsa, baby carrots, green olives, dark raisins, halved chicken breast, chicken stock, and ground cinnamon. Bring the mix to a simmer, stir once.
3. Cover the mixture tightly, bake in the oven until the chicken stock has been completely absorbed, approximately 25 minutes. Sprinkle fresh cilantro or parsley, mix. Serve immediately.

Nutrition: Calories – 143; Protein - 102g; Carbohydrates - 66g. Fat - 18g. Sodium - 97mg

605. Spicy Chicken with Minty Couscous

Preparation time: 15 minutes
Cooking time: 25 minutes
Servings: 2
Ingredients:
- 2 small chicken breasts, sliced
- 1 red chili pepper, finely chopped
- 1 garlic clove, crushed
- ginger root, 2 cm long peeled and grated
- 1 teaspoon ground cumin
- ½ teaspoon turmeric
- 2 Tablespoons extra-virgin olive oil
- 1 pinch sea salt
- ¾ cup couscous
- Small bunch mint leaves, finely chopped
- 2 lemons, grate the rind and juice them

Directions:
1. In a large bowl, place the chicken breast slices and chopped chili pepper. Sprinkle with the crushed garlic, ginger, cumin, turmeric, and a pinch of salt. Add the grated rind of both lemons and the juice from 1 lemon. Pour 1 tablespoon of the olive oil over the chicken, coat evenly.
2. Cover the dish with plastic and refrigerate within 1 hour. After 1 hour, coat a skillet with olive oil and fry the chicken. As the chicken is cooking, pour the couscous into a bowl and pour hot water over it, let it absorb the water (approximately 5 minutes).
3. Fluff the couscous. Add some chopped mint, the other tablespoon of olive oil, and juice from the second lemon. Top the couscous with the chicken. Garnish with chopped mint. Serve immediately.

Nutrition: Calories – 166; Protein - 106g; Carbohydrates - 52g; Sugars - 0.1g; Fat - 17g; Sodium - 108mg

606. Chicken, Pasta and Snow Peas

Preparation time: 15 minutes
Cooking time: 20 minutes
Servings: 2
Ingredients:
- 1-pound chicken breasts
- 2 ½ cups penne pasta
- 1 cup snow peas, trimmed and halved
- 1 teaspoon olive oil
- 1 standard jar Tomato and Basil pasta sauce
- Fresh ground pepper

Directions:
5. In a medium frying pan, heat the olive oil. Flavor the chicken breasts with salt and pepper. Cook the chicken breasts until cooked through (approximately 5 – 7 minutes each side).
6. Cook the pasta, as stated in the instruction of the package. Cook the snow peas with the pasta. Scoop 1 cup of the pasta water. Drain the pasta and peas, set aside.
7. Once the chicken is cooked, slice diagonally. Return back the chicken in the frying pan. Add the pasta sauce. If the mixture seems dry, add some of the pasta water to the desired consistency. Heat, then divide into bowls. Serve immediately.

Nutrition: Calories – 140; Protein - 34g; Carbohydrates - 52g; Fat - 17g; Sodium - 118mg

607. Chicken with Noodles

Preparation time: 15 minutes
Cooking time: 30 minutes
Servings: 6
Ingredients:
- 4 chicken breasts, skinless, boneless
- 1-pound pasta (angel hair, or linguine, or ramen)
- ½ teaspoon sesame oil
- 1 Tablespoon canola oil
- 2 Tablespoons chili paste
- 1 onion, diced
- 2 garlic cloves, chopped coarsely
- ½ cup of soy sauce
- ½ medium cabbage, sliced
- 2 carrots, chopped coarsely

Directions:
5. Cook your pasta in a large pot. Mix the canola oil, sesame oil, and chili paste and heat for 25 seconds in a large pot. Add the onion, cook for 2 minutes. Put the garlic and fry within 20 seconds. Add the chicken, cook on each side 5 - 7 minutes, until cooked through.
6. Remove the mix from the pan, set aside. Add the cabbage, carrots, cook until the vegetables are tender. Pour everything back into the pan. Add the noodles. Pour in the soy sauce and combine thoroughly. Heat for 5 minutes. Serve immediately.

Nutrition: Calories – 110; Protein - 30g; Carbohydrates - 32g; Sugars - 0.1g; Fat - 18g; Sodium - 121mg

608. Honey Crusted Chicken

Preparation time: 10 minutes
Cooking time: 25 minutes
Servings: 2
Ingredients:
- 1 teaspoon paprika
- 8 saltine crackers, 2 inches square
- 2 chicken breasts, each 4 ounces
- 4 tsp. honey

Directions:
1. Set the oven to heat at 375 degrees F. Grease a baking dish with cooking oil. Smash the crackers in a Zip lock bag and toss them with paprika in a bowl. Brush chicken with honey and add it to the crackers.
2. Mix well and transfer the chicken to the baking dish. Bake the chicken for 25 minutes until golden brown. Serve.

Nutrition: Calories 219; Fat 17 g; Sodium 456 mg; Carbs 12.1 g; Protein 31 g

609. Paella with Chicken, Leeks, and Tarragon

Preparation time: 10 minutes
Cooking time: 20 minutes
Servings: 2
Ingredients:
- 1 teaspoon extra-virgin olive oil
- 1 small onion, sliced
- 2 leeks (whites only), thinly sliced
- 3 garlic cloves, minced
- 1-pound boneless, skinless chicken breast, cut into strips 1/2-inch-wide and 2 inches long
- 2 large tomatoes, chopped
- 1 red pepper, sliced
- 2/3 cup long-grain brown rice
- 1 teaspoon tarragon, or to taste
- 2 cups fat-free, unsalted chicken broth
- 1 cup frozen peas
- 1/4 cup chopped fresh parsley
- 1 lemon, cut into 4 wedges

Directions:
1. Preheat a nonstick pan with olive oil over medium heat. Toss in leeks, onions, chicken strips, and garlic. Sauté for 5 minutes. Stir in red pepper slices and tomatoes. Stir and cook for 5 minutes.
2. Add tarragon, broth, and rice. Let it boil, then reduce the heat to a simmer. Continue cooking for 10 minutes, then add peas and continue cooking until the liquid is thoroughly cooked. Garnish with parsley and lemon. Serve.

Nutrition: Calories 388; Fat 15.2 g; Sodium 572 mg; Carbs 5.4 g; Protein 27 g

610. Southwestern Chicken and Pasta

Preparation time: 10 minutes
Cooking time: 10 minutes

Servings: 2

Ingredients:

- 1 cup uncooked whole-wheat rigatoni
- 2 chicken breasts, cut into cubes
- 1/4 cup of salsa
- 1 1/2 cups of canned unsalted tomato sauce
- 1/8 tsp. garlic powder
- 1 tsp. cumin
- 1/2 tsp. chili powder
- 1/2 cup canned black beans, drained
- 1/2 cup fresh corn
- 1/4 cup Monterey Jack and Colby cheese, shredded

Directions:

1. Fill a pot with water up to ¾ full and boil it. Add pasta to cook until it is al dente, then drain the pasta while rinsing under cold water. Preheat a skillet with cooking oil, then cook the chicken for 10 minutes until golden from both sides.
2. Add tomato sauce, salsa, cumin, garlic powder, black beans, corn, and chili powder. Cook the mixture while stirring, then toss in the pasta. Serve with 2 tablespoons cheese on top. Enjoy.

Nutrition: Calories 245; Fat 16.3 g; Sodium 515 mg; Carbs 19.3 g; Protein 33.3 g

611. Stuffed Chicken Breasts

Preparation time: 15 minutes
Cooking time: 30 minutes
Servings: 4

Ingredients:

- 3 tbsp. seedless raisins
- 1/2 cup of chopped onion
- 1/2 cup of chopped celery
- 1/4 tsp. garlic, minced
- 1 bay leaf
- 1 cup apple with peel, chopped
- 2 tbsp. chopped water chestnuts
- 4 large chicken breast halves, 5 ounces each
- 1 tablespoon olive oil
- 1 cup fat-free milk
- 1 teaspoon curry powder
- 2 tablespoons all-purpose (plain) flour
- 1 lemon, cut into 4 wedges

Directions:

1. Set the oven to heat at 425 degrees F. Grease a baking dish with cooking oil. Soak raisins in warm water until they swell. Grease a heated skillet with cooking spray.
2. Add celery, garlic, onions, and bay leaf. Sauté for 5 minutes. Discard the bay leaf, then toss in apples. Stir cook for 2 minutes. Drain the soaked raisin and pat them dry to remove excess water.
3. Add raisins and water chestnuts to the apple mixture. Pull apart the chicken's skin and stuff the apple raisin mixture between the skin and the chicken. Preheat olive oil in another skillet and sear the breasts for 5 minutes per side.
4. Place the chicken breasts in the baking dish and cover the dish. Bake for 15 minutes until temperature reaches 165 degrees F. Prepare sauce by mixing milk, flour, and curry powder in a saucepan.

5. Stir cook until the mixture thickens, about 5 minutes. Pour this sauce over the baked chicken. Bake again in the covered dish for 10 minutes. Serve.

Nutrition: Calories 357; Fat 32.7 g; Sodium 277 mg; Carbs 17.7 g; Protein 31.2 g

612. Buffalo Chicken Salad Wrap

Preparation time: 10 minutes
Cooking time: 10 minutes
Servings: 4

Ingredients:

- 3-4 ounces chicken breasts
- 2 whole chipotle peppers
- 1/4 cup white wine vinegar
- 1/4 cup low-calorie mayonnaise
- 2 stalks celery, diced
- 2 carrots, cut into matchsticks
- 1 small yellow onion, diced
- 1/2 cup thinly sliced rutabaga or another root vegetable
- 4 ounces spinach, cut into strips
- 2 whole-grain tortillas (12-inch diameter)

Directions:

1. Set the oven or a grill to heat at 375 degrees F. Bake the chicken first for 10 minutes per side. Blend chipotle peppers with mayonnaise and wine vinegar in the blender. Dice the baked chicken into cubes or small chunks.
2. Mix the chipotle mixture with all the ingredients except tortillas and spinach. Spread 2 ounces of spinach over the tortilla and scoop the stuffing on top. Wrap the tortilla and cut it into half. Serve.

Nutrition: Calories 300; Fat 16.4 g; Sodium 471 mg; Carbs 8.7 g; Protein 38.5 g

613. Chicken with Mushrooms

Preparation time: 15 minutes
Cooking time: 6 hours & 10 minutes
Servings: 2

Ingredients:

- 2 chicken breasts, skinless and boneless
- 1 cup mushrooms, sliced
- 1 onion, sliced
- 1 cup chicken stock
- 1/2 tsp. thyme, dried
- Pepper
- Salt

Directions:

1. Add all ingredients to the slow cooker. Cook on low within 6 hours. Serve and enjoy.

Nutrition: Calories: 313; Fat: 11.3g; Protein: 44.3g; Carbs: 6.9g; Sodium 541 mg

614. Baked Chicken

Preparation time: 15 minutes
Cooking time: 35 minutes

Servings: 4
Ingredients:
- 2 lbs. chicken tenders
- 1 large zucchini
- 1 cup grape tomatoes
- 2 tbsp. olive oil
- 3 dill sprigs
- For topping:
- 2 tbsp. feta cheese, crumbled
- 1 tbsp. olive oil
- 1 tbsp. fresh lemon juice
- 1 tbsp. fresh dill, chopped

Directions:
1. Warm oven to 200 C/ 400 F. Drizzle the olive oil on a baking tray, then place chicken, zucchini, dill, and tomatoes on the tray. Season with salt. Bake chicken within 30 minutes.
2. Meanwhile, in a small bowl, stir all topping ingredients. Place chicken on the serving tray, then top with veggies and discard dill sprigs. Sprinkle topping mixture on top of chicken and vegetables. Serve and enjoy.

Nutrition: Calories: 557; Fat: 28.6g; Protein: 67.9g; Carbs: 5.2g; Sodium 760 mg

615. Garlic Pepper Chicken

Preparation time: 15 minutes
Cooking time: 21 minutes
Servings: 2
Ingredients:
- 2 chicken breasts, cut into strips
- 2 bell peppers, cut into strips
- 5 garlic cloves, chopped
- 3 tbsp. water
- 2 tbsp. olive oil
- 1 tbsp. paprika
- 2 tsp. black pepper
- 1/2 tsp. salt

Directions:
1. Warm-up olive oil in a large saucepan over medium heat. Add garlic and sauté for 2-3 minutes. Add peppers and cook for 3 minutes. Add chicken and spices and stir to coat. Add water and stir well. Bring to boil. Cover and simmer for 10-15 minutes. Serve and enjoy.

Nutrition: Calories: 462; Fat: 25.7g; Protein: 44.7g; Carbs: 14.8g; Sodium 720 mg

616. Mustard Chicken Tenders

Preparation time: 15 minutes
Cooking time: 20 minutes
Servings: 4
Ingredients:
- 1 lb. chicken tenders
- 2 tbsp. fresh tarragon, chopped
- 1/2 cup whole grain mustard
- 1/2 tsp. paprika
- 1 garlic clove, minced
- 1/2 oz. fresh lemon juice
- 1/2 tsp. pepper
- 1/4 tsp. kosher salt

Directions:
1. Warm oven to 425 F. Add all ingredients except chicken to the large bowl and mix well. Put the chicken in the bowl, then stir until well coated. Place chicken on a baking dish and cover. Bake within 15-20 minutes. Serve and enjoy.

Nutrition: Calories: 242; Fat: 9.5g; Protein: 33.2g; Carbs: 3.1g; Sodium 240 mg

617. Salsa Chicken Chili

Preparation time: 15 minutes
Cooking time: 20 minutes
Servings: 8
Ingredients:
- 2 1/2 lbs. chicken breasts, skinless and boneless
- 1/2 tsp. cumin powder
- 3 garlic cloves, minced
- 1 onion, diced
- 16 oz. salsa
- 1 tsp. oregano
- 1 tbsp. olive oil

Directions:
1. Add oil into the instant pot and set the pot on sauté mode. Add onion to the pot and sauté until softened, about 3 minutes. Add garlic and sauté for a minute. Add oregano and cumin and sauté for a minute. Add half salsa and stir well. Place chicken and pour remaining salsa over chicken.
2. Seal pot with the lid and select manual, and set timer for 10 minutes. Remove chicken and shred. Move it back to the pot, then stir well to combine. Serve and enjoy.

Nutrition: Calories: 308; Fat: 12.4g; Protein: 42.1g; Carbs: 5.4g; Sodium 656 mg

618. Lemon Garlic Chicken

Preparation time: 15 minutes
Cooking time: 12 minutes
Servings: 3
Ingredients:
- 3 chicken breasts, cut into thin slices
- 2 lemon zest, grated
- ¼ cup olive oil
- 4 garlic cloves, minced
- Pepper
- Salt

Directions:
1. Warm-up olive oil in a pan over medium heat. Add garlic to the pan and sauté for 30 seconds. Put the chicken in the pan and sauté within 10 minutes. Add lemon zest and lemon juice and bring to boil. Remove from heat and season with pepper and salt. Serve and enjoy.

Nutrition: Calories: 439; Fat: 27.8g; Protein: 42.9g; Carbs: 4.9g; Sodium 306 mg

619. Simple Mediterranean Chicken

Preparation time: 15 minutes
Cooking time: 15 minutes
Servings: 12
Ingredients:

- 2 chicken breasts, skinless and boneless
- 1 ½ cup grape tomatoes, cut in half
- ½ cup olives
- 2 tbsp. olive oil
- 1 tsp. Italian seasoning
- ¼ tsp. pepper
- ¼ tsp. salt

Directions:

1. Season chicken with Italian seasoning, pepper, and salt. Warm-up olive oil in a pan over medium heat. Add season chicken to the pan and cook for 4-6 minutes on each side. Transfer chicken on a plate.
2. Put tomatoes plus olives in the pan and cook for 2-4 minutes. Pour olive and tomato mixture on top of the chicken and serve.

Nutrition: Calories: 468; Fat: 29.4g; Protein: 43.8g; Carbs: 7.8g; Sodium 410 mg

620. Roasted Chicken Thighs

Preparation time: 15 minutes
Cooking time: 55 minutes
Servings: 4
Ingredients:

- 8 chicken thighs
- 3 tbsp. fresh parsley, chopped
- 1 tsp. dried oregano
- 6 garlic cloves, crushed
- ¼ cup capers, drained
- 10 oz. roasted red peppers, sliced
- 2 cups grape tomatoes
- 1 ½ lbs. potatoes, cut into small chunks
- 4 tbsp. olive oil
- Pepper
- Salt

Directions:

1. Warm oven to 200 400 F. Season chicken with pepper and salt. Heat-up 2 tablespoons of olive oil in a pan over medium heat. Add chicken to the pan and sear until lightly golden brown from all the sides.
2. Transfer chicken onto a baking tray. Add tomato, potatoes, capers, oregano, garlic, and red peppers around the chicken. Season with pepper and salt and drizzle with remaining olive oil. Bake in preheated oven for 45-55 minutes. Garnish with parsley and serve.

Nutrition: Calories: 848; Fat: 29.1g; Protein: 91.3g; Carbs: 45.2g; Sodium 110 mg

621. Mediterranean Turkey Breast

Preparation time: 15 minutes
Cooking time: 4 minutes & 30 minutes
Servings: 6
Ingredients:

- 4 lbs. turkey breast
- 3 tbsp. flour
- ¾ cup chicken stock
- 4 garlic cloves, chopped
- 1 tsp. dried oregano
- ½ fresh lemon juice
- ½ cup sun-dried tomatoes, chopped
- ½ cup olives, chopped
- 1 onion, chopped
- ¼ tsp. pepper
- ½ tsp. salt

Directions:

1. Add turkey breast, garlic, oregano, lemon juice, sun-dried tomatoes, olives, onion, pepper, and salt to the slow cooker. Add half stock. Cook on high within 4 hours.
2. Whisk remaining stock and flour in a small bowl and add to slow cooker. Cover and cook for 30 minutes more. Serve and enjoy.

Nutrition: Calories: 537; Fat: 9.7g; Protein: 79.1g; Carbs: 29.6g; Sodium 330 mg

622. Olive Capers Chicken

Preparation time: 15 minutes
Cooking time: 16 minutes
Servings: 4
Ingredients:

- 2 lbs. chicken
- 1/3 cup chicken stock
- oz. Capers
- 6 oz. olives
- 1/4 cup fresh basil
- 1 tbsp. olive oil
- 1 tsp. oregano
- 2 garlic cloves, minced
- 2 tbsp. red wine vinegar
- 1/8 tsp. pepper
- 1/4 tsp. salt

Directions:

1. Put olive oil in your instant pot and set the pot on sauté mode. Add chicken to the pot and sauté for 3-4 minutes. Add remaining ingredients and stir well. Seal pot with the lid and select manual, and set timer for 12 minutes. Serve and enjoy.

Nutrition: Calories: 433; Fat: 15.2g; Protein: 66.9g; Carbs: 4.8g; Sodium 244 mg

623. Chicken with Potatoes Olives & Sprouts

Preparation time: 15 minutes

Cooking time: 35 minutes
Servings: 4
Ingredients:

- 1 lb. chicken breasts, skinless, boneless, and cut into pieces
- ¼ cup olives, quartered
- 1 tsp. oregano
- 1 ½ tsp. Dijon mustard
- 1 lemon juice
- 1/3 cup vinaigrette dressing
- 1 medium onion, diced
- 3 cups potatoes cut into pieces
- 4 cups Brussels sprouts, trimmed and quartered
- ¼ tsp. pepper
- ¼ tsp. salt

Directions:

1. Warm-up oven to 400 F. Place chicken in the center of the baking tray, then place potatoes, sprouts, and onions around the chicken.
2. In a small bowl, mix vinaigrette, oregano, mustard, lemon juice, and salt and pour over chicken and veggies. Sprinkle olives and season with pepper.
3. Bake in preheated oven for 20 minutes. Transfer chicken to a plate. Stir the vegetables and roast for 15 minutes more. Serve and enjoy.

Nutrition: Calories: 397; Fat: 13g; Protein: 38.3g; Carbs: 31.4g; Sodium 175 mg

624. Garlic Mushroom Chicken

Preparation time: 15 minutes
Cooking time: 15 minutes
Servings: 4
Ingredients:

- 4 chicken breasts, boneless and skinless
- 3 garlic cloves, minced
- 1 onion, chopped
- 2 cups mushrooms, sliced
- 1 tbsp. olive oil
- ½ cup chicken stock
- ¼ tsp. pepper
- ½ tsp. salt

Directions:

1. Season chicken with pepper and salt. Warm oil in a pan on medium heat, then put season chicken in the pan and cook for 5-6 minutes on each side. Remove and place on a plate.
2. Add onion and mushrooms to the pan and sauté until tender, about 2-3 minutes. Add garlic and sauté for a minute. Add stock and bring to boil. Stir well and cook for 1-2 minutes. Pour over chicken and serve.

Nutrition: Calories: 331; Fat: 14.5g; Protein: 43.9g; Carbs: 4.6; Sodium 420 mg

625. Grilled Chicken

Preparation time: 15 minutes
Cooking time: 15 minutes
Servings: 4
Ingredients:

- 4 chicken breasts, skinless and boneless
- 1 ½ tsp. dried oregano
- 1 tsp. paprika
- 5 garlic cloves, minced
- ½ cup fresh parsley, minced
- ½ cup olive oil
- ½ cup fresh lemon juice
- Pepper
- Salt

Directions:

1. Add lemon juice, oregano, paprika, garlic, parsley, and olive oil to a large zip-lock bag. Season chicken with pepper and salt and add to bag. Seal bag and shake well to coat chicken with marinade. Let sit chicken in the marinade for 20 minutes.
2. Remove chicken from marinade and grill over medium-high heat for 5-6 minutes on each side. Serve and enjoy.

Nutrition: Calories: 512; Fat: 36.5g; Protein: 43.1g; Carbs: 3g; Sodium 110mg

626. Delicious Lemon Chicken Salad

Preparation time: 15 minutes
Cooking time: 5 minutes
Servings: 4
Ingredients:

- 1 lb. chicken breast, cooked and diced
- 1 tbsp. fresh dill, chopped
- 2 tsp. olive oil
- 1/4 cup low-fat yogurt
- 1 tsp. lemon zest, grated
- 2 tbsp. onion, minced
- ¼ tsp. pepper
- ¼ tsp. salt

Directions:

1. Put all you're fixing into the large mixing bowl and toss well. Season with pepper and salt. Cover and place in the refrigerator. Serve chilled and enjoy.

Nutrition: Calories: 165; Fat: 5.4g; Protein: 25.2g; Carbs: 2.2g; Sodium 153mg

627. Healthy Chicken Orzo

Preparation time: 15 minutes
Cooking time: 15 minutes
Servings: 4
Ingredients:

- 1 cup whole wheat orzo
- 1 lb. chicken breasts, sliced
- ½ tsp. red pepper flakes
- ½ cup feta cheese, crumbled
- ½ tsp. oregano
- 1 tbsp. fresh parsley, chopped
- 1 tbsp. fresh basil, chopped
- ¼ cup pine nuts
- 1 cup spinach, chopped
- ¼ cup white wine
- ½ cup olives, sliced

- 1 cup grape tomatoes, cut in half
- ½ tbsp. garlic, minced
- 2 tbsp. olive oil
- ½ tsp. pepper
- ½ tsp. salt

Directions:
1. Add water in a small saucepan and bring to boil. Heat 1 tablespoon of olive oil in a pan over medium heat. Season chicken with pepper and salt and cook in the pan for 5-7 minutes on each side. Remove from pan and set aside.
2. Add orzo in boiling water and cook according to the packet directions. Heat remaining olive oil in a pan on medium heat, then put garlic in the pan and sauté for a minute. Stir in white wine and cherry tomatoes and cook on high for 3 minutes.
3. Add cooked orzo, spices, spinach, pine nuts, and olives and stir until well combined. Add chicken on top of orzo and sprinkle with feta cheese. Serve and enjoy.

Nutrition: Calories: 518; Fat: 27.7g; Protein: 40.6g; Carbs: 26.2g; Sodium 121mg

628. The Ultimate Faux-Tisserie Chicken

Preparation time: 15 minutes
Cooking time: 35 minutes
Servings: 5
Ingredients:
- 1 c. low sodium broth
- 2 tbsps. Olive oil
- ½ quartered medium onion
- 2 tbsps. Favorite seasoning
- 2 ½ lbs. whole chicken
- Black pepper
- 5 large fresh garlic cloves

Directions:
1. Massage the chicken with 1 tablespoon of olive oil and sprinkle pepper on top. Place onion wedges and garlic cloves inside the chicken. Take a butcher's twin and secure the legs
2. Set your pot to Sauté mode. Put olive oil in your pan on medium heat, allow the oil to heat up. Add chicken and sear both sides for 4 minutes per side. Sprinkle your seasoning over the chicken, remove the chicken and place a trivet at the bottom of your pot
3. Sprinkle seasoning over the chicken, making sure to rub it. Transfer the chicken to the trivet with the breast side facing up, lock up the lid. Cook on HIGH pressure for 25 minutes. Allow it to rest and serve!

Nutrition: Calories: 1010; Fat: 64 g; Carbs: 47 g; Protein: 60 g; Sodium: 209 mg

629. Oregano Chicken Thighs

Preparation time: 15 minutes
Cooking time: 20 minutes
Servings: 6
Ingredients:
- 12 chicken thighs

- 1 tsp. dried parsley
- ¼ tsp. pepper and salt.
- ½ c. extra virgin essential olive oil
- 4 minced garlic cloves
- 1 c. chopped oregano
- ¼ c. low-sodium veggie stock

Directions:
1. In your food processor, mix parsley with oregano, garlic, salt, pepper, and stock and pulse. Put chicken thighs within the bowl, add oregano paste, toss, cover, and then leave aside within the fridge for 10 minutes.
2. Heat the kitchen grill over medium heat, add chicken pieces, close the lid and cook for twenty or so minutes with them. Divide between plates and serve!

Nutrition: Calories: 254; Fat: 3 g; Carbs: 7 g; Protein: 17 g; Sugars: 0.9 g; Sodium: 730 mg

630. Pesto Chicken Breasts with Summer Squash

Preparation time: 15 minutes
Cooking time: 10 minutes
Servings: 4
Ingredients:
- 4 medium boneless, skinless chicken breast halves
- 1 tbsp. olive oil
- 2 tbsps. Homemade pesto
- 2 c. finely chopped zucchini
- 2 tbsps. Finely shredded Asiago

Directions:
1. Cook your chicken in hot oil on medium heat within 4 minutes in a large nonstick skillet. Flip the chicken then put the zucchini.
2. Cook within 4 to 6 minutes more or until the chicken is tender and no longer pink (170 F), and squash is crisp-tender, stirring squash gently once or twice. Transfer chicken and squash to 4 dinner plates. Spread pesto over chicken; sprinkle with Asiago.

Nutrition: Calories: 230; Fat: 9 g; Carbs: 8 g; Protein: 30 g; Sodium: 578 mg

631. Chicken, Tomato and Green Beans

Preparation time: 15 minutes
Cooking time: 25 minutes
Servings: 4
Ingredients:
- 6 oz. low-sodium canned tomato paste
- 2 tbsps. Olive oil
- ¼ tsp. black pepper
- 2 lbs. trimmed green beans
- 2 tbsps. Chopped parsley
- 1 ½ lbs. boneless, skinless, and cubed chicken breasts
- 25 oz. no-salt-added canned tomato sauce

Directions:
1. Heat a pan with 50 % with the oil over medium heat, add chicken, stir, cover, and cook within 5 minutes on both sides and transfer to a bowl. Heat inside the same pan

while using rest through the oil over medium heat, add green beans, stir and cook for 10 minutes.

2. Return chicken for that pan, add black pepper, tomato sauce, tomato paste, and parsley, stir, cover, cook for 10 minutes more, divide between plates and serve. Enjoy!

Nutrition: Calories: 190; Fat: 4 g; Carbs: 12 g; Protein: 9 g; Sodium: 168 mg

632. Chicken Tortillas

Preparation time: 15 minutes
Cooking time: 5 minutes
Servings: 4
Ingredients:
- 6 oz. boneless, skinless, and cooked chicken breasts
- Black pepper
- 1/3 c. fat-free yogurt
- 4 heated up whole-wheat tortillas
- 2 chopped tomatoes

Directions:
1. Heat-up a pan over medium heat, add one tortilla during those times, heat up, and hang them on the working surface. Spread yogurt on each tortilla, add chicken and tomatoes, roll, divide between plates and serve. Enjoy!

Nutrition: Calories: 190; Fat: 2 g; Carbs: 12 g; Protein: 6 g; Sodium: 300 mg

633. Pumpkin and Black Beans Chicken

Preparation time: 15 minutes
Cooking time: 25 minutes
Servings: 4
Ingredients:
- 1 tbsp. essential olive oil
- 1 tbsp. Chopped cilantro
- 1 c. coconut milk
- 15 oz. canned black beans, drained
- 1 lb. skinless and boneless chicken breasts
- 2 c. water
- ½ c. pumpkin flesh

Directions:
1. Heat a pan when using oil over medium-high heat, add the chicken and cook for 5 minutes. Add the river, milk, pumpkin, and black beans toss, cover the pan, reduce heat to medium and cook for 20 mins. Add cilantro, toss, divide between plates and serve. Enjoy!

Nutrition: Calories: 254; Fat: 6 g; Carbs: 16 g; Protein: 22 g; Sodium: 92 mg

634. Chicken Thighs and Apples Mix

Preparation time: 15 minutes
Cooking time: 60 minutes
Servings: 4
Ingredients:
- **3 cored and sliced apples**

- 1 tbsp. apple cider vinegar treatment
- ¾ c. natural apple juice
- ¼ tsp. pepper and salt
- 1 tbsp. grated ginger
- 8 chicken thighs
- 3 tbsps. Chopped onion

Directions:
1. In a bowl, mix chicken with salt, pepper, vinegar, onion, ginger, and apple juice, toss well, cover, keep within the fridge for ten minutes, transfer with a baking dish, and include apples. Introduce inside the oven at 400 0F for just 1 hour. Divide between plates and serve. Enjoy!

Nutrition: Calories: 214; Fat: 3 g; Carbs: 14 g; Protein: 15 g; Sodium: 405 mg

635. Thai Chicken Thighs

Preparation time: 15 minutes
Cooking time: 1 hour & 5minutes
Servings: 6
Ingredients:
- ½ c. Thai chili sauce
- 1 chopped green onions bunch
- 4 lbs. chicken thighs

Directions:
1. Heat a pan over medium-high heat. Add chicken thighs, brown them for 5 minutes on both sides Transfer to some baking dish, then add chili sauce and green onions and toss.
2. Introduce within the oven and bake at 4000F for 60 minutes. Divide everything between plates and serve. Enjoy!

Nutrition: Calories: 220; Fat: 4 g; Carbs: 12 g; Protein: 10 g; Sodium: 870 mg

636. Falling "Off" The Bone Chicken

Preparation time: 15 minutes
Cooking time: 40 minutes
Servings: 4
Ingredients:
- 6 peeled garlic cloves
- 1 tbsp. organic extra virgin coconut oil
- 2 tbsps. Lemon juice
- 1 ½ c. pacific organic bone chicken broth
- ¼ tsp. freshly ground black pepper
- ½ tsp. sea flavored vinegar
- 1 whole organic chicken piece
- 1 tsp. paprika
- 1 tsp. dried thyme

Directions:
1. Take a small bowl and toss in the thyme, paprika, pepper, and flavored vinegar and mix them. Use the mixture to season the chicken properly. Pour down the oil in your instant pot and heat it to shimmering; toss in the chicken with breast downward and let it cook for about 6-7 minutes
2. After the 7 minutes, flip over the chicken pour down the broth, garlic cloves, and lemon juice. Cook within 25

minutes on a high setting. Remove the dish from the cooker and let it stand for about 5 minutes before serving.

Nutrition: Calories: 664; Fat: 44 g; Carbs: 44 g; Protein: 27 g; Sugars: 0.1 g; Sodium: 800 mg

637. Feisty Chicken Porridge

Preparation time: 15 minutes
Cooking time: 30 minutes
Servings: 4
Ingredients:
- 1 ½ c. fresh ginger
- 1 lb. cooked chicken legs
- Green onions
- Toasted cashew nuts
- 5 c. chicken broth
- 1 cup jasmine rice
- 4 c. water

Directions:
1. Place the rice in your fridge and allow it to chill 1 hour before cooking. Take the rice out and add them to your Instant Pot. Pour broth and water. Lock up the lid and cook on Porridge mode.
2. Separate the meat from the chicken legs and add the meat to your soup. Stir well over sauté mode. Season with a bit of flavored vinegar and enjoy with a garnish of nuts and onion

Nutrition: Calories: 206; Fat: 8 g; Carbs: 8 g; Protein: 23 g; Sugars: 0 g; Sodium: 950 mg

638. Parmesan and Chicken Spaghetti Squash

Preparation time: 15 minutes
Cooking time: 20 minutes
Servings: 6
Ingredients:
- 16 oz. mozzarella
- 1 spaghetti squash piece
- 1 lb. cooked cube chicken
- 1 c. Marinara sauce

Directions:
1. Split up the squash in halves and remove the seeds. Arrange or put one cup of water in your pot, then put a trivet on top.
2. Add the squash halves to the trivet. Cook within 20 minutes at HIGH pressure. Remove the squashes and shred them using a fork into spaghetti portions
3. Pour sauce over the squash and give it a nice mix. Top them up with the cubed-up chicken and top with mozzarella. Broil for 1-2 minutes and broil until the cheese has melted

Nutrition: Calories: 237; Fat: 10 g; Carbs: 32 g; Protein: 11 g; Sodium: 500 mg

639. Apricot Chicken

Preparation time: 15 minutes

Cooking time: 6 minutes
Servings: 4
Ingredients:
- 1 bottle creamy French dressing
- ¼ c. flavorless oil
- White cooked rice
- 1 large jar Apricot preserve
- 4 lbs. boneless and skinless chicken
- 1 package onion soup mix

Directions:
1. Rinse and pat dry the chicken. Dice into bite-size pieces. In a large bowl, mix the apricot preserve, creamy dressing, and onion soup mix. Stir until thoroughly combined. Place the chicken in the bowl. Mix until coated.
2. In a large skillet, heat the oil. Place the chicken in the oil gently. Cook 4 – 6 minutes on each side, until golden brown. Serve over rice.

Nutrition: Calories: 202; Fat: 12 g; Carbs: 75 g; Protein: 20 g; Sugars: 10 g; Sodium: 630 mg

640. Oven-Fried Chicken Breasts

Preparation time: 15 minutes
Cooking time: 30 minutes
Servings: 8
Ingredients:
- ½ pack Ritz crackers
- 1 c. plain non-fat yogurt
- 8 boneless, skinless, and halved chicken breasts

Directions:
1. Preheat the oven to 350 0F. Rinse and pat dry the chicken breasts. Pour the yogurt into a shallow bowl. Dip the chicken pieces in the yogurt, then roll in the cracker crumbs. Place the chicken in a single layer in a baking dish. Bake within 15 minutes per side. Serve.

Nutrition: Calories: 200; Fat: 13 g; Carbs: 98 g; Protein: 19 g; Sodium: 217 mg

641. Rosemary Roasted Chicken

Preparation time: 15 minutes
Cooking time: 20 minutes
Servings: 8
Ingredients:
- 8 rosemary springs
- 1 minced garlic clove
- Black pepper
- 1 tbsp. chopped rosemary
- 1 chicken
- 1 tbsp. organic olive oil

Directions:
1. In a bowl, mix garlic with rosemary, rub the chicken with black pepper, the oil and rosemary mix, place it inside roasting pan, introduce inside the oven at 350 0F, and roast for sixty minutes and 20 min. Carve chicken, divide between plates and serve using a side dish. Enjoy!

Nutrition: Calories: 325; Fat: 5 g; Carbs: 15 g; Protein: 14 g; Sodium: 950 mg

642. Artichoke and Spinach Chicken

Preparation time: 15 minutes
Cooking time: 5 minutes
Servings: 4
Ingredients:
- 10 oz. baby spinach
- ½ tsp. crushed red pepper flakes
- 14 oz. chopped artichoke hearts
- 28 oz. no-salt-added tomato sauce
- 2 tbsps. Essential olive oil
- 4 boneless and skinless chicken breasts

Directions:
1. Heat-up a pan with the oil over medium-high heat, add chicken and red pepper flakes and cook for 5 minutes on them. Add spinach, artichokes, and tomato sauce, toss, cook for ten minutes more, divide between plates and serve. Enjoy!

Nutrition: Calories: 212; Fat: 3 g; Carbs: 16 g; Protein: 20 g; Sugars: 5 g; Sodium: 418 mg

643. Creamy Chicken Fried Rice

Preparation time: 15 minutes
Cooking time: 45 minutes
Servings: 4
Ingredients:
- 2 pounds of chicken; white and dark meat (diced into cubes)
- 2 Tablespoons butter or margarine
- 1 ½ cups instant rice
- 1 cup mixed frozen vegetables
- 1 can condensed cream of chicken soup
- 1 cup of water
- 1 cube instant chicken bouillon
- Salt and pepper to taste

Directions:
1. Take the vegetables out of the freezer. Set aside. Warm large, deep skillet over medium heat, add the butter or margarine. Place the chicken in the skillet, season with salt and pepper. Fry until both sides are brown.
2. Remove the chicken, then adjust the heat and add the rice. Add the water and bouillon. Cook the rice, then add the chicken, the vegetables. Mix in the soup, then simmer until the vegetables are tender. Serve immediately.

Nutrition: Calories - 119 Protein - 22g Carbohydrates - 63g Fat - 18g Sodium - 180mg

644. Chicken Tikka

Preparation time: 15 minutes
Cooking time: 20 minutes
Servings: 6

Ingredients:
- 4 chicken breasts, skinless, boneless; cubed
- 2 large onion, cubed
- 10 Cherry tomatoes
- 1/3 cup plain non-fat yogurt
- 4 garlic cloves, crushed
- 1 ½ inch fresh ginger, peeled and chopped
- 1 small onion, grated
- 1 ½ teaspoon chili powder
- 1 Tablespoon ground coriander
- 1 teaspoon salt
- 2 tablespoons of coriander leaves

Directions:
1. In a large bowl, combine the non-fat yogurt, crushed garlic, ginger, chili powder, coriander, salt, and pepper. Add the cubed chicken, stir until the chicken is coated. Cover with plastic film, place in the fridge. Marinate 2 – 4 hours. Heat the broiler or barbecue.
2. After marinating the chicken, get some skewers ready. Alternate pieces of chicken cubes, cherry tomatoes, and cubed onions onto the skewers.
3. Grill within 6 – 8 minutes on each side. Once the chicken is cooked through, pull the meat and vegetables off the skewers onto plates. Garnish with coriander. Serve immediately.

Nutrition: Calories - 117 Protein - 19g Carbohydrates - 59g Fat - 19g Sodium - 203mg

645. Honey Spiced Cajun Chicken

Preparation time: 15 minutes
Cooking time: 20 minutes
Servings: 4
Ingredients:
- 2 chicken breasts, skinless, boneless
- 1 Tablespoon butter or margarine
- 1 pound of linguini
- 3 large mushrooms, sliced
- 1 large tomato, diced
- 2 Tablespoons regular mustard
- 4 Tablespoons honey
- 3 ounces low-fat table cream
- Parsley, roughly chopped

Directions:
1. Wash and dry the chicken breasts. Warm 1 tablespoon of butter or margarine in a large pan. Add the chicken breasts. Season with salt and pepper. Cook on each side 6 – 10 minutes, until cooked thoroughly. Pull the chicken breasts from the pan. Set aside.
2. Cook the linguine as stated to instructions on the package in a large pot. Save 1 cup of the pasta water. Drain the linguine. Add the mushrooms, tomatoes to the pan from cooking the chicken. Heat until they are tender.
3. Add the honey, mustard, and cream. Combine thoroughly. Add the chicken and linguine to the pan. Stir until coated. Garnish with parsley. Serve immediately.

Nutrition: Calories - 112 Protein - 12g Carbohydrates - 56g Fat - 20g Sodium - 158mg

646. Italian Chicken

Preparation time: 15 minutes
Cooking time: 35 minutes
Servings: 4
Ingredients:
- 4 chicken breasts, skinless boneless
- 1 large jar of pasta sauce, low sodium
- 1 Tablespoon flavorless oil (olive, canola, or sunflower)
- 1 large onion, diced
- 1 large green pepper, diced
- ½ teaspoon garlic salt
- Salt and pepper to taste
- 1 cup low-fat mozzarella cheese, grated
- Spinach leaves, washed, dried, rough chop

Directions:
1. Wash the chicken breasts, pat dry. In a large pot, heat the oil. Add the onion, cook, until it sweats and becomes translucent. Add the chicken. Season with salt, pepper, and garlic salt. Cook the chicken. 6 – 10 minutes on each side.
2. Add the peppers. Cook for 2 minutes. Pour the pasta sauce over the chicken. Mix well. Simmer on low for 20 minutes. Serve on plates, sprinkle the cheese over each piece. Garnish with spinach.

Nutrition: Calories - 142 Protein - 17g Carbohydrates - 51g Fat - 15g Sodium - 225mg

647. Lemon-Parsley Chicken Breast

Preparation time: 15 minutes
Cooking time: 15 minutes
Servings: 2
Ingredients:
- 2 chicken breasts, skinless, boneless
- 1/3 cup white wine
- 1/3 cup lemon juice
- 2 garlic cloves, minced
- 3 Tablespoons bread crumbs
- 2 Tablespoons flavorless oil (olive, canola, or sunflower)
- ¼ cup fresh parsley

Directions:
1. Mix the wine, lemon juice, plus garlic in a measuring cup. Pound each chicken breast until they are ¼ inch thick. Coat the chicken with bread crumbs, and heat the oil in a large skillet.
2. Fry the chicken within 6 minutes on each side, until they turn brown. Stir in the wine mixture over the chicken. Simmer for 5 minutes. Pour any extra juices over the chicken. Garnish with parsley.

Nutrition: Calories - 117 Protein - 14g Carbohydrates - 74 g Fat - 12g Sodium - 189mg

648. Teriyaki Chicken Wings

Preparation time: 15 minutes
Cooking time: 30 minutes
Servings: 6

Ingredients:
- 3 pounds of chicken wings (15 – 20)
- 1/3 cup lemon juice
- ¼ cup of soy sauce
- ¼ cup of vegetable oil
- 3 tablespoons chili sauce
- 1 garlic clove, finely chopped
- ¼ teaspoon fresh ground pepper
- ¼ teaspoon celery seed
- Dash liquid mustard

Directions:
1. Prepare the marinade. Combine lemon juice, soy sauce, chili sauce, oil, celery seed, garlic, pepper, and mustard. Stir well, set aside. Rinse and dry the chicken wings.
2. Pour marinade over the chicken wings. Coat thoroughly. Refrigerate for 2 hours. After 2 hours. Preheat the broiler in the oven. Drain off the excess sauce.
3. Place the wings on a cookie sheet with parchment paper. Broil on each side for 10 minutes. Serve immediately.

Nutrition: Calories 96 Protein - 15g Carbohydrates - 63g Fat - 15g Sodium-145mg

649. Hot Chicken Wings

Preparation time: 15 minutes
Cooking time: 25 minutes
Servings: 4
Ingredients:
- 10 - 20 chicken wings
- ½ stick margarine
- 1 bottle Durkee hot sauce
- 2 Tablespoons honey
- 10 shakes Tabasco sauce
- 2 Tablespoons cayenne pepper

Directions:
1. Warm canola oil in a deep pot. Deep-fry the wings until cooked, approximately 20 minutes. Mix the hot sauce, honey, Tabasco, and cayenne pepper in a medium bowl. Mix well.
2. Place the cooked wings on paper towels. Drain the excess oil. Mix the chicken wings in the sauce until coated evenly.

Nutrition: Calories - 102 Protein - 23g Carbohydrates - 55g Sugars - 0.1g Fat - 14g Sodium-140mg

650. Crispy Cashew Chicken

Preparation time: 15 minutes
Cooking time: 30 minutes
Servings: 5
Ingredients:
- 2 chicken breasts, skinless, boneless
- 2 egg whites
- 1 cup cashew nuts
- ¼ cup bread crumbs
- 2 cups of peanut oil or vegetable oil
- ¼ cup of corn starch
- 1 teaspoon brown sugar
- 2 teaspoons salt

- 1 teaspoon dry sherry

Directions:
1. Warm oven to 400 F. Put the cashews in a blender. Pulse until they are finely chopped. Place in a shallow bowl and stir in the bread crumbs.
2. Wash the chicken breasts. Pat them dry. Cut into small cubes. In a separate shallow bowl, mix the salt, corn starch, brown sugar, and sherry. In a separate bowl, beat the egg white.
3. Put the oil into a large, deep pot. Heat to high temp. Place the chicken pieces on a plate. Arrange the bowls in a row; flour, eggs, cashews & bread crumbs. Prepare a baking tray with parchment paper.
4. Dunk the chicken pieces in the flour, then the egg, and then the cashew mixture. Shake off the excess mixture. Gently place the chicken in the oil. Fry on each side for 2 minutes. Place on the baking tray.
5. Once done, slide the baking tray into the oven. Cook for an additional 4 minutes, flip, cook for an additional 4 minutes, until golden brown. Serve immediately, or cold, with your favorite low-fat dip.

Nutrition: Calories - 86 Protein - 21g Carbohydrates - 50g Sugars - 0.1g Fat - 16g Sodium-139mg

651. Chicken Tortellini Soup

Preparation time: 15 minutes
Cooking time: 30 minutes
Servings: 5
Ingredients:
- 2 chicken breasts, boneless, skinless; diced into cubes
- 1 Tablespoon flavorless oil (olive oil, canola, sunflower)
- 1 teaspoon butter
- 2 cups cheese tortellini
- 2 cups frozen broccoli
- 2 cans cream of chicken soup
- 4 cups of water
- 1 large onion, diced
- 2 garlic cloves, minced
- 2 large carrots, sliced
- 1 celery stick, sliced
- 1 teaspoon Oregano
- ½ teaspoon Basil

Directions:
1. Pull the broccoli out of the freezer. Set in a bowl. Rinse and pat dry the chicken breasts. Dice into cubes. In a large pot, heat the oil. Fry the cubes of chicken breast. Pull from the pot, place on paper to drain off the oil.
2. Add the teaspoon of butter to the hot pot. Sauté the onion, garlic, carrots, and celery, broccoli. Once the vegetable el dente, add the chicken soup and water. Stir the ingredients until they are combined. Bring it to a simmer.
3. Add the chicken and tortellini back to the pot. Cook on low within 10 minutes, or until the tortellini is cooked. Serve immediately.

Nutrition: Calories - 79 Protein - 15g Carbohydrates - 55g Sugars - 0g Fat - 13g Sodium-179mg

652. Chicken Divan

Preparation time: 15 minutes
Cooking time: 30 minutes
Servings: 4
Ingredients:
- 1/2-pound cooked chicken, boneless, skinless, diced in bite-size pieces
- 1 cup broccoli, cooked, diced into bite-size pieces
- 1 cup extra sharp cheddar cheese, grated
- 1 can mushroom soup
- ½ cup of water
- 1 cup croutons

Directions:
1. Warm oven to 350 F. In a large pot, heat the soup and water. Add the chicken, broccoli, and cheese. Combine thoroughly. Pour into a greased baking dish. Place the croutons over the mixture. Bake within 30 minutes or until the casserole is bubbling, and the croutons are golden brown.

Nutrition: Calories - 380 Protein - 25g Carbohydrates - 10g Sugars - 1g Fat - 22g Sodium-397mg

653. Sweet Potato-Turkey Meatloaf

Preparation time: 15 minutes
Cooking time: 25 minutes
Servings: 4
Ingredients:
- 1 large sweet potato, peeled and cubed
- 1-pound ground turkey (breast)
- 1 large egg
- 1 small sweet onion, finely chopped
- 2 cloves garlic, minced
- 2 slices whole-wheat bread, crumbs
- ¼ cup honey barbecue sauce
- ¼ cup ketchup
- 2 Tablespoons Dijon Mustard
- 1 Tablespoon fresh ground pepper
- ½ Tablespoon salt

Directions:
1. Warm oven to 350 F. Grease a baking dish. In a large pot, boil a cup of lightly salted water, add the sweet potato. Cook until tender. Drain the water. Mash the potato.
2. Mix the honey barbecue sauce, ketchup, and Dijon mustard in a small bowl. Mix thoroughly. In a large bowl, mix the turkey and the egg. Add the sweet onion, garlic. Pour in the combined sauces. Add the bread crumbs. Season the mixture with salt and pepper.
3. Add the sweet potato. Combine thoroughly with your hands. If the mixture feels wet, add more bread crumbs. Shape the mixture into a loaf. Place in the loaf pan. Bake for 25 – 35 minutes until the meat is cooked through. Broil for 5 minutes. Slice and serve.

Nutrition: Calories - 133 Protein - 85g Carbohydrates - 50g Fat - 34g Sodium - 202mg

654. Oaxacan Chicken

Preparation time: 15 minutes
Cooking time: 28 minutes
Servings: 2
Ingredients:

- 1 4-ounce chicken breast, skinned and halved
- ½ cup uncooked long-grain rice
- 1 teaspoon of extra-virgin olive oil
- ½ cup low-sodium salsa
- ½ cup chicken stock, mixed with 2 Tablespoons water
- ¾ cup baby carrots
- 2 tablespoons green olives, pitted and chopped
- 2 Tablespoons dark raisins
- ½ teaspoon ground Cinnamon
- 2 Tablespoons fresh cilantro or parsley, coarsely chopped

Directions:

1. Warm oven to 350 F. In a large saucepan that can go in the oven, heat the olive oil. Add the rice. Sauté the rice until it begins to pop, approximately 2 minutes.
2. Add the salsa, baby carrots, green olives, dark raisins, halved chicken breast, chicken stock, and ground cinnamon. Bring the mix to a simmer, stir once.
3. Cover the mixture tightly, bake in the oven until the chicken stock has been completely absorbed, approximately 25 minutes. Sprinkle fresh cilantro or parsley, mix. Serve immediately.

Nutrition: Calories - 143 Protein - 102g Carbohydrates - 66g Fat - 18g Sodium - 97mg

655. Spicy Chicken with Minty Couscous

Preparation time: 15 minutes
Cooking time: 25 minutes
Servings: 2
Ingredients:

- 2 small chicken breasts, sliced
- 1 red chili pepper, finely chopped
- 1 garlic clove, crushed
- ginger root, 2 cm long peeled and grated
- 1 teaspoon ground cumin
- ½ teaspoon turmeric
- 2 Tablespoons extra-virgin olive oil
- 1 pinch sea salt
- ¾ cup couscous
- Small bunch mint leaves, finely chopped
- 2 lemons, grate the rind and juice them

Directions:

1. In a large bowl, place the chicken breast slices and chopped chili pepper. Sprinkle with the crushed garlic, ginger, cumin, turmeric, and a pinch of salt. Add the grated rind of both lemons and the juice from 1 lemon. Pour 1 tablespoon of the olive oil over the chicken, coat evenly.
2. Cover the dish with plastic and refrigerate within 1 hour. After 1 hour, coat a skillet with olive oil and fry the chicken. As the chicken is cooking, pour the couscous into a bowl and pour hot water over it, let it absorb the water (approximately 5 minutes).

3. Fluff the couscous. Add some chopped mint, the other tablespoon of olive oil, and juice from the second lemon. Top the couscous with the chicken. Garnish with chopped mint. Serve immediately.

Nutrition: Calories - 166 Protein - 106g Carbohydrates - 52g Sugars - 0.1g Fat - 17g Sodium - 108mg

656. Chicken, Pasta and Snow Peas

Preparation time: 15 minutes
Cooking time: 20 minutes
Servings: 2
Ingredients:

- 1-pound chicken breasts
- 2 ½ cups penne pasta
- 1 cup snow peas, trimmed and halved
- 1 teaspoon olive oil
- 1 standard jar Tomato and Basil pasta sauce
- Fresh ground pepper

Directions:

1. In a medium frying pan, heat the olive oil. Flavor the chicken breasts with salt and pepper. Cook the chicken breasts until cooked through (approximately 5 – 7 minutes each side).
2. Cook the pasta, as stated in the instruction of the package. Cook the snow peas with the pasta. Scoop 1 cup of the pasta water. Drain the pasta and peas, set aside.
3. Once the chicken is cooked, slice diagonally. Return back the chicken in the frying pan. Add the pasta sauce. If the mixture seems dry, add some of the pasta water to the desired consistency. Heat, then divide into bowls. Serve immediately.

Nutrition: Calories - 140 Protein - 34g Carbohydrates - 52g Fat - 17g Sodium - 118mg

657. Chicken with Noodles

Preparation time: 15 minutes
Cooking time: 30 minutes
Servings: 6
Ingredients:

- 4 chicken breasts, skinless, boneless
- 1-pound pasta (angel hair, or linguine, or ramen)
- ½ teaspoon sesame oil
- 1 Tablespoon canola oil
- 2 Tablespoons chili paste
- 1 onion, diced
- 2 garlic cloves, chopped coarsely
- ½ cup of soy sauce
- ½ medium cabbage, sliced
- 2 carrots, chopped coarsely

Directions:

1. Cook your pasta in a large pot. Mix the canola oil, sesame oil, and chili paste and heat for 25 seconds in a large pot. Add the onion, cook for 2 minutes. Put the garlic and fry within 20 seconds. Add the chicken, cook on each side 5 - 7 minutes, until cooked through.
2. Remove the mix from the pan, set aside. Add the cabbage, carrots, cook until the vegetables are tender.

Pour everything back into the pan. Add the noodles. Pour in the soy sauce and combine thoroughly. Heat for 5 minutes. Serve immediately.

Nutrition: Calories - 110 Protein - 30g Carbohydrates - 32g Sugars - 0.1g Fat - 18g Sodium - 121mg

658. Southwestern Chicken and Pasta

Preparation time: 10 minutes
Cooking time: 10 minutes
Servings: 2
Ingredients:
- 1 cup uncooked whole-wheat rigatoni
- 2 chicken breasts, cut into cubes
- 1/4 cup of salsa
- 1 1/2 cups of canned unsalted tomato sauce
- 1/8 tsp. garlic powder
- 1 tsp. cumin
- 1/2 tsp. chili powder
- 1/2 cup canned black beans, drained
- 1/2 cup fresh corn
- 1/4 cup Monterey Jack and Colby cheese, shredded

Directions:
1. Fill a pot with water up to ¾ full and boil it. Add pasta to cook until it is al dente, then drain the pasta while rinsing under cold water. Preheat a skillet with cooking oil, then cook the chicken for 10 minutes until golden from both sides.
2. Add tomato sauce, salsa, cumin, garlic powder, black beans, corn, and chili powder. Cook the mixture while stirring, then toss in the pasta. Serve with 2 tablespoons cheese on top. Enjoy.

Nutrition: Calories 245 Fat 16.3 g Sodium 515 mg Carbs 19.3 g Protein 33.3 g

659. Stuffed Chicken Breasts

Preparation time: 15 minutes
Cooking time: 30 minutes
Servings: 4
Ingredients:
- 3 tbsp. seedless raisins
- 1/2 cup of chopped onion
- 1/2 cup of chopped celery
- 1/4 tsp. garlic, minced
- 1 bay leaf
- 1 cup apple with peel, chopped
- 2 tbsp. chopped water chestnuts
- 4 large chicken breast halves, 5 ounces each
- 1 tablespoon olive oil
- 1 cup fat-free milk
- 1 teaspoon curry powder
- 2 tablespoons all-purpose (plain) flour
- 1 lemon, cut into 4 wedges

Directions:
1. Set the oven to heat at 425 degrees F. Grease a baking dish with cooking oil. Soak raisins in warm water until they swell. Grease a heated skillet with cooking spray.

2. Add celery, garlic, onions, and bay leaf. Sauté for 5 minutes. Discard the bay leaf, then toss in apples. Stir cook for 2 minutes. Drain the soaked raisin and pat them dry to remove excess water.
3. Add raisins and water chestnuts to the apple mixture. Pull apart the chicken's skin and stuff the apple raisin mixture between the skin and the chicken. Preheat olive oil in another skillet and sear the breasts for 5 minutes per side.
4. Place the chicken breasts in the baking dish and cover the dish. Bake for 15 minutes until temperature reaches 165 degrees F. Prepare sauce by mixing milk, flour, and curry powder in a saucepan.
5. Stir cook until the mixture thickens, about 5 minutes. Pour this sauce over the baked chicken. Bake again in the covered dish for 10 minutes. Serve.

Nutrition: Calories 357 Fat 32.7 g Sodium 277 mg Carbs 17.7 g Protein 31.2 g

660. Buffalo Chicken Salad Wrap

Preparation time: 10 minutes
Cooking time: 10 minutes
Servings: 4
Ingredients:
- 3-4 ounces chicken breasts
- 2 whole chipotle peppers
- 1/4 cup white wine vinegar
- 1/4 cup low-calorie mayonnaise
- 2 stalks celery, diced
- 2 carrots, cut into matchsticks
- 1 small yellow onion, diced
- 1/2 cup thinly sliced rutabaga or another root vegetable
- 4 ounces spinach, cut into strips
- 2 whole-grain tortillas (12-inch diameter)

Directions:
1. Set the oven or a grill to heat at 375 degrees F. Bake the chicken first for 10 minutes per side. Blend chipotle peppers with mayonnaise and wine vinegar in the blender. Dice the baked chicken into cubes or small chunks.
2. Mix the chipotle mixture with all the ingredients except tortillas and spinach. Spread 2 ounces of spinach over the tortilla and scoop the stuffing on top. Wrap the tortilla and cut it into half. Serve.

Nutrition: Calories 300 Fat 16.4 g Sodium 471 mg Carbs 8.7 g Protein 38.5 g

661. Chicken Sliders

Preparation time: 10 minutes
Cooking time: 10 minutes
Servings: 4
Ingredients:
- 10 ounces ground chicken breast
- 1 tablespoon black pepper
- 1 tablespoon minced garlic
- 1 tablespoon balsamic vinegar
- 1/2 cup minced onion
- 1 fresh chili pepper, minced

- 1 tablespoon fennel seed, crushed
- 4 whole-wheat mini buns
- 4 lettuce leaves
- 4 tomato slices

Directions:
1. Combine all the ingredients except the wheat buns, tomato, and lettuce. Mix well and refrigerate the mixture for 1 hour. Divide the mixture into 4 patties.
2. Broil these patties in a greased baking tray until golden brown. Place the chicken patties in the wheat buns along with lettuce and tomato. Serve.

Nutrition: Calories 224 Fat 4.5 g Sodium 212 mg Carbs 10.2 g Protein 67.4 g

662. White Chicken Chili

Preparation time: 20 minutes
Cooking time: 15 minutes
Servings: 4
Ingredients:
- 1 can white chunk chicken
- 2 cans low-sodium white beans, drained
- 1 can low-sodium diced tomatoes
- 4 cups of low-sodium chicken broth
- 1 medium onion, chopped
- 1/2 medium green pepper, chopped
- 1 medium red pepper, chopped
- 2 garlic cloves, minced
- 2 teaspoons chili powder
- 1 teaspoon ground cumin
- 1 teaspoon dried oregano
- Cayenne pepper, to taste
- 8 tablespoons shredded reduced-fat Monterey Jack cheese
- 3 tablespoons chopped fresh cilantro

Directions:
1. In a soup pot, add beans, tomatoes, chicken, and chicken broth. Cover this soup pot and let it simmer over medium heat. Meanwhile, grease a nonstick pan with cooking spray. Add peppers, garlic, and onions. Sauté for 5 minutes until soft.
2. Transfer the mixture to the soup pot. Add cumin, chili powder, cayenne pepper, and oregano. Cook for 10 minutes, then garnish the chili with cilantro and 1 tablespoon cheese. Serve.

Nutrition: Calories 225 Fat 12.9 g Sodium 480 mg Carbs 24.7 g Protein 25.3g

663. Salsa Chicken Chili

Preparation time: 15 minutes
Cooking time: 20 minutes
Servings: 8
Ingredients:
- 2 1/2 lbs. chicken breasts, skinless and boneless
- 1/2 tsp. cumin powder
- 3 garlic cloves, minced
- 1 onion, diced
- 16 oz. salsa
- 1 tsp. oregano
- 1 tbsp. olive oil

Directions:
1. Add oil into the instant pot and set the pot on sauté mode. Add onion to the pot and sauté until softened, about 3 minutes. Add garlic and sauté for a minute. Add oregano and cumin and sauté for a minute. Add half salsa and stir well. Place chicken and pour remaining salsa over chicken.
2. Seal pot with the lid and select manual and set timer for 10 minutes. Remove chicken and shred. Move it back to the pot, then stir well to combine. Serve and enjoy.

Nutrition: Calories: 308 Fat: 12.4g Protein: 42.1g Carbs: 5.4g Sodium 656 mg

664. Honey Crusted Chicken

Preparation time: 10 minutes
Cooking time: 25 minutes
Servings: 2
Ingredients:
- 1 teaspoon paprika
- 8 saltine crackers, 2 inches square
- 2 chicken breasts, each 4 ounces
- 4 tsp. honey

Directions:
1. Set the oven to heat at 375 degrees F. Grease a baking dish with cooking oil. Smash the crackers in a Zip lock bag and toss them with paprika in a bowl. Brush chicken with honey and add it to the crackers.
2. Mix well and transfer the chicken to the baking dish. Bake the chicken for 25 minutes until golden brown. Serve.

Nutrition: Calories 219 Fat 17 g Sodium 456 mg Carbs 12.1 g Protein 31 g

665. Paella with Chicken, Leeks, and Tarragon

Preparation time: 10 minutes
Cooking time: 20 minutes
Servings: 2
Ingredients:
- 1 teaspoon extra-virgin olive oil
- 1 small onion, sliced
- 2 leeks (whites only), thinly sliced
- 3 garlic cloves, minced
- 1-pound boneless, skinless chicken breast, cut into strips 1/2-inch-wide and 2 inches long
- 2 large tomatoes, chopped
- 1 red pepper, sliced
- 2/3 cup long-grain brown rice
- 1 teaspoon tarragon, or to taste
- 2 cups fat-free, unsalted chicken broth
- 1 cup frozen peas
- 1/4 cup chopped fresh parsley
- 1 lemon, cut into 4 wedges

Directions:
1. Preheat a nonstick pan with olive oil over medium heat. Toss in leeks, onions, chicken strips, and garlic. Sauté for 5 minutes. Stir in red pepper slices and tomatoes. Stir and cook for 5 minutes.

2. Add tarragon, broth, and rice. Let it boil, then reduce the heat to a simmer. Continue cooking for 10 minutes, then add peas and continue cooking until the liquid is thoroughly cooked. Garnish with parsley and lemon. Serve.

Nutrition: Calories 388 Fat 15.2 g Sodium 572 mg Carbs 5.4 g Protein 27 g

666. Olive Capers Chicken

Preparation time: 15 minutes
Cooking time: 16 minutes
Servings: 4
Ingredients:
- 2 lbs. chicken
- 1/3 cup chicken stock
- oz. Capers
- 6 oz. olives
- 1/4 cup fresh basil
- 1 tbsp. olive oil
- 1 tsp. oregano
- 2 garlic cloves, minced
- 2 tbsp. red wine vinegar
- 1/8 tsp. pepper
- 1/4 tsp. salt

Directions:
1. Put olive oil in your instant pot and set the pot on sauté mode. Add chicken to the pot and sauté for 3-4 minutes. Add remaining ingredients and stir well. Seal pot with the lid and select manual and set timer for 12 minutes. Serve and enjoy.

Nutrition: Calories: 433 Fat: 15.2g Protein: 66.9g Carbs: 4.8g Sodium 244 mg

667. Chicken with Mushrooms

Preparation time: 15 minutes
Cooking time: 6 hours & 10 minutes
Servings: 2
Ingredients:
- 2 chicken breasts, skinless and boneless
- 1 cup mushrooms, sliced
- 1 onion, sliced
- 1 cup chicken stock
- 1/2 tsp. thyme, dried
- Pepper
- Salt

Directions:
1. Add all ingredients to the slow cooker. Cook on low within 6 hours. Serve and enjoy.

Nutrition: Calories: 313 Fat: 11.3g Protein: 44.3g Carbs: 6.9g Sodium 541 mg

668. Baked Chicken

Preparation time: 15 minutes
Cooking time: 35 minutes
Servings: 4
Ingredients:

- 2 lbs. chicken tenders
- 1 large zucchini
- 1 cup grape tomatoes
- 2 tbsp. olive oil
- 3 dill sprigs
- For topping:
- 2 tbsp. feta cheese, crumbled
- 1 tbsp. olive oil
- 1 tbsp. fresh lemon juice
- 1 tbsp. fresh dill, chopped

Directions:
1. Warm oven to 200 C/ 400 F. Drizzle the olive oil on a baking tray, then place chicken, zucchini, dill, and tomatoes on the tray. Season with salt. Bake chicken within 30 minutes.
2. Meanwhile, in a small bowl, stir all topping ingredients. Place chicken on the serving tray, then top with veggies and discard dill sprigs. Sprinkle topping mixture on top of chicken and vegetables. Serve and enjoy.

Nutrition: Calories: 557 Fat: 28.6g Protein: 67.9g Carbs: 5.2g Sodium 760 mg

669. Garlic Pepper Chicken

Preparation time: 15 minutes
Cooking time: 21 minutes
Servings: 2
Ingredients:
- 2 chicken breasts, cut into strips
- 2 bell peppers, cut into strips
- 5 garlic cloves, chopped
- 3 tbsp. water
- 2 tbsp. olive oil
- 1 tbsp. paprika
- 2 tsp. black pepper
- 1/2 tsp. salt

Directions:
1. Warm-up olive oil in a large saucepan over medium heat. Add garlic and sauté for 2-3 minutes. Add peppers and cook for 3 minutes. Add chicken and spices and stir to coat. Add water and stir well. Bring to boil. Cover and simmer for 10-15 minutes. Serve and enjoy.

Nutrition: Calories: 462 Fat: 25.7g Protein: 44.7g Carbs: 14.8g Sodium 720 mg

670. Mustard Chicken Tenders

Preparation time: 15 minutes
Cooking time: 20 minutes
Servings: 4
Ingredients:
- 1 lb. chicken tenders
- 2 tbsp. fresh tarragon, chopped
- 1/2 cup whole grain mustard
- 1/2 tsp. paprika
- 1 garlic clove, minced
- 1/2 oz. fresh lemon juice
- 1/2 tsp. pepper

- 1/4 tsp. kosher salt

Directions:
1. Warm oven to 425 F. Add all ingredients except chicken to the large bowl and mix well. Put the chicken in the bowl, then stir until well coated. Place chicken on a baking dish and cover. Bake within 15-20 minutes. Serve and enjoy.

Nutrition: Calories: 242 Fat: 9.5g Protein: 33.2g Carbs: 3.1g Sodium 240 mg

671. Healthy Chicken Orzo

Preparation time: 15 minutes
Cooking time: 15 minutes
Servings: 4
Ingredients:
- 1 cup whole wheat orzo
- 1 lb. chicken breasts, sliced
- ½ tsp. red pepper flakes
- ½ cup feta cheese, crumbled
- ½ tsp. oregano
- 1 tbsp. fresh parsley, chopped
- 1 tbsp. fresh basil, chopped
- ¼ cup pine nuts
- 1 cup spinach, chopped
- ¼ cup white wine
- ½ cup olives, sliced
- 1 cup grape tomatoes, cut in half
- ½ tbsp. garlic, minced
- 2 tbsp. olive oil
- ½ tsp. pepper
- ½ tsp. salt

Directions:
1. Add water in a small saucepan and bring to boil. Heat 1 tablespoon of olive oil in a pan over medium heat. Season chicken with pepper and salt and cook in the pan for 5-7 minutes on each side. Remove from pan and set aside.
2. Add orzo in boiling water and cook according to the packet directions. Heat remaining olive oil in a pan on medium heat, then put garlic in the pan and sauté for a minute. Stir in white wine and cherry tomatoes and cook on high for 3 minutes.
3. Add cooked orzo, spices, spinach, pine nuts, and olives and stir until well combined. Add chicken on top of orzo and sprinkle with feta cheese. Serve and enjoy.

Nutrition: Calories: 518 Fat: 27.7g Protein: 40.6g Carbs: 26.2g Sodium 121mg

672. Lemon Garlic Chicken

Preparation time: 15 minutes
Cooking time: 12 minutes
Servings: 3
Ingredients:
- 3 chicken breasts, cut into thin slices
- 2 lemon zest, grated
- ¼ cup olive oil
- 4 garlic cloves, minced
- Pepper
- Salt

Directions:
1. Warm-up olive oil in a pan over medium heat. Add garlic to the pan and sauté for 30 seconds. Put the chicken in the pan and sauté within 10 minutes. Add lemon zest and lemon juice and bring to boil. Remove from heat and season with pepper and salt. Serve and enjoy.

Nutrition: Calories: 439 Fat: 27.8g Protein: 42.9g Carbs: 4.9g Sodium 306 mg

673. Simple Mediterranean Chicken

Preparation time: 15 minutes
Cooking time: 15 minutes
Servings: 12
Ingredients:
- 2 chicken breasts, skinless and boneless
- 1 ½ cup grape tomatoes, cut in half
- ½ cup olives
- 2 tbsp. olive oil
- 1 tsp. Italian seasoning
- ¼ tsp. pepper
- ¼ tsp. salt

Directions:
1. Season chicken with Italian seasoning, pepper, and salt. Warm-up olive oil in a pan over medium heat. Add season chicken to the pan and cook for 4-6 minutes on each side. Transfer chicken on a plate.
2. Put tomatoes plus olives in the pan and cook for 2-4 minutes. Pour olive and tomato mixture on top of the chicken and serve.

Nutrition: Calories: 468 Fat: 29.4g Protein: 43.8g Carbs: 7.8g Sodium 410 mg

674. Roasted Chicken Thighs

Preparation time: 15 minutes
Cooking time: 55 minutes
Servings: 4
Ingredients:
- 8 chicken thighs
- 3 tbsp. fresh parsley, chopped
- 1 tsp. dried oregano
- 6 garlic cloves, crushed
- ¼ cup capers, drained
- 10 oz. roasted red peppers, sliced
- 2 cups grape tomatoes
- 1 ½ lbs. potatoes, cut into small chunks
- 4 tbsp. olive oil
- Pepper
- Salt

Directions:
1. Warm oven to 200 400 F. Season chicken with pepper and salt. Heat-up 2 tablespoons of olive oil in a pan over medium heat. Add chicken to the pan and sear until lightly golden brown from all the sides.
2. Transfer chicken onto a baking tray. Add tomato, potatoes, capers, oregano, garlic, and red peppers around the chicken. Season with pepper and salt and drizzle with

remaining olive oil. Bake in preheated oven for 45-55 minutes. Garnish with parsley and serve.

Nutrition: Calories: 848 Fat: 29.1g Protein: 91.3g Carbs: 45.2g Sodium 110 mg

675. Mediterranean Turkey Breast

Preparation time: 15 minutes
Cooking time: 4 minutes & 30 minutes
Servings: 6
Ingredients:
- 4 lbs. turkey breast
- 3 tbsp. flour
- ¾ cup chicken stock
- 4 garlic cloves, chopped
- 1 tsp. dried oregano
- ½ fresh lemon juice
- ½ cup sun-dried tomatoes, chopped
- ½ cup olives, chopped
- 1 onion, chopped
- ¼ tsp. pepper
- ½ tsp. salt

Directions:
1. Add turkey breast, garlic, oregano, lemon juice, sun-dried tomatoes, olives, onion, pepper, and salt to the slow cooker. Add half stock. Cook on high within 4 hours.
2. Whisk remaining stock and flour in a small bowl and add to slow cooker. Cover and cook for 30 minutes more. Serve and enjoy.

Nutrition: Calories: 537 Fat: 9.7g Protein: 79.1g Carbs: 29.6g Sodium 330 mg

676. Fruity Chicken Salad

Preparation time: 10 minutes
Cooking time: 30 minutes
Servings: 4
Ingredients:
- 1 whole chicken, chopped
- 8 black tea bags
- 4 scallions, chopped
- 2 celery ribs, chopped
- 1 cup mandarin orange, chopped
- ½ cup fat free yogurt
- 1 cup cashews, toasted and chopped
- Black pepper to the taste

Directions:
1. Put chicken pieces in a pot, add water to cover, also add tea bags, bring to a boil over medium heat and cook for 25 minutes until chicken is tender.
2. Discard liquid and tea bags but reserve about 4 ounces.
3. Transfer chicken to a cutting board, leave aside to cool down, discard bones, shred meat and put it in a bowl.
4. Add celery, orange pieces, cashews, scallion and reserved liquid and toss everything.
5. Add salt, pepper, mayo and yogurt, toss to coat well and keep in the fridge until you serve it.

Nutrition: Calories 150, fat 3, fiber 3, carbs 7, protein 6

677. Chicken Corn Chili

Preparation time: 10 minutes
Cooking time: 1 hour and 10 minutes
Servings: 6
Ingredients:
- 1 cup white flour
- 1 tablespoon lemon juice
- Salt and black pepper to the taste
- 4 pounds chicken breast, skinless, boneless and cubed
- 4 ounces olive oil
- 4 ounces celery, chopped
- 1 tablespoon garlic, minced
- 8 ounces onion, chopped
- 5 ounces red bell pepper, chopped
- 7 ounces poblano pepper, chopped
- ¼ teaspoon cumin, ground
- 2 cups corn
- A pinch of cayenne pepper
- 1-quart chicken stock
- 1 teaspoon chili powder
- 16 ounces canned beans, drained
- ¼ cup cilantro, chopped

Directions:
1. Put flour in a bowl, add chicken pieces and toss well.
2. Heat up a pan with the oil over medium high heat, add chicken, cook for 5 minutes on each side, transfer to a bowl and leave aside.
3. Heat up the pan again over medium high heat, add onion, celery, garlic, bell pepper, poblano pepper and corn, stir and cook for 2 minutes more.
4. Add stock, cumin, chili powder, beans, cayenne, cumin, salt, pepper, chicken pieces and lemon juice, stir, bring to a simmer, reduce heat to medium low, cover and cook for 1 hour.
5. Add cilantro, stir, divide into bowls and serve right away!

Nutrition: Calories 345, Fat 2, Fiber 3, Carbs 9, Protein 4

678. Chicken Noodles Soup

Preparation time: 10 minutes
Cooking time: 15 minutes
Servings: 4
Ingredients:
- 4 cups chicken stock
- 1 teaspoon ginger, grated
- 1 tablespoon lemon juice
- 1 chicken breast, skinless, boneless, cooked and cut into medium pieces
- 2 garlic cloves, minced
- A pinch of sea salt
- Black pepper to the taste
- ½ cup egg noodles
- 2 carrots, chopped
- 1/3 cup parsley, chopped

Directions:
1. In a pot, mix chicken, stock, ginger, lemon juice, garlic, salt, pepper, carrots and noodles, stir, bring to a boil over medium high heat and simmer for 15 minutes.
2. Add parsley, stir, ladle into bowls serve right away.

Nutrition: Calories 145, Fat 2, Fiber 1, Carbs 7, Protein 21

679. Sweet Chicken and Peaches

Preparation time: 10 minutes
Cooking time: 1 hour and 10 minutes
Servings: 4
Ingredients:

- 6 green tea and peach tea bags
- 1 whole chicken, cut into medium pieces
- ¾ cup water
- 1/3 cup honey
- Salt and black pepper to the taste
- ¼ cup olive oil
- 4 peaches, halved

Directions:
1. Put the water in a pot, bring to a simmer over medium heat, add tea bags, reduce heat to low and simmer for 10 minutes.
2. Discard tea bags, add pepper and honey, whisk really well and leave aside.
3. Rub chicken pieces with the oil, season with salt and pepper, place on preheated grill over medium high heat, brush with tea marinade, cover grill and cook for 15 minutes.
4. Brush chicken with some more marinade, cook for 15 minutes more and then flip again.
5. Brush again with the tea marinade, cover and cook for 20 minutes more.
6. Divide chicken pieces on plates and keep warm.
7. Brush peaches with what's left of the tea and honey marinade, place them on your grill and cook for 4 minutes.
8. Flip again and cook for 3 minutes more.
9. Divide between plates next to chicken pieces and serve.

Nutrition: Calories 500, fat 1, fiber 3, carbs 15, protein 10

680. Pineapple Glazed Chicken

Preparation time: 10 minutes
Cooking time: 1 hour and 10 minutes
Servings: 4
Ingredients:

- ½ cup apricot preserves
- ½ cup pineapple preserves
- 1 tablespoon low sodium soy sauce
- 1 onion, chopped
- ¼ teaspoon red pepper flakes
- 1 tablespoon vegetable oil
- Black pepper to the taste
- 6 chicken legs

Directions:
1. In a bowl, mix soy sauce, pepper flakes, apricot and pineapple preserves and whisk really well.
2. Heat up a pan with the oil over medium high heat, add chicken pieces, cook them for 5 minutes on each side and transfer to a bowl.
3. Spread onion on the bottom of a baking dish and add chicken pieces on top.

4. Season with black pepper, drizzle the tea glaze on top, cover dish, introduce in the oven at 350 degrees F and bake for 30 minutes.
5. Uncover dish and bake for 20 minutes more.
6. Divide chicken on plates and keep warm.
7. Pour cooking juices into a pan, heat up over medium high heat, cook until sauce is reduced and drizzle it over chicken pieces.

Nutrition: Calories 198, Fat 1, Fiber 1, Carbs 4, Protein 19

681. Salsa Chicken

Preparation time: 50 minutes
Cooking time: 5 minutes
Servings: 4
Ingredients:

- 1 pound chicken breast, boneless and skinless
- 16 ounce scanned salsa Verde
- Black pepper to the taste
- A pinch of sea salt
- 1 tablespoon olive oil
- 1 and ½ cups fat free Monterey jack cheese, shredded
- ¼ cup cilantro, chopped
- Wild rice, cooked for serving
- Juice from 1 lime

Directions:
1. Mix chicken with salt, pepper, and oil and toss to coat.
2. Spread salsa in a baking dish, add chicken on top, introduce in the oven at 400 degrees F and bake for 40 minutes.
3. Take chicken out of the oven, add cheese, introduce everything in preheated broiler and broil for 3 minutes.
4. Add lime juice, divide between plates, sprinkle cilantro and serve with white rice.

Nutrition: Calories 150, fat 1, fiber 4, carbs 20, proteins

682. Pear Chicken Casserole

Preparation time: 10 minutes
Cooking time: 5 minutes
Servings: 8
Ingredients:

- 2 tablespoons olive oil
- 2 pounds chicken breasts, skinless and boneless
- 2 carrots, chopped
- Black pepper to the taste
- 1 yellow onion, chopped
- 1 teaspoon Cajun seasoning
- ¼ cup flour
- ½ cup orange juice
- 1 can low sodium chicken stock
- 1 cup peas
- ½ cup parsley, chopped
- 2 tablespoons dill, chopped
- ½ cup fat free yogurt
- 2 and ½ cups cornflakes

Directions:
1. Put water in a pot, add chicken, bring to a boil over medium heat, simmer for 10 minutes, drain and leave aside for now.

2. Heat up a pan with the oil over medium high heat, add onion, carrots and pepper, stir and cook for 10 minutes.
3. Add Cajun seasoning and flour, stir and cook for 1 minute.
4. Add stock and orange juice stirring all the time and bring to a boil.
5. Add chicken, dill, peas and half of the parsley, stir and take off heat.
6. Add yogurt, stir, transfer everything to a baking dish, introduce in the oven at 375 degrees F and bake for 15 minutes.
7. Meanwhile, in a bowl, mix cornflakes with the rest of the parsley and stir.
8. Take chicken out of the oven, sprinkle cornflakes all over, introduce in the oven again and bake for 6 more minutes.
9. Take dish out of the oven, leave aside for 10 minutes, divide between plates and serve.

Nutrition: Calories 130, fat 3, fiber 3, carbs 9, protein 5

683. Poached Chicken with Rice

Preparation time: 10 minutes
Cooking time: 40 minutes
Servings: 4
Ingredients:
- ½ tablespoon ginger, finely grated
- 3 garlic cloves, minced
- 1 tablespoon low sodium soy sauce
- 1 teaspoon black peppercorns
- 8 chicken legs
- 4 pak choi, halved
- Black pepper to the taste
- 2 bunches spring onions, chopped
- 3 tablespoons sesame oil
- Brown rice, already cooked for serving

Directions:
1. In a pan, mix ginger with half of the soy sauce, garlic, peppercorns and chicken.
2. Add water to cover, season with black pepper to the taste, place on stove, bring to a boil over medium high heat, reduce temperature to low and simmer for 30 minutes.
3. Heat up a pan with the oil over medium high heat, add onions, stir and cook for 1 minute.
4. Take pan off heat, add soy sauce, stir well to make a relish and leave aside for now.
5. Take chicken out of the pan and also leave aside to cool down on a plate.
6. Add pak choi to chicken liquid, place on stove again on medium heat and cook for 4 minutes.
7. Strain pak choi, discard solids and reserve cooking liquid.
8. Discard skin and bones from chicken legs, shred meat and divide in bowls.
9. Add rice on the side, pak choi, the relish you've made and some of the reserved cooking liquid.

Nutrition: Calories 200, fat 2, fiber 4, carbs 7, protein 10

684. Hawaiian Chicken

Preparation time: 4 hours and 10 minutes

Cooking time: 12 minutes
Servings: 4
Ingredients:
- 2 tablespoons tomato paste
- ¼ cup canned pineapple juice
- 2 tablespoons low sodium soy sauce
- 2 garlic cloves, minced
- 1 and ½ teaspoons ginger, grated
- 4 chicken breast halves, skinless and boneless
- Cooking spray
- Black pepper to the taste
- ¼ cup cilantro, chopped
- 2 cups brown rice, already cooked

Directions:
1. In a bowl, mix pineapple juice with tomato paste, soy sauce, garlic and ginger and stir well.
2. Reserve ¼ cup of mix, transfer the rest to a zip-top bag, add chicken, seal bag, shake and keep in the fridge for 4 hours.
3. Heat up a pan after you've sprayed some cooking oil in it over medium high heat, add marinated chicken and season with black pepper to the taste.
4. Add the reserved marinade, stir and cook chicken for 6 minutes on each side.
5. Add rice and cilantro, stir gently, take off heat and divide between plates.

Nutrition: Calories 140, fat 1, fiber 4, carbs 9, protein 12

685. Fruity Chicken Bites

Preparation time: 10 minutes
Cooking time: 10 minutes
Servings: 4
Ingredients:
- 20 ounces canned pineapple slices
- A drizzle of olive oil
- 3 cups chicken thighs, boneless, skinless and cut into medium pieces
- 1 tablespoon smoked tea rub

Directions:
1. Heat up a pan over medium high heat, add pineapple slices, grill them for a few minutes on each side, transfer to a cutting board, cool them down and cut into medium cubes.
2. Heat up a pan with a drizzle of oil over medium high heat, rub chicken pieces with smoked tea rub, place them in the pan and cook them for 10 minutes flipping from time to time.
3. Arrange chicken cubes on a platter, add a pineapple piece on top and stick a toothpick in each.
4. Serve right away!

Nutrition: Calories 120, Fat 3, Fiber 1, Carbs 5, Protein 2

686. Chicken Tortillas

Preparation time: 15 minutes
Cooking time: 5 minutes
Servings: 4
Ingredients:
- 6 oz. boneless, skinless, and cooked chicken breasts
- Black pepper

- 1/3 c. fat-free yogurt
- 4 heated up whole-wheat tortillas
- 2 chopped tomatoes

Directions:
1. Heat-up a pan over medium heat, add one tortilla during those times, heat up, and hang them on the working surface. Spread yogurt on each tortilla, add chicken and tomatoes, roll, divide between plates and serve. Enjoy!

Nutrition: Calories: 190 Fat: 2 g Carbs: 12 g Protein: 6 g Sodium: 300 mg

687. Chicken with Potatoes Olives & Sprouts

Preparation time: 15 minutes
Cooking time: 35 minutes
Servings: 4
Ingredients:
- lb. chicken breasts, skinless, boneless, and cut into pieces
- ¼ cup olives, quartered
- tsp. oregano
- 1 ½ tsp. Dijon mustard
- 1 lemon juice
- 1/3 cup vinaigrette dressing
- 1 medium onion, diced
- cups potatoes cut into pieces
- cups Brussels sprouts, trimmed and quartered
- ¼ tsp. pepper
- ¼ tsp. salt

Directions:
1. Warm-up oven to 400 F. Place chicken in the center of the baking tray, then place potatoes, sprouts, and onions around the chicken.
2. In a small bowl, mix vinaigrette, oregano, mustard, lemon juice, and salt and pour over chicken and veggies. Sprinkle olives and season with pepper.
3. Bake in preheated oven for 20 minutes. Transfer chicken to a plate. Stir the vegetables and roast for 15 minutes more. Serve and enjoy.

Nutrition: Calories: 397 Fat: 13g Protein: 38.3g Carbs: 31.4g Sodium 175 mg

688. Garlic Mushroom Chicken

Preparation time: 15 minutes
Cooking time: 15 minutes
Servings: 4
Ingredients:
- 4 chicken breasts, boneless and skinless
- 3 garlic cloves, minced
- onion, chopped
- cups mushrooms, sliced
- tbsp. olive oil
- ½ cup chicken stock
- ¼ tsp. pepper
- ½ tsp. salt

Directions:

1. Season chicken with pepper and salt. Warm oil in a pan on medium heat, then put season chicken in the pan and cook for 5-6 minutes on each side. Remove and place on a plate.
2. Add onion and mushrooms to the pan and sauté until tender, about 2-3 minutes. Add garlic and sauté for a minute. Add stock and bring to boil. Stir well and cook for 1-2 minutes. Pour over chicken and serve.

Nutrition: Calories: 331 Fat: 14.5g Protein: 43.9g Carbs: 4.6g Sodium 420 mg

689. Grilled Chicken

Preparation time: 15 minutes
Cooking time: 15 minutes
Servings: 4
Ingredients:
- 4 chicken breasts, skinless and boneless
- ½ tsp. dried oregano
- 1 tsp. paprika
- 5 garlic cloves, minced
- ½ cup fresh parsley, minced
- ½ cup olive oil
- ½ cup fresh lemon juice
- Pepper
- Salt

Directions:
1. Add lemon juice, oregano, paprika, garlic, parsley, and olive oil to a large zip-lock bag. Season chicken with pepper and salt and add to bag. Seal bag and shake well to coat chicken with marinade. Let sit chicken in the marinade for 20 minutes.
2. Remove chicken from marinade and grill over medium-high heat for 5-6 minutes on each side. Serve and enjoy.

Nutrition: Calories: 512 Fat: 36.5g Protein: 43.1g Carbs: 3g Sodium 110mg

690. Delicious Lemon Chicken Salad

Preparation time: 15 minutes
Cooking time: 5 minutes
Servings: 4
Ingredients:
- lb. chicken breast, cooked and diced
- tbsp. fresh dill, chopped
- tsp. olive oil
- 1/4 cup low-fat yogurt
- tsp. lemon zest, grated
- tbsp. onion, minced
- ¼ tsp. pepper
- ¼ tsp. salt

Directions:
1. Put all you're fixing into the large mixing bowl and toss well. Season with pepper and salt. Cover and place in the refrigerator. Serve chilled and enjoy.

Nutrition: Calories: 165 Fat: 5.4g Protein: 25.2g Carbs: 2.2g Sodium 153mg

691. Feisty Chicken Porridge

Preparation time: 15 minutes
Cooking time: 30 minutes
Servings: 4
Ingredients:
- ½ c. fresh ginger
- 1 lb. cooked chicken legs
- Green onions
- Toasted cashew nuts
- 5 c. chicken broth
- 1 cup jasmine rice
- 4 c. water

Directions:
1. Place the rice in your fridge and allow it to chill 1 hour before cooking. Take the rice out and add them to your Instant Pot. Pour broth and water. Lock up the lid and cook on Porridge mode.
2. Separate the meat from the chicken legs and add the meat to your soup. Stir well over sauté mode. Season with a bit of flavored vinegar and enjoy with a garnish of nuts and onion.

Nutrition: Calories: 206 Fat: 8 g Carbs: 8 g Protein: 23 g Sugars: 0 g Sodium: 950 mg

692. The Ultimate Faux-Tisserie Chicken

Preparation time: 15 minutes
Cooking time: 35 minutes
Servings: 5
Ingredients:
- c. low sodium broth
- tbsps. Olive oil
- ½ quartered medium onion
- tbsps. Favorite seasoning
- 2 ½ lbs. whole chicken
- Black pepper
- large fresh garlic cloves

Directions:
1. Massage the chicken with 1 tablespoon of olive oil and sprinkle pepper on top. Place onion wedges and garlic cloves inside the chicken. Take a butcher's twin and secure the legs
2. Set your pot to Sauté mode. Put olive oil in your pan on medium heat, allow the oil to heat up. Add chicken and sear both sides for 4 minutes per side. Sprinkle your seasoning over the chicken, remove the chicken and place a trivet at the bottom of your pot
3. Sprinkle seasoning over the chicken, making sure to rub it. Transfer the chicken to the trivet with the breast side facing up, lock up the lid. Cook on HIGH pressure for 25 minutes. Allow it to rest and serve!

Nutrition: Calories: 1010 Fat: 64 g Carbs: 47 g Protein: 60 g Sodium: 209 mg

693. Oregano Chicken Thighs

Preparation time: 15 minutes
Cooking time: 20 minutes

Servings: 6
Ingredients:
- 12 chicken thighs
- tsp. dried parsley
- ¼ tsp. pepper and salt.
- ½ c. extra virgin essential olive oil
- 4 minced garlic cloves
- c. chopped oregano
- ¼ c. low-sodium veggie stock

Directions:
1. In your food processor, mix parsley with oregano, garlic, salt, pepper, and stock and pulse. Put chicken thighs within the bowl, add oregano paste, toss, cover, and then leave aside within the fridge for 10 minutes.
2. Heat the kitchen grill over medium heat, add chicken pieces, close the lid and cook for twenty or so minutes with them. Divide between plates and serve!

Nutrition: Calories: 254 Fat: 3 g Carbs: 7 g Protein: 17 g Sugars: 0.9 g Sodium: 730 mg

694. Pesto Chicken Breasts with Summer Squash

Preparation time: 15 minutes
Cooking time: 10 minutes
Servings: 4
Ingredients:
- 4 medium boneless, skinless chicken breast halves
- tbsp. olive oil
- tbsps. Homemade pesto
- c. finely chopped zucchini
- 2 tbsps. Finely shredded Asiago

Directions:
1. Cook your chicken in hot oil on medium heat within 4 minutes in a large nonstick skillet. Flip the chicken then put the zucchini.
2. Cook within 4 to 6 minutes more or until the chicken is tender and no longer pink (170 F), and squash is crisp-tender, stirring squash gently once or twice. Transfer chicken and squash to 4 dinner plates. Spread pesto over chicken, sprinkle with Asiago.

Nutrition: Calories: 230 Fat: 9 g Carbs: 8 g Protein: 30 g Sodium: 578 mg

695. Chicken, Tomato and Green Beans

Preparation time: 15 minutes
Cooking time: 25 minutes
Servings: 4
Ingredients:
- 6 oz. low-sodium canned tomato paste
- 2 tbsps. Olive oil
- ¼ tsp. black pepper
- 2 lbs. trimmed green beans
- 2 tbsps. Chopped parsley
- ½ lbs. boneless, skinless, and cubed chicken breasts
- 25 oz. no-salt-added canned tomato sauce

Directions:

1. Heat a pan with 50 % with the oil over medium heat, add chicken, stir, cover, and cook within 5 minutes on both sides and transfer to a bowl. Heat inside the same pan while using rest through the oil over medium heat, add green beans, stir and cook for 10 minutes.
2. Return chicken for that pan, add black pepper, tomato sauce, tomato paste, and parsley, stir, cover, cook for 10 minutes more, divide between plates and serve. Enjoy!

Nutrition: Calories: 190 Fat: 4 g Carbs: 12 g Protein: 9 g Sodium: 168 mg

696. Artichoke and Spinach Chicken

Preparation time: 15 minutes
Cooking time: 5 minutes
Servings: 4
Ingredients:
- 10 oz. baby spinach
- ½ tsp. crushed red pepper flakes
- 14 oz. chopped artichoke hearts
- 28 oz. no-salt-added tomato sauce
- 2 tbsps. Essential olive oil
- 4 boneless and skinless chicken breasts

Directions:
1. Heat-up a pan with the oil over medium-high heat, add chicken and red pepper flakes and cook for 5 minutes on them. Add spinach, artichokes, and tomato sauce, toss, cook for ten minutes more, divide between plates and serve. Enjoy!

Nutrition: Calories: 212 Fat: 3 g Carbs: 16 g Protein: 20 g Sugars: 5 g Sodium: 418 mg

697. Pumpkin and Black Beans Chicken

Preparation time: 15 minutes
Cooking time: 25 minutes
Servings: 4
Ingredients:
- tbsp. essential olive oil   tbsp. Chopped cilantro
- 1 c. coconut milk
- 15 oz. canned black beans, drained
- 1 lb. skinless and boneless chicken breasts
- c. water
- ½ c. pumpkin flesh

Directions:
1. Heat a pan when using oil over medium-high heat, add the chicken and cook for 5 minutes. Add the river, milk, pumpkin, and black beans toss, cover the pan, reduce heat to medium and cook for 20 mins. Add cilantro, toss, divide between plates and serve. Enjoy!

Nutrition: Calories: 254 Fat: 6 G Carbs: 16 G Protein: 22 G Sodium: 92 Mg

698. Chicken Thighs and Apples Mix

Preparation time: 15 minutes
Cooking time: 60 minutes
Servings: 4
Ingredients:
- 3 cored and sliced apples
- tbsp. apple cider vinegar treatment
- ¾ c. natural apple juice
- ¼ tsp. pepper and salt
- 1 tbsp. grated ginger
- 8 chicken thighs
- tbsps. Chopped onion

Directions:
1. In a bowl, mix chicken with salt, pepper, vinegar, onion, ginger, and apple juice, toss well, cover, keep within the fridge for ten minutes, transfer with a baking dish, and include apples. Introduce inside the oven at 400 0F for just 1 hour. Divide between plates and serve. Enjoy!

Nutrition: Calories: 214 Fat: 3 G Carbs: 14 G Protein: 15 G Sodium: 405 Mg

699. Thai Chicken Thighs

Preparation time: 15 minutes
Cooking time: 1 hour & 5minutes
Servings: 6
Ingredients:
- ½ c. Thai chili sauce
- chopped green onions bunch
- 4 lbs. chicken thighs

Directions:
1. Heat a pan over medium-high heat. Add chicken thighs, brown them for 5 minutes on both sides Transfer to some baking dish, then add chili sauce and green onions and toss.
2. Introduce within the oven and bake at 4000F for 60 minutes. Divide everything between plates and serve. Enjoy!

Nutrition: Calories: 220 Fat: 4 g Carbs: 12 g Protein: 10 g Sodium: 870 mg

700. Falling "Off" The Bone Chicken

Preparation time: 15 minutes
Cooking time: 40 minutes
Servings: 4
Ingredients:
- 6 peeled garlic cloves
- tbsp. organic extra virgin coconut oil
- tbsps. Lemon juice
- ½ c. pacific organic bone chicken broth
- ¼ tsp. freshly ground black pepper
- ½ tsp. sea flavored vinegar
- 1 whole organic chicken piece
- 1 tsp. paprika

- 1 tsp. dried thyme

Directions:
1. Take a small bowl and toss in the thyme, paprika, pepper, and flavored vinegar and mix them. Use the mixture to season the chicken properly. Pour down the oil in your instant pot and heat it to shimmering; toss in the chicken with breast downward and let it cook for about 6-7 minutes 2. After the 7 minutes, flip over the chicken pour down the broth, garlic cloves, and lemon juice. Cook within 25 minutes on a high setting. Remove the dish from the cooker and let it stand for about 5 minutes before serving.

Nutrition: Calories: 664 Fat: 44 G Carbs: 44 G Protein: 27 G Sugars: 0.1 G Sodium: 800 Mg

MEAT

701. Pork Tenderloin with Apples and Balsamic Vinegar

Preparation time: 10 Minutes
Cooking Time: 25 minutes
Servings: 4
Ingredients:
- 1 tablespoon olive oil
- 1-pound pork tenderloin, trimmed from fat
- Freshly ground black pepper
- 2 cups chopped onion
- 2 cups chopped apple
- 1 ½ tablespoons fresh rosemary, chopped
- 1 cup low sodium chicken broth
- 1 ½ tablespoons balsamic vinegar

Directions:
1. Heat the oven to 4500F.
2. Heat the oil in a large skillet over medium flame.
3. Sear the pork and season with black pepper. Cook the pork for 3 minutes until all sides turn light brown. Remove from the heat and place in a baking pan.
4. Roast the pork for 15 minutes.
5. Meanwhile, place the onion, apples, and rosemary on the skillet where the pork is seared. Continue stirring for 5 minutes. Pour in broth and balsamic vinegar and allow to simmer until the sauce thickens.
6. Serve the roasted pork with the onion and apple sauce.

Nutrition: Calories: 240; Protein: 26g; Carbs: 17g; Fat: 6g; Saturated Fat: 1g; Sodium: 83mg

702. Pork Tenderloin with Apples and Blue Cheese

Preparation time: 10 Minutes
Cooking Time: 25 minutes
Servings: 4
Ingredients:
- 1-pound pork tenderloin, trimmed from fat
- ½ teaspoon white pepper
- 2 teaspoons black pepper
- ¼ teaspoon cayenne pepper
- 1 teaspoon paprika
- 2 apples, sliced
- ½ cup unsweetened apple juice
- ¼ cup crumbled blue cheese

Directions:

1. Heat the oven to 3500F.
2. Season the tenderloin with white pepper, black pepper, cayenne pepper, and paprika.
3. Heat a non-stick pan over medium flame and sear the meat for 3 minutes on each side. Transfer to a baking dish and roast in the oven for 20 minutes or until the internal temperature is at 1550F. Remove from the oven to cool.
4. While the pork is roasting, prepare the sauce. Using the same skillet used to sear the meat, sauté the apples for 3 minutes. Add the apple juice and allow the sauce to thicken for at least 10 minutes.
5. Serve the pork with the apple sauce and sprinkle with blue cheese on top.

Nutrition: Calories: 235; Protein: 26g; Carbs: 17; Fat: 3g; Saturated Fat: 1g; Sodium: 145mg

703. Pork Tenderloin with Fennel Sauce

Preparation time: 10 Minutes
Cooking Time: 30 minutes
Servings: 4
Ingredients:
- 4 pork tenderloin fillets, trimmed from fat and cut into 4 portions
- 1 tablespoon olive oil
- 1 teaspoon fennel seeds
- 1 fennel bulb, cored and sliced thinly
- 1 sweet onion, sliced thinly
- ½ cup dry white wine
- 12 ounces low sodium chicken broth
- 1 orange, sliced for garnish

Directions:
1. Place the pork slices in between wax paper and pound with a mallet to about ¼-inch thick.
2. Heat oil in a skillet and fry the fennel seeds for 3 minutes or until fragrant.
3. Stir in the pork and cook on all sides for 3 minutes or until golden brown. Remove the pork from the skillet and set aside.
4. Using the same skillet, add the fennel bulb slices and onion. Sauté for 5 minutes then set aside.
5. Add the wine and chicken broth in the skillet and bring to a boil until the sauce reduces in half.
6. Return the pork to the skillet and cook for another 5 minutes.
7. Serve the pork with sauce and vegetables.

Nutrition: Calories: 276; Protein: 29g; Carbs: 13g; Fat: 12g; Saturated Fat: 3 g; Sodium: 122mg

704. Spicy Beef Kebabs

Preparation time: 10 Minutes
Cooking Time: 10 minutes
Servings: 8
Ingredients:

- 2 yellow onions, minced
- 2 tablespoons fresh lemon juice
- 1 ½ pounds lean ground beef, minced
- ¼ cup bulgur, soaked in water for 30 minutes then rinsed
- ¼ cup chopped pine nuts
- 2 cloves of garlic, minced
- 1 teaspoon ground cumin
- ½ teaspoon ground cinnamon
- ½ teaspoon ground cardamom
- ½ teaspoon freshly ground black pepper
- 16 wooden skewers, soaked in water for 30 minutes

Directions:

1. In a mixing bowl, combine all ingredients except for the skewers. Mix well unto
2. Form a sausage from the meat mixture and thread it into the skewers. If the sausage is crumbly, add a tablespoon of water at a time until it holds well together. Refrigerate the skewered meat sausages until ready to cook.
3. Heat the grill to 3500F and place the grill rack 6 inches from the heat source.
4. Place the skewered kebabs on the grill and broil for 5 minutes on each side.
5. Serve with yogurt if desired.

Nutrition: Calories: 219; Protein: 23g; Carbs: 3g; Fat: 12g; Saturated Fat: 3g; Sodium: 53mg

705. Spicy Beef Curry

Preparation time: 10 Minutes
Cooking Time: 40 minutes
Servings: 6
Ingredients:

- 1 medium serrano pepper, cut into thirds
- 4 cloves of garlic, minced
- 1 2-inch piece ginger, peeled and chopped
- 1 yellow onion, chopped
- 2 tablespoon ground coriander
- 2 teaspoons ground cumin
- ½ teaspoon ground turmeric
- 2 teaspoons garam masala
- 1 tablespoon olive oil
- pounds beef, cut into chunks
- 1 cup ripe tomatoes, diced
- 2 cups water
- 1 cup fresh cilantro for garnish

Directions:

1. In a food processor, pulse the serrano peppers, garlic, ginger, onion, coriander, cumin, turmeric, and garam masala until well-combined.
2. Heat oil over medium heat in a skillet and sauté the spice mixture for 2 minutes or until fragrant.
3. Stir in the beef and allow to cook while stirring constantly for three minutes or until the beef turns brown.

4. Stir in the tomatoes and sauté for another three minutes.
5. Add in the water and bring to a boil.
6. Once boiling, turn the heat to low and allow to simmer for thirty minutes or until the meat is tender.
7. Add cilantro last before serving.

Nutrition: Calories: 181; Protein: 16g; Carbs: 5g; Fat: 8g; Saturated Fat: 2g; Sodium: 74mg

706. Pork Tenderloin with Apples and Sweet Potatoes

Preparation time: 10 Minutes
Cooking Time: 30 minutes
Servings: 4
Ingredients:

- ¾ cup apple cider
- ¼ cup apple cider vinegar
- 2 tablespoons maple syrup
- ¼ teaspoon smoked paprika powder
- 1 teaspoon grated ginger
- ¼ teaspoon ground black pepper
- 2 teaspoons olive oil
- 1 12-ounce pork tenderloin
- 1 large sweet potato, cut into cubes
- 1 large apple, cored and into cubes

Directions:

1. Preheat the oven to 3750F.
2. In a bowl, combine the apple cider, apple cider vinegar, maple syrup, smoked paprika, ginger, and black pepper. Set aside.
3. Heat the oil in a large skillet and sear the meat for 3 minutes on both sides.
4. Transfer the pork in a baking dish and place the sweet potatoes and apples around the pork. Pour in the apple cider sauce.
5. Place inside the oven and cook for 20 minutes.

Nutrition: Calories: 267; Protein: 23.5g; Carbs: 31 g; Fat: 5g; Saturated Fat: 0.5g; Sodium: 69mg

707. Pork Medallions with Five Spice Powder

Preparation time: 10 Minutes
Cooking Time: 25 minutes
Servings: 4
Ingredients:

- 1 tablespoon olive oil
- 3 cloves of garlic, minded
- 1-pound pork tenderloin, fat trimmed
- 2 tablespoon low-sodium soy sauce
- 1 tablespoon green onion, minced
- ¾ teaspoon five spice powder
- ½ cup water
- ¼ cup dry white wine
- 1/3 cup chopped onion
- ½ head green cabbage, thinly sliced and wilted
- 1 tablespoon chopped fresh parsley

Directions:

1. In a bowl, combine the olive oil, garlic, pork tenderloin, soy sauce, green onion, and five spice powder. Mix until well combined and allow to marinate in the fridge for at least two hours.
2. Heat the oven to 4000F.
3. Remove the pork from the marinade and pat dry.
4. On a skillet, sear the meat on all sides until slightly brown before transferring into a heat-proof baking dish.
5. Place inside the oven and roast the pork for 20 minutes.
6. Meanwhile, pour the water, dry white wine, and onions in the skillet where you seared the pork and deglaze. Allow to simmer until the sauce has reduced.
7. Serve the pork medallions with wilted cabbages and drizzle the sauce on top.

Nutrition: Calories: 219; Protein: 25g; Carbs: 5g; Fat: 11g; Saturated Fat: 2g; Sodium: 296mg

708. Grilled Pork Fajitas

Preparation time: 10 Minutes
Cooking Time: 15 minutes
Servings: 8
Ingredients:
- ½ teaspoon paprika
- ½ teaspoon oregano
- ¼ teaspoon ground coriander
- ¼ teaspoon garlic powder
- 1 tablespoon chili powder
- 1-pound pork tenderloin, fat trimmed and cut into large strips
- 1 onion, sliced
- 8 whole wheat flour tortillas, warmed
- 4 medium tomatoes, chopped
- 4 cups shredded lettuce

Directions:
1. In a bowl, mix the paprika, oregano, coriander, garlic powder, and chili powder.
2. Sprinkle the spice mixture on the pork tenderloin strips and toss to coat the meat with the spices.
3. Prepare the grill and heat to 4000F.
4. Place the meat and onion in a grill basket and broil for 20 minutes or until all sides have browned.
5. Assemble the fajitas by placing in the center of the tortillas the grilled pork and onions. Add in the tomatoes and lettuce before rolling the fajitas.

Nutrition: Calories: 250; Protein: 20g; Carbs: 29g; Fat: 6g; Saturated Fat: 2g; Sodium: 234mg

709. New York Strip Steak with Mushroom Sauce

Preparation time: 10 Minutes
Cooking Time: 20 minutes
Servings: 2
Ingredients:
- 2 New York Strip steaks -4 ounces each, trimmed from fat
- 3 cloves of garlic, minced
- 2 ounces shiitake mushrooms, sliced
- 2 ounces button mushrooms, sliced

- ¼ teaspoon thyme
- ¼ teaspoon rosemary
- ¼ cup low sodium beef broth

Directions:
1. Heat the grill to 3500F.
2. Position the grill rack 6 inches from the heat source.
3. Grill the steaks for 10 minutes on each side or until slightly pink on the inside.
4. Meanwhile, prepare the sauce. In a small nonstick pan, water sauté the garlic, mushrooms, thyme and rosemary for a minute. Pour in the broth and bring to a boil. Allow the sauce to simmer until the liquid is reduced.
5. Top the steaks with the mushroom sauce.
6. Serve warm.

Nutrition: Calories: 270; Protein: 23g; Carbs: 4g; Fat: 6g; Saturated Fat: 2g; Sodium: 96 mg

710. Pork Chops with Black Currant Jam

Preparation time: 10 Minutes
Cooking Time: 20 minutes
Servings: 6
Ingredients:
- ¼ cup black currant jam
- 2 tablespoons Dijon mustard
- 1 teaspoon olive oil
- 6 center cut pork loin chops, trimmed from fat
- 1/3 cup wine vinegar
- 1/8 teaspoon ground black pepper
- 6 orange slices

Directions:
1. In a small bowl, mix together the jam and mustard. Set aside.
2. In a nonstick pan, heat the oil over medium flames and sear the pork chops for 5 minutes on each side or until all sides turn brown.
3. Brush the pork chops with the mustard mixture and turn the flame to low. Cook for two more minutes on each side. Set aside.
4. Using the same frying pan, pour in the wine vinegar to deglaze the pan. Season with ground black pepper and allow to simmer for at least 5 minutes or until the vinegar has reduced.
5. Pour over the pork chops and garnish with orange slices on top.

Nutrition: Calories: 198; Protein: 25g; Carbs: 11g; Fat: 6g; Saturated Fat: 2g; Sodium: 188mg

711. Pork Medallion with Herbes de Provence

Preparation time: 10 Minutes
Cooking Time: 15 minutes
Servings: 2
Ingredients:
- 8 ounces of pork medallion, trimmed from fat
- Freshly ground black pepper to taste
- ½ teaspoon Herbes de Provence
- ¼ cup dry white wine

Directions:
1. Season the meat with black pepper.
2. Place the meat in between sheets of wax paper and pound on a mallet until about ¼ inch thick.
3. In a nonstick skillet, sear the pork over medium heat for 5 minutes on each side or until the meat is slightly brown.
4. Remove meat from the skillet and sprinkle with Herbes de Provence.
5. Using the same skillet, pour the wine and scrape the sides to deglaze. Allow to simmer until the wine is reduced.
6. Pour the wine sauce over the pork.
7. Serve immediately.

Nutrition: Calories: 120; Protein: 24g; Carbs: 1g; Fat: 2g; Saturated Fat: 0.5g; Sodium: 62mg

712. Simple Beef Brisket and Tomato Soup

Preparation time: 10 Minutes
Cooking Time: 3 hours
Servings: 8

Ingredients:
- 1 tablespoon olive oil
- 2 ½ pounds beef brisket, trimmed of fat and cut into 8 equal parts
- A dash of ground black pepper
- 1 ½ cups chopped onions
- 4 cloves of garlic, smashed
- 1 teaspoon dried thyme
- 1 cup ripe roma tomatoes, chopped
- ¼ cup red wine vinegar
- 1 cup beef stock, low sodium or home made

Directions:
1. In a heavy pot, heat the oil over medium-high heat.
2. Season the brisket with ground black pepper and place in the pot.
3. Cook while stirring constantly until the beef turns brown on all sides.
4. Stir in the onions and cook until fragrant. Add in the garlic and thyme and cook for another minute until fragrant.
5. Pour in the rest of the ingredients and bring to a boil.
6. Cook until the beef is tender. This may take about 3 hours or more.

Nutrition: Calories: 229; Protein: 31g; Carbs: 6g; Fat: 9g; Saturated Fat: 3g; Sodium: 184mg

713. Beef Stew with Fennel and Shallots

Preparation time: 10 Minutes
Cooking Time: 40 minutes
Servings: 6

Ingredients:
- 1 tablespoon olive oil
- 1-pound boneless lean beef stew meat, trimmed from fat and cut into cubes
- ½ fennel bulb, trimmed and sliced thinly
- 3 large shallots, chopped

- ¾ teaspoons ground black pepper
- 2 fresh thyme sprigs
- 1 bay leaf
- 3 cups low sodium beef broth
- ½ cup red wine
- 4 large carrots, peeled and cut into chunks
- 4 large white potatoes, peeled and cut into chunks
- 3 portobello mushrooms, cleaned and cut into chunks
- 1/3 cup Italian parsley, chopped

Directions:
1. Heat oil in a pot over medium heat and stir in the beef cubes for 5 minutes or until all sides turn brown.
2. Stir in the fennel, shallots, black pepper, and thyme for one minute or until the ingredients become fragrant.
3. Stir in the bay leaf, broth, red wine, carrots, white potatoes and mushrooms.
4. Bring to a boil and cook for 30 minutes or until everything is tender.
5. Stir in the parsley last.

Nutrition: Calories: 244; Protein: 21g; Carbs: 22g; Fat: 8g; Saturated Fat: 2g; Sodium: 184mg

714. Rustic Beef and Barley Soup

Preparation time: 10 Minutes
Cooking Time: 40 minutes
Servings: 6

Ingredients:
- 1 teaspoon olive oil
- 1-pound beef round steak, sliced into strips
- 2 cups yellow onion, chopped
- 1 cup diced celery
- 4 cloves of garlic, chopped
- 1 cup diced roma tomatoes
- ½ cup diced sweet potato
- ½ cup diced mushrooms
- 1 cup diced carrots
- ¼ cup uncooked barley
- 3 cups low sodium vegetable stock
- 1 teaspoon dried sage
- 1 paprika
- A dash of black pepper to taste
- 1 cup chopped kale

Directions:
1. In a large pot, heat the oil over medium flame and stir in the beef. Cook for 5 minutes while stirring constantly until all sides turn brown.
2. Stir in the onion, celery, and garlic until fragrant.
3. Add in the rest of the ingredients except for the kale.
4. Bring to a boil and cook for 30 minutes until everything is tender.
5. Stir in the kale last and cook for another 5 minutes.

Nutrition: Calories per Serving: 246; Protein: 21g; Carbs: 24g; Fat: 4g; Saturated Fat: 1g; Sodium: 13mg

715. Beef Stroganoff

Preparation time: 10 Minutes

Cooking Time: 25 minutes
Servings: 4
Ingredients:
- ½ cup chopped onion
- ½ pound boneless beef round steak, cut into ¾ inch thick
- 4 cups pasta noodles
- ½ cup fat-free cream of mushroom soup
- ½ cup water
- ½ teaspoon paprika
- ½ cup fat-free sour cream

Directions:
1. In a non-stick frying pan, sauté the onions over low to medium heat without oil while stirring constantly for about 5 minutes.
2. Stir in the beef and cook for another 5 minutes until the beef is tender and turn brown on all sides. Set aside.
3. In a large pot, fill it with water until ¾ full and bring to a boil. Cook the noodles until done according to package instructions. Drain the noodles and set aside.
4. In a saucepan, whisk the mushroom soup and water. Bring to a boil over medium heat and stir constantly until the sauce has reduced. Add in paprika and sour cream.
5. Assemble the stroganoff by placing the pasta in a bowl and pouring over the sauce. Top with the meat.
6. Serve warm.

Nutrition: Calories: 273; Protein: 20g; Carbs: 37g; Fat: 5g; Saturated Fat: 2g; Sodium: 193mg

716. Curried Pork Tenderloin in Apple Cider

Preparation time: 10 Minutes
Cooking Time: 26 minutes
Servings: 6
Ingredients:
- 16 ounces pork tenderloin, cut into 6 pieces
- 1 ½ tablespoons curry powder
- 1 tablespoon extra-virgin olive oil
- 2 medium onions, chopped
- 2 cups apple cider, organic and unsweetened
- 1 tart apple, peeled and chopped into chunks

Directions:
1. In a bowl, season the pork with the curry powder and set aside.
2. Heat oil in a pot over medium flame.
3. Sauté the onions for one minute until fragrant.
4. Stir in the seasoned pork tenderloin and cook for 5 minutes or until lightly golden.
5. Add in the apple cider and apple chunks.
6. Close the lid and bring to a boil.
7. Allow to simmer for 20 minutes.

Nutrition: Calories: 244; Protein: 24g; Carbs: 18g; Fat: 8g; Saturated Fat: 2g; Sodium: 70mg

717. Pork and Roasted Tomatoes Mix

Preparation time: 10 Minutes
Cooking Time: 15 minutes
Servings: 6

Ingredients:
- 1/2 c. chopped yellow onion
- 2 c. chopped zucchinis
- 1 lb. ground pork meat
- ¾ c. shredded low-fat cheddar cheese
- Black pepper
- 15 oz. no-salt-added, chopped and canned roasted tomatoes

Directions:
1. Heat up a pan over medium-high heat, add pork, onion, black pepper and zucchini, stir and cook for 7 minutes.
2. Add roasted tomatoes, stir, bring to a boil, cook over medium heat for 8 minutes, divide into bowls, sprinkle cheddar on the top and serve.
3. Enjoy!

Nutrition: Calories: 270, Fat: 5 g, Carbs: 10 g, Protein: 12 g, Sugars: 8 g, Sodium: 390 mg

718. Provence Pork Medallions

Preparation time: 10 Minutes
Cooking Time: 20 minutes
Servings: 4
Ingredients:
- 1 tsp. Herb de Provence
- Pepper.
- 1/2 c. dry white wine
- 16 oz. pork tenderloins
- Salt

Directions:
1. Season pork lightly with salt and pepper.
2. Place the pork between two pieces of parchment paper and pound with a mallet.
3. You need to have 1/4-inch thick meat.
4. In a large non-stick frying pan, cook the pork over medium-high heat for 2-3 minutes per side.
5. Remove from the heat and sprinkle with herb de Provence. Remove the pork from skillet and place aside. Keep warm.
6. Place the skillet over heat again. Add the wine and cook, stirring to scrape down the bits.
7. Cook until reduced slightly and pour over pork. Serve.

Nutrition: Calories: 105.7, Fat: 1.7 g, Carbs: 0.8 g, Protein: 22.6 g, Sugars: 0 g, Sodium: 67 mg

719. Garlic Pork Shoulder

Preparation time: 10 Minutes
Cooking Time: 4 hours
Servings: 6
Ingredients:
- 2 tsps. Sweet paprika
- 4 lbs. pork shoulder
- 3 tbsps. Extra virgin essential olive oil
- Black pepper
- 3 tbsps. Minced garlic

Directions:
1. In a bowl, mix extra virgin extra virgin olive oil with paprika, black pepper and oil and whisk well.

2. Brush pork shoulder with this mix, arrange inside a baking dish and introduce inside oven at 425 0F for twenty or so minutes.
3. Reduce heat to 325 0F F and bake for 4 hours.
4. Slice the meat, divide it between plates and serve having a side salad.
5. Enjoy!

Nutrition: Calories: 321, Fat: 6 g, Carbs: 12 g, Protein: 18 g, Sugars: 0 g, Sodium: 470 mg

720. Grilled Flank Steak with Lime Vinaigrette

Preparation time: 10 Minutes
Cooking Time: 10 minutes
Servings: 6
Ingredients:
- 2 tablespoons lime juice, freshly squeezed
- 2 tablespoons extra virgin olive oil
- ½ teaspoon ground black pepper
- ¼ cup chopped fresh cilantro
- 1 tablespoon ground cumin
- ¼ teaspoon red pepper flakes
- ¾ pound flank steak

Directions:
1. Heat the grill to low medium heat
2. In a food processor, place all ingredients except for the cumin, red pepper flakes, and flank steak. Pulse until smooth. This will be the vinaigrette sauce. Set aside.
3. Season the flank steak with ground cumin and red pepper flakes and allow to marinate for at least 10 minutes.
4. Place the steak on the grill rack and cook for 5 minutes on each side. Cut into the center to check the doneness of the meat. You can also insert a meat thermometer to check the internal temperature.
5. Remove from the grill and allow to stand for 5 minutes.
6. Slice the steak to 2 inches long and toss the vinaigrette to flavor the meat.
7. Serve with salad if desired.

Nutrition: Calories per Serving: 103; Protein: 13g; Carbs: 1g; Fat: 5g; Saturated Fat: 1g; Sodium: 73mg

721. Asian Pork Tenderloin

Preparation time: 10 Minutes
Cooking Time: 15 minutes
Servings: 4
Ingredients:
- 2 tablespoons sesame seeds
- 1 teaspoon ground coriander
- 1/8 teaspoon cayenne pepper
- 1/8 teaspoon celery seed
- ½ teaspoon minced onion
- ¼ teaspoon ground cumin
- 1/8 teaspoon ground cinnamon
- 1 tablespoon sesame oil
- 1-pound pork tenderloin sliced into 4 equal portions

Directions:
1. Preheat the oven to 4000F.

2. In a skillet, toast the sesame seeds over low heat and set aside. Allow the sesame seeds to cool.
3. In a bowl, combine the rest of the ingredients expect for the pork tenderloin. Stir in the toasted sesame seeds.
4. Place the pork tenderloin in a baking dish and rub the spices on both sides.
5. Place the baking dish with the pork in the oven and bake for 15 minutes or until the internal temperature of the meat reaches to 1700F.
6. Serve warm.

Nutrition: Calories: 248; Protein: 26g; Carbs: 0g; Fat: 16g; Saturated Fat: 5g; Sodium: 57mg

722. Roast and Mushrooms

Preparation time: 10 Minutes
Cooking Time: 20 minutes
Servings: 4
Ingredients:
- 1 tsp. Italian seasoning
- 12 oz. low-sodium beef stock
- 3 1/2 lbs. pork roast
- 4 oz. sliced mushrooms

Directions:
1. In a roasting pan, combine the roast with mushrooms, stock and Italian seasoning, and toss
2. Introduce inside the oven and bake at 350F for starters hour and 20 minutes.
3. Slice the roast, divide it along while using mushroom mix between plates and serve.
4. Enjoy!

Nutrition: Calories: 310, Fat: 16 g, Carbs: 10 g, Protein: 22 g, Sugars: 4 g, Sodium: 600 mg

723. Pork and Celery Mix

Preparation time: 10 Minutes
Cooking Time: 30 minutes
Servings: 8
Ingredients:
- 3 tsps. Fenugreek powder
- Black pepper
- 1 tbsp. organic olive oil
- 1 1/2 c. coconut cream
- 26 oz. chopped celery leaves and stalks
- 1 lb. cubed pork meat
- 1 tbsp. chopped onion

Directions:
1. Heat up a pan while using oil over medium-high heat, add the pork as well as the onion, black pepper and fenugreek, toss and brown for 5 minutes.
2. Add the celery too because coconut cream, toss, cook over medium heat for twenty minutes, divide everything into bowls and serve.
3. Enjoy!

Nutrition: Calories: 340, Fat: 5 g, Carbs: 8 g, Protein: 14 g, Sugars: 2.1 g, Sodium: 200 mg

724. Pork and Dates Sauce

Preparation time: 10 Minutes
Cooking Time: 40 minutes
Servings: 6
Ingredients:
- 2 tbsps. Water
- 2 tbsps. Mustard
- 1/3 c. pitted dates
- Black pepper
- 1/4 tsp. onion powder
- 1/4 c. coconut amino
- 1 1/2 lbs. pork tenderloin
- 1/4 tsp. smoked paprika

Directions:
1. In your blender, mix dates with water, coconut amino, mustard, paprika, pepper and onion powder and blend well.
2. Put pork tenderloin within the roasting pan, add the dates sauce, toss to coat perfectly, introduce everything inside the oven at 400F, bake for 40 minutes, slice the meat, divide it as well since the sauce between plates and serve.
3. Enjoy!

Nutrition: Calories: 240, Fat: 8 g, Carbs: 13 g, Protein: 24 g, Sugars: 0 g, Sodium: 433 mg

725. Pork Roast and Cranberry Roast

Preparation time: 10 Minutes
Cooking Time: 30 minutes
Servings: 4
Ingredients:
- 2 minced garlic cloves
- 1/2 tsp. grated ginger
- Black pepper
- 1/2 c. low-sodium veggie stock
- 1 1/2 lbs. pork loin roast
- 1 tbsp. coconut flour
- 1/2 c. cranberries
- Juice of 1/2 lemon

Directions:
1. Put the stock in the little pan, get hot over medium-high heat, add black pepper, ginger, garlic, cranberries, fresh freshly squeezed lemon juice along using the flour, whisk well and cook for ten minutes.
2. Put the roast in the pan, add the cranberry sauce at the very top, introduce inside oven and bake at 375F for an hour and 20 minutes.
3. Slice the roast, divide it along using the sauce between plates and serve.
4. Enjoy!

Nutrition: Calories: 330, Fat: 13 g, Carbs: 13 g, Protein: 25 g, Sugars: 7 g, Sodium: 150 mg

726. Easy Pork Chops

Preparation time: 10 Minutes

Cooking Time: 10 minutes
Servings: 4
Ingredients:
- 1 c. low-sodium chicken stock
- 1 tsp. sweet paprika
- 4 boneless pork chops
- 1/4 tsp. black pepper
- 1 tbsp. extra-virgin olive oil

Directions:
1. Heat up a pan while using the oil over medium-high heat, add pork chops, brown them for 5 minutes on either sides, add paprika, black pepper and stock, toss, cook for fifteen minutes more, divide between plates and serve by using a side salad.
2. Enjoy!

Nutrition: Calories: 272, Fat: 4 g, Carbs: 14 g, Protein: 17 g, Sugars: 0.2 g, Sodium: 68 mg

727. Beef & Vegetable Stir-Fry

Preparation time: 20 Minutes
Cooking Time: 30 minutes
Servings: 4
Ingredients:
- 1 lb. thinly sliced skirt steak
- 2 tbsps. sesame seeds
- ¾ c. stir-fry sauce
- 1 thinly sliced red bell pepper
- 2 thinly sliced scallions
- 2 tbsps. canola oil
- 1/4 tsp. ground black pepper
- 1 sliced broccoli head
- 11/2 c. fluffy brown rice

Directions:
1. Prepare the Stir-Fry Sauce.
2. Heat the canola oil in a large wok or skillet over medium-high heat. Season the steak with the black pepper and cook for 4 minutes, until crispy on the outside and pink on the inside. Remove the steak from the skillet and place the broccoli and peppers in the hot oil. Stir-fry for 4 minutes, stirring or tossing occasionally, until crisp and slightly tender.
3. Place the steak back in the skillet with the vegetables. Pour the stir-fry sauce over the steak and vegetables and let simmer for 3 minutes. Remove from the heat.
4. Serve the stir-fry over rice and top with the scallions and sesame seeds.
5. For leftovers, divide the stir-fry evenly into microwaveable airtight containers and store in the refrigerator for up to 5 days. Reheat in the microwave on high for 2 to 3 minutes, until heated through.

Nutrition: Calories: 408, Fat: 18 g, Carbs: 36 g, Protein: 31 g, Sugars: 5.5 g, Sodium: 197 mg

728. Simple Veal Chops

Preparation time: 10 Minutes
Cooking Time: 10 minutes
Servings: 4
Ingredients:
- 3 tbsps. essential olive oil

- Zest of 1 grated lemon
- 3 tbsps. whole-wheat flour
- 1 1/2 c. whole-wheat breadcrumbs
- Black pepper
- 1 tbsp. milk
- 4 veal rib chops
- 2 eggs

Directions:
1. Put whole-wheat flour within a bowl.
2. In another bowl, mix eggs with milk and whisk
3. In 1 / 3 bowl, mix the breadcrumbs with lemon zest.
4. Season veal chops with black pepper, dredge them in flour, and dip inside egg mix then in breadcrumbs.
5. Heat up a pan because of the oil over medium-high heat, add veal chops, cook for 2 main minutes on both sides and transfer to some baking sheet, introduce them inside oven at 350 0F, bake for quarter-hour, divide between plates and serve utilizing a side salad.
6. Enjoy!

Nutrition: Calories: 270, Fat: 6 g, Carbs: 10 g, Protein: 16 g, Sugars: 0 g, Sodium: 320 mg

729. Beef and Barley Farmers Soup

Preparation time: 10 Minutes
Cooking Time: 20 minutes
Servings: 4
Ingredients:
- 1 diced onion
- 15 g sunflower oil
- 15 g balsamic vinegar
- 900 g Campbell's red and white vegetable beef soup bowl
- 2 thinly sliced green onion stalks
- 1 diced carrot
- 340 g cubed lean beef
- 1 Julienned celery stalk
- 1 Minced Garlic Clove
- 85 g pot barley

Directions:
1. Throw a cast iron pan or a deep saucepan on medium heat with the oil and cubed beef to allow the two to cook. Wait till beef is properly browned on all sides, and then add in the diced vegetables. Cover and cook for an additional 3-5 minutes, stirring occasionally.
2. Add in a combination of the broth, vinegar, and barley; reduce flame and bring to a boil. Continue to cook for about 20 minutes, or until thickened to preferred consistency.
3. Top with chopped green onions and serve!

Nutrition: Calories: 279, Fat: 7.6 g, Carbs: 28.91 g, Protein: 24.82 g, Sugars: 3 g, Sodium: 590 mg

730. Simple Pork and Capers

Preparation time: 10 Minutes
Cooking Time: 10 minutes
Servings: 2
Ingredients:

- 8 oz. cubed pork
- 1 c. low-sodium chicken stock
- Black pepper
- 2 tbsps. Organic extra virgin olive oil
- 1 minced garlic oil
- 2 tbsps. Capers

Directions:
1. Heat up a pan with the oil over medium-high heat, add the pork season with black pepper and cook for 4 minutes on both sides.
2. Add garlic, capers and stock, stir and cook for 7 minutes more.
3. Divide everything between plates and serve.
4. Enjoy!

Nutrition: Calories: 224, Fat: 12 g, Carbs: 12 g, Protein: 10 g, Sugars: 5 g, Sodium: 5 mg

731. A "Boney" Pork Chop

Preparation time: 20 Minutes
Cooking Time: 30 minutes
Servings: 4
Ingredients:
- 1 c. baby carrots
- Flavored vinegar
- 3 tbsps. Worcestershire sauce
- Ground pepper
- 1 chopped onion
- 4 ¾ bone-in thick pork chops
- 1/4 c. divided butter
- 1 c. vegetables

Directions:
1. Take a bowl and add pork chops, season with pepper and flavored vinegar
2. Take a skillet and place it over medium heat, add 2 teaspoon of butter and melt it
3. Toss the pork chops and brown them
4. Each side should take about 3-5 minutes
5. Set your pot to sauté mode and add 2 tablespoon of butter, add carrots and sauté them
6. Pour broth and Worcestershire
7. Add pork chops and lock up the lid
8. Cook on HIGH pressure for 13 minutes
9. Release the pressure naturally
10. Enjoy!

Nutrition: Calories: 715, Fat: 37.4 g, Carbs: 2 g, Protein: 20.7 g, Sugars: 0 g, Sodium: 276 mg

732. Beef Pot

Preparation time: 10 Minutes
Cooking Time: 40 minutes
Servings: 2
Ingredients:
- 4 tbsps. Sour cream
- 1/4 shredded cabbage head
- 1 tsp. butter
- 2 peeled and sliced carrots
- 1 chopped onion
- 10 oz. boiled and sliced beef tenderloin

- 1 tbsp. flour

Directions:
1. Sauté the cabbage, carrots and onions in butter.
2. Spray a pot with cooking spray.
3. In layers place the sautéed vegetables, then beef, then another layer of vegetables.
4. Beat the sour cream with flour until smooth and pour over the beef.
5. Cover and bake at 400F for 40 minutes.

Nutrition: Calories: 210, Fat: 30 g, Carbs: 4 g, Protein: 14 g, Sugars: 1 g, Sodium: 600 mg

733. Beef with Cucumber Raito

Preparation time: 10 Minutes
Cooking Time: 30 minutes
Servings: 2

Ingredients:
- 1/2 tsp. lemon-pepper seasoning
- 1/4 c. coarsely shredded unpeeled cucumber
- Black pepper and salt
- 1 tbsp. finely chopped red onion
- 1/4 tsp. sugar
- 1 lb. sliced de-boned beef sirloin steak
- 8 oz. plain fat-free yogurt
- 1 tbsp. snipped fresh mint

Directions:
1. Preheat broiler.
2. In a small bowl combine yogurt, cucumber, onion, snipped mint, and sugar. Season to taste with salt and pepper; set aside
3. Trim fat from meat. Sprinkle meat with lemon-pepper seasoning.
4. Place meat on the unheated rack of a broiler pan. Broil 3 to 4 inches from heat, turning meat over after half of the broiling time.
5. Allow 15 to 17 minutes for medium-rare (145 degree F) and 20 to 22 minutes for medium (160 degree F).
6. Cut steak across the grain into thin slices.
7. Serve and enjoy.

Nutrition: Calories: 176, Fat: 3 g, Carbs: 5 g, Protein: 28 g, Sugars: 8.9 g, Sodium: 88.3 mg

734. Bistro Beef Tenderloin

Preparation time: 10 Minutes
Cooking Time: 45 minutes
Servings: 12

Ingredients:
- 2 tbsps. Extra-virgin olive oil
- 2 tbsps. Dijon mustard
- 1 tsp. kosher salt
- 2/3 c. chopped mixed fresh herbs
- 3 lbs. trimmed beef tenderloin
- 1/2 tsp. freshly ground pepper

Directions:
1. Preheat oven to 400F.
2. Tie kitchen string around tenderloin in three places so it doesn't flatten while roasting.

3. Rub the tenderloin with oil; pat on salt and pepper. Place in a large roasting pan.
4. Roast until a thermometer inserted into the thickest part of the tenderloin registers 140F for medium-rare, about 45 minutes, turning two or three times during roasting to ensure even cooking.
5. Transfer to a cutting board; let rest for 10 minutes. Remove the string.
6. Place herbs on a large plate. Coat the tenderloin evenly with mustard; then roll in the herbs, pressing gently to adhere. Slice and serve.

Nutrition: Calories: 280, Fat: 20.6 g, Carbs: 0.9 g, Protein: 22.2 g, Sugars: 0 g, Sodium: 160 mg

735. The Surprising No "Noodle" Lasagna

Preparation time: 10 Minutes
Cooking Time: 10 minutes
Servings: 8

Ingredients:
- 1/2 c. Parmesan cheese
- 2 minced garlic cloves
- 8 oz. sliced mozzarella
- 1 lb. ground beef
- 25 oz. marinara sauce
- 1 small sized onion
- 1 1/2 c. ricotta cheese
- 1 large sized egg

Directions:
1. Set your pot to Sauté mode and add garlic, onion and ground beef
2. Take a small bowl and add ricotta and parmesan with egg and mix
3. Drain the grease and transfer the beef to a 1 and a 1/2 quart soufflé dish
4. Add marinara sauce to the browned meat and reserve half
5. Top the remaining meat sauce with half of your mozzarella cheese
6. Spread half of the ricotta cheese over the mozzarella layer
7. Top with the remaining meat sauce
8. Add a final layer of mozzarella cheese on top
9. Spread any remaining ricotta cheese mix over the mozzarella
10. Carefully add this mixture to your Soufflé Dish
11. Pour 1 cup of water to your pot
12. Place it over a trivet
13. Lock up the lid and cook on HIGH pressure for 10 minutes
14. Release the pressure naturally over 10 minutes
15. Serve and enjoy!

Nutrition: Calories: 607, Fat: 23 g, Carbs: 65 g, Protein: 33 g, Sugars: 0.31 g, Sodium: 128 mg

736. Lamb Chops with Kale

Preparation time: 10 Minutes
Cooking Time: 35 minutes
Servings: 4

Ingredients:
- 1 tbsp. olive oil
- 1 sliced yellow onion
- 1 c. torn kale
- 2 tbsps. low-sodium tomato paste
- 1/4 tsp. black pepper
- 1/2 c. low-sodium veggie stock
- 1 lb. lamb chops

Directions:
1. Grease a roasting pan with the oil, arrange the lamb chops inside, also add the kale and the other ingredients and toss gently.
2. Bake everything at 390F for 35 minutes, divide between plates and serve.

Nutrition: Calories: 275, Fat: 11.8 g, Carbs: 7.3 g, Protein: 33.6 g, Sugars: 0.1 g, Sodium: 280 mg

737. Beef with Mushrooms

Preparation time: 15 Minutes
Cooking Time: 8 hours
Servings: 8

Ingredients:
- 2 c. salt-free tomato paste
- 2 c. sliced fresh mushrooms
- 2 c. low-fat, low-sodium beef broth
- 2 lbs. cubed lean beef stew meat
- 1 c. chopped fresh parsley leaves
- Freshly ground black pepper
- 4 minced garlic cloves

Directions:
1. In a slow cooker add all ingredients except lemon juice and, stir to combine.
2. Set the slow cooker on low.
3. Cover and cook for about 8 hours.
4. Serve hot with the drizzling of lemon juice

Nutrition: Calories: 260, Fat: 12 g, Carbs: 18 g, Protein: 44 g, Sugars: 4 g, Sodium: 480 mg

738. Lemony Braised Beef Roast

Preparation time: 15 Minutes
Cooking Time: 6-8 hours
Servings: 6

Ingredients:
- 1 tbsp. minced fresh rosemary
- 1/2 c. low-fat, low-sodium beef broth
- Freshly ground black pepper
- 2 lbs. lean beef pot roast
- 1 sliced onion
- 2 minced garlic cloves
- 1/4 c. fresh lemon juice
- 1 tsp. ground cumin

Directions:
1. In a large slow cooker, add all ingredients and mix well.
2. Set the slow cooker on low.
3. Cover and cook for about 6-8 hours.

Nutrition: Calories: 344, Fat: 2.8 g, Carbs: 18 g, Protein: 32 g, Sugars: 2.4 g, Sodium: 278 mg

739. Grilled Fennel-Cumin Lamb Chops

Preparation time: 10 Minutes
Cooking Time: 30 minutes
Servings: 2

Ingredients:
- 1/4 tsp. salt
- 1 minced large garlic clove
- 1/8 tsp. cracked black pepper
- ¾ tsp. crushed fennel seeds
- 1/4 tsp. ground coriander
- 4-6 sliced lamb rib chops
- ¾ tsp. ground cumin

Directions:
1. Trim fat from chops. Place the chops on a plate.
2. In a small bowl combine the garlic, fennel seeds, cumin, salt, coriander, and black pepper. Sprinkle the mixture evenly over chops; rub in with your fingers. Cover the chops with plastic wrap and marinate in the refrigerator at least 30 minutes or up to 24 hours.
3. Grill chops on the rack of an uncovered grill directly over medium coals until chops are desired doneness.

Nutrition: Calories: 239, Fat: 12 g, Carbs: 2 g, Protein: 29 g, Sugars: 0 g, Sodium: 409 mg

740. Beef Heart

Preparation time: 40 Minutes
Cooking Time: 30 minutes
Servings: 4

Ingredients:
- 1 chopped large onion
- 1 c. water
- 2 peeled and chopped tomatoes
- 1 boiled beef heart
- 2 tbsps. tomato paste

Directions:
1. Boil the beef heart until half-done.
2. Sauté the onions with tomatoes until soft.
3. Cut the beef heart into cubes and add to tomato and onion mixture. Add water and tomato paste. Stew on low heat for 30 minutes.

Nutrition: Calories: 138, Fat: 3 g, Carbs: 0.1 g, Protein: 24.2 g, Sugars: 0 g, Sodium: 50.2 mg

741. Jerk Beef and Plantain Kabobs

Preparation time: 10 Minutes
Cooking Time: 15 minutes
Servings: 4

Ingredients:
- 2 peeled and sliced ripe plantains
- 2 tbsps. Red wine vinegar
- Lime wedges
- 1 tbsp. cooking oil

- 1 sliced medium red onion
- 12 oz. sliced boneless beef sirloin steak
- 1 tbsp. Jamaican jerk seasoning

Directions:
1. Trim fat from meat. Cut into 1-inch pieces. In a small bowl, stir together red wine vinegar, oil, and jerk seasoning. Toss meat cubes with half of the vinegar mixture. On long skewers, alternately thread meat, plantain chunks, and onion wedges, leaving a 1/4-inch space between pieces.
2. Brush plantains and onion wedges with remaining vinegar mixture.
3. Place skewers on the rack of an uncovered grill directly over medium coals. Grill for 12 to 15 minutes or until meat is desired doneness, turning occasionally.
4. Serve with lime wedges.

Nutrition: Calories: 260, Fat: 7 g, Carbs: 21 g, Protein: 26 g, Sugars: 2.5 g, Sodium: 358 mg

742. Authentic Pepper Steak

Preparation time: 5 Minutes
Cooking Time: 30 minutes
Servings: 4
Ingredients:
- 1 tbsp. sesame oil
- 80 oz. sliced mushroom
- 1 c. water
- 1 sliced red pepper piece
- 1 pack onion soup mix
- 1 lb. de-boned beef eye of round steak
- 1 tbsp. minced garlic

Directions:
1. Add the listed ingredients to your Instant Pot
2. Lock up the lid and cook on HIGH pressure for 20 minutes
3. Release the pressure naturally over 10 minutes
4. Serve the pepper steak and enjoy!

Nutrition: Calories: 222, Fat: 15 g, Carbs: 5 g, Protein: 36 g, Sugars: 1.56 g, Sodium: 556 mg

743. Lamb Chops with Rosemary

Preparation time: 5 Minutes
Cooking Time: 15 minutes
Servings: 4
Ingredients:
- 1 lb. lamb chops
- 1/2 tsp. freshly ground black pepper
- 1 tbsp. olive oil
- 5 garlic cloves
- 1 tbsp. chopped fresh rosemary

Directions:
1. Adjust oven rack to the top third of the oven. Preheat broiler. Line a baking sheet with foil.
2. Place the garlic, rosemary, pepper, and olive oil into a small bowl and stir well to combine.

3. Place the lamb chops on a baking sheet and brush half of the garlic-rosemary mixture equally between the chops, coating well. Place the sheet beneath broiler and broil 4–5 minutes.
4. Remove from oven and carefully flip over the chops. Divide the remaining garlic-rosemary mixture evenly between the chops and spread to coat. Return pan to oven and broil for another 3 minutes.
5. Remove from oven and serve immediately.

Nutrition: Calories: 185, Fat: 9 g, Carbs: 1 g, Protein: 23 g, Sugars: 0 g, Sodium: 72.8 mg

744. Cane Wrapped Around In Prosciutto

Preparation time: 3 Minutes
Cooking Time: 5 minutes
Servings: 4
Ingredients:
- 80 oz. sliced prosciutto
- 1 lb. thick asparagus

Directions:
1. The first step here is to prepare your instant pot by pouring in about 2 cups of water
2. Take the asparagus and wrap them up in prosciutto spears. Once all of the asparagus are wrapped, gently place the processed asparaguses in the cooking basket inside your pot in layers. Turn up the heat to a high temperature and when there is a pressure build up, take down the heat and let it cook for about 2-3 minutes at the high pressure. Once the timer runs out, gently open the cover of the pressure cooker
3. Take out the steamer basket from the pot instantly and toss the asparaguses on a plate to serve
4. Eat warm or let them come down to room temperature

Nutrition: Calories: 212, Fat: 14 g, Carbs: 11 g, Protein: 12 g, Sugars: 367.6 g, Sodium: 0 mg

745. Beef Veggie Pot Meal

Preparation time: 45-50 Minutes
Cooking Time: 40 minutes
Servings: 2-3
Ingredients:
- 1 tsp. butter
- 1/4 shredded cabbage head
- 2 peeled and sliced carrots
- 1 tbsp. flour
- 4 tbsps. sour cream
- 1 chopped onion
- 10 oz. sliced and boiled beef tenderloin

Directions:
1. In a saucepan; add the butter, cabbage, carrots, and onions.
2. Cook on medium-high heat until the veggies get softened.
3. Add the beef meat and stir the mix.
4. In a mixing bowl, beat the cream with flour until smooth.
5. Add the sauce over the beef.
6. Cover and cook for 40 minutes.

7. Serve warm.

Nutrition: Calories: 245.5, Fat: 10.2 g, Carbs: 18.4 g, Protein: 19.0 g, Sugars: 5.5 g, Sodium: 188.2 mg

746. Braised Beef Shanks

Preparation time: 10 Minutes
Cooking Time: 4-6 hours
Servings: 2
Ingredients:
- Freshly ground black pepper
- 5 minced garlic cloves
- 11/2 lbs. lean beef shanks
- 2 sprigs fresh rosemary
- 1 c. low-fat, low-sodium beef broth
- 1 tbsp. fresh lime juice

Directions:
1. In a slow cooker, add all ingredients and mix. Set the slow cooker on low.
2. Cover and cook for 4-6 hours.

Nutrition: Calories: 50, Fat: 1 g, Carbs: 0.8 g, Protein: 8 g, Sugars: 0 g, Sodium: 108 mg

747. Pork and Capers

Preparation time: 10 minutes
Cooking time: 15 minutes
Servings: 2
Ingredients:
- 2 tablespoons olive oil
- 1 cup low-sodium chicken stock
- 2 tablespoons capers
- 1 garlic clove, minced
- 8 ounces pork, cubed
- Black pepper to the taste

Directions:
1. Heat up a pan with the oil over medium-high heat, add the pork season with black pepper and cook for 4 minutes on each side.
2. Add garlic, capers and stock, stir and cook for 7 minutes more.
3. Divide everything between plates and serve.
4. Enjoy!

Nutrition: Calories 224, Fat 12, Fiber 6, Carbs 12, Protein 10

748. Pork and Red Peppers Mix

Preparation time: 10 minutes
Cooking time: 1 hour
Servings: 4
Ingredients:
- 3 red bell peppers, chopped
- 1 and ½ pounds pork meat, cubed
- ¼ cup low-sodium tomato sauce
- Black pepper to the taste
- 2 pounds Portobello mushrooms, sliced
- 2 yellow onions, chopped

- 1 tablespoon olive oil

Directions:
1. Heat up a pan with the oil over medium-high heat, add the pork and brown it for 5 minutes.
2. Add bell peppers, mushrooms and onions, stir and cook for 5 minutes more.
3. Add tomato sauce and black pepper, toss, introduce in the oven and bake at 350 degrees F for 50 minutes.
4. Divide everything between plates and serve.
5. Enjoy!

Nutrition: Calories 130, Fat 12, Fiber 1, Carbs 3, Protein 9

749. Garlic Pork and Kale

Preparation time: 10 minutes
Cooking time: 20 minutes
Servings: 4
Ingredients:
- 1 cup yellow onion, chopped
- 1 and ½ pound pork meat, cut into strips
- ½ cup red bell pepper, chopped
- Black pepper to the taste
- 1 tablespoon olive oil
- 4 pounds kale, chopped
- 1 teaspoon garlic, minced
- ¼ cup red hot chili pepper, chopped
- 1 cup low-sodium veggie stock

Directions:
1. Heat up a pan with the oil over medium-high heat, add pork strips and cook them for 6 minutes
2. Add onions, bell pepper, black pepper and garlic, stir and cook for 4 minutes more.
3. Add kale, stock and chili pepper, toss, cook for 10 minutes, divide between plates and serve.
4. Enjoy!

Nutrition: Calories 350, Fat 4, Fiber 7, Carbs 8, Protein 16

750. Italian Pork Soup

Preparation time: 10 minutes
Cooking time: 30 minutes
Servings: 10
Ingredients:
- 64 ounces low-sodium veggie stock
- 1 tablespoon olive oil
- 1 cup coconut cream
- 10 ounces spinach
- 1 and ½ pounds pork meat, cubed
- 1 pound radishes, chopped
- 2 garlic cloves, minced
- Black pepper to the taste
- A pinch of red pepper flakes, crushed
- 1 yellow onion, chopped

Directions:
1. Heat up a pot with the oil over medium-high heat, add the meat, onion and garlic, stir and brown for 5 minutes.
2. Add stock, spinach, radishes, black pepper, pepper flakes and cream, stir, bring to a simmer, reduce heat to medium and cook for 25 minutes.
3. Ladle into bowls and serve.
4. Enjoy!

Nutrition: Calories 301, fat 16, fiber 2, carbs 8, protein 17

751. Pork, Shallots and Watercress Soup

Preparation time: 10 minutes
Cooking time: 30 minutes
Servings: 4
Ingredients:
- 6 cups low-sodium chicken stock
- 2 teaspoons coconut aminos
- 6 and ½ cups watercress
- Black pepper to the taste
- 1 pound pork meat, cubed
- 1 tablespoon olive oil
- 3 shallots, chopped
- 3 egg whites, whisked

Directions:
1. Heat up a pot with the oil over medium-high heat, add the meat and some black pepper and brown it for 5 minutes.
2. Add shallots and aminos, toss and cook for 3 minutes more.
3. Add the stock, stir, bring to a simmer and cook over medium heat for 15 minutes more.
4. Add egg whites and the watercress, toss, cook for 6 minutes more, ladle into bowls and serve.
5. Enjoy!

Nutrition: Calories 260, Fat 5, Fiber 5, Carbs 8, Protein 16

752. Pork and Fennel Mix

Preparation time: 10 minutes
Cooking time: 30 minutes
Servings: 4
Ingredients:
- 12 ounces pork meat, cubed
- 2 fennel bulbs, sliced
- Black pepper to the taste
- 2 tablespoons olive oil
- 4 figs, cut halved
- 1/8 cup apple cider vinegar

Directions:
1. Heat up a pan with the oil over medium-high heat, add the pork and brown for 5 minutes on each side.
2. Add fennel, black pepper, figs and cider vinegar, toss, reduce heat to medium, cook for 20 minutes more, divide everything between plates and serve.
3. Enjoy!

Nutrition: Calories 260, Fat 3, Fiber 3, Carbs 8, Protein 16

753. Pork Casserole with Cabbage

Preparation time: 10 minutes
Cooking time: 40 minutes
Servings: 4
Ingredients:

- 17 ounces pork meat, cubed
- 1 green cabbage, shredded
- Salt and black pepper to the taste
- 1 small yellow onion, chopped
- 2 garlic cloves, minced
- 1 tablespoon olive oil
- ½ cup low-fat parmesan, grated
- ½ cup coconut cream.

Directions:
1. Heat up a pot with the oil over medium-high heat, add onion, stir and cook for 2 minutes.
2. Add garlic and the meat and brown for 5 minutes.
3. Add the cabbage, toss and cook everything for 10 minutes more.
4. Add black pepper and coconut cream and toss.
5. Sprinkle parmesan on top, introduce the pan in the oven and bake at 350 degrees F for 20 minutes.
6. Enjoy!

Nutrition: Calories 260, Fat 7, Fiber 4, Carbs 12, Protein 17

754. French Pork Mix

Preparation time: 1 hour
Cooking time: 5 hours and 10 minutes
Servings: 8
Ingredients:
- 3 tablespoons olive oil+ a drizzle
- 2 tablespoons onion, chopped
- 1 tablespoon parsley flakes
- 1 and ½ cups red grapes juice, unsweetened
- 1 teaspoon thyme, dried
- Black pepper to the taste
- 1/3 cup almond flour
- 4 pounds pork meat, cubed
- 24 small white onions
- 2 garlic cloves, minced
- 1 pound mushrooms, roughly chopped

Directions:
1. In a bowl, mix the grape juice with olive oil, minced onion, thyme, parsley, pepper and pork, toss and keep in the fridge for 1 hour.
2. Drain meat, dredge it in flour and reserve 1 cup of marinade.
3. Heat up a pan with a drizzle of oil over medium-high heat, add the onions and cook them for 5 minutes.
4. Add the garlic, the mushrooms and the meat, cook everything for 5 minutes and transfer to a slow cooker.
5. Add black pepper and reserved marinade, cover the pot and cook on High for 5 hours.
6. Divide everything between plates and serve.
7. Enjoy!

Nutrition: Calories 325, Fat 11, Fiber 1, Carbs 7, Protein 16

755. Easy Pork and Okra Stew

Preparation time: 10 minutes
Cooking time: 30 minutes
Servings: 9
Ingredients:
- 1 pound pork meat, cubed

- 1 green bell pepper, chopped
- 2 yellow onions, chopped
- Black pepper to the taste
- 1 cup parsley, chopped
- 8 green onions, chopped
- ¼ cup olive oil
- 1 cup low-sodium veggie stock
- 6 garlic cloves
- 20 ounces canned tomatoes, no-salt-added and chopped
- 20 ounces okra, chopped

Directions:
1. Heat up a pot with the oil over medium-high heat, add the meat and brown it for 5 minutes.
2. Add yellow onions, bell pepper, green onions, parsley and black pepper, stir and cook for 4 minutes more.
3. Add stock, garlic, tomatoes and okra, stir, bring to a simmer, cook for 20 minutes over medium heat, divide into bowls and serve.
4. Enjoy!

Nutrition: Calories 314, Fat 12, Fiber 4, Carbs 13, Protein 17

756. Burgundy Stew

Preparation time: 10 minutes
Cooking time: 3 hours and 5 minutes
Servings: 6
Ingredients:
- 2 pounds pork roast, cubed
- A drizzle of olive oil
- 15 ounces canned tomatoes, no-salt-added and chopped
- 4 carrots, chopped
- Black pepper to the taste
- ½ pounds mushrooms, sliced
- 2 celery ribs, chopped
- 2 yellow onions, chopped
- 1 cup low-sodium veggie stock
- 1 tablespoon thyme, chopped
- ½ teaspoon mustard powder

Directions:
1. Heat up a Dutch oven with the oil over medium-high heat, add the meat and brown it for 5 minutes.
2. Add tomatoes, carrot, black pepper, mushrooms, celery, onions, stock, thyme and mustard powder, toss, introduce in the oven and bake at 325 degrees F for 3 hours.
3. Divide everything between plates and serve.
4. Enjoy!

Nutrition: Calories 265, Fat 13, Fiber 4, Carbs 7, Protein 18

757. Pork Roast with Mushrooms

Preparation time: 10 minutes
Cooking time: 1 hour and 20 minutes
Servings: 4
Ingredients:
- 3 and ½ pounds pork roast
- 4 ounces mushrooms, sliced
- 12 ounces low-sodium beef stock
- 1 teaspoon Italian seasoning

Directions:
1. In a roasting pan, combine the roast with mushrooms, stock and Italian seasoning, and toss, introduce in the oven and bake at 350 degrees F for 1 hour and 20 minutes.
2. Slice the roast, divide it and the mushroom mix between plates and serve.
3. Enjoy!

Nutrition: Calories 310, Fat 16, Fiber 2, Carbs 10, Protein 22

758. Pork Meatloaf

Preparation time: 10 minutes
Cooking time: 50 minutes
Servings: 6
Ingredients:
- 1 cup white mushrooms, chopped
- 3 pounds pork, ground
- 2 tablespoons parsley, chopped
- 2 garlic cloves, minced
- ½ cup yellow onion, chopped
- ¼ cup red bell pepper, chopped
- ½ cup almond flour
- 1/3 cup low-fat parmesan, grated
- 3 eggs
- Black pepper to the taste
- 1 teaspoon balsamic vinegar

Directions:
1. In a bowl, mix the pork with the black pepper, bell pepper, mushrooms, garlic, onion, parsley, almond flour, parmesan, vinegar and eggs, stir very well, transfer this into a loaf pan and bake in the oven at 375 degrees F for 50 minutes.
2. Leave meatloaf to cool down, slice and serve it.
3. Enjoy!

Nutrition: Calories 274, Fat 14, Fiber 3, Carbs 8, Protein 24

759. Garlic Meatballs Salad

Preparation time: 10 minutes
Cooking time: 15 minutes
Servings: 6
Ingredients:
- 17 ounces pork ground
- 1 yellow onion, grated
- 1 egg, whisked
- ¼ cup parsley, chopped
- Black pepper to the taste
- 2 garlic cloves, minced
- ¼ cup mint, chopped
- 2 and ½ teaspoons oregano, dried
- ¼ cup olive oil
- 7 ounces cherry tomatoes, halved
- 1 cucumber, thinly sliced
- 1 cup baby spinach
- 1 and ½ tablespoons lemon juice
- A drizzle of avocado oil

Directions:

1. In a bowl, combine the pork with the onion, egg, parsley, black pepper, mint, garlic and oregano, stir well and shape medium meatballs out of this mix.
2. Heat up a pan with the olive oil over medium-high heat, add the meatballs and cook them for 5 minutes on each side.
3. In a salad bowl, combine the meatballs with the tomatoes, cucumber, spinach, lemon juice and avocado oil, toss and serve.
4. Enjoy!

Nutrition: Calories 220, Fat 4, Fiber 6, Carbs 8, Protein 12

760. Meatballs and Sauce

Preparation time: 10 minutes
Cooking time: 32 minutes
Servings: 6
Ingredients:
- 2 pounds pork, ground
- Black pepper to the taste
- ½ teaspoon garlic powder
- 1 tablespoon coconut aminos
- ¼ cup low sodium veggie
- ¾ cup almond flour
- 1 tablespoon parsley, chopped
- For the sauce:
- 1 cup yellow onion, chopped
- 2 cups mushrooms, sliced
- 2 tablespoons olive oil
- 1 teaspoon coconut aminos
- ½ cup coconut cream
- Black pepper to the taste

Directions:
1. In a bowl, mix the pork with black pepper, garlic powder, 1 tablespoons coconut aminos, stock, almond flour and parsley, stir well, shape medium meatballs out of this mix, arrange them on a baking sheet, introduce in the oven at 375 degrees F and bake for 20 minutes.
2. Meanwhile, heat up a pan with the oil over medium heat, add mushrooms, stir and cook for 4 minutes.
3. Add onions, 1 teaspoon coconut aminos, cream and black pepper, stir and cook for 5 minutes more.
4. Add the meatballs, toss gently, cook for 1-2 minutes more, divide everything into bowls and serve.
5. Enjoy!

Nutrition: Calories 435, Fat 23, Fiber 4, Carbs 6, Protein 32

761. Stir Fry Ground Pork

Preparation time: 10 minutes
Cooking time: 25 minutes
Servings: 10
Ingredients:
- 3 garlic cloves, minced
- 1 pound pork, ground
- ½ cup tomato sauce, no-salt-added
- 1 yellow onion, chopped
- 2 habanero peppers, chopped
- 1 teaspoon curry powder
- 1 teaspoon thyme, dried

- 2 teaspoons coriander, ground
- ½ teaspoon allspice, ground
- 2 teaspoons cumin, ground
- ½ teaspoon turmeric powder
- Black pepper to the taste
- 1 teaspoon garlic powder
- 2 tablespoons olive oil

Directions:
1. Heat up a pan with the oil over medium-high heat, add the onion and the garlic, stir and cook for 5 minutes.
2. Add habanero peppers, curry powder, thyme, coriander, allspice, cumin, turmeric, black pepper and garlic powder, stir and cook for 5 minutes more.
3. Add the pork and the tomato sauce, toss, cook for 15 minutes more, divide everything into bowls and serve.
4. Enjoy!

Nutrition: Calories 267, Fat 23, Fiber 6, Carbs 12, Protein 22

762. Citrus Pork

Preparation time: 10 minutes
Cooking time: 30 minutes
Servings: 4
Ingredients:
- Zest of 2 limes, grated
- Zest of 1 orange, grated
- Juice of 1 orange
- Juice of 2 limes
- 4 teaspoons garlic, minced
- ¾ cup olive oil
- 1 cup cilantro, chopped
- 1 cup mint, chopped
- Black pepper to the taste
- 4 pork loin steaks

Directions:
1. In your food processor, mix lime zest and juice with orange zest and juice, garlic, oil, cilantro, mint and pepper and blend well.
2. Put the steaks in a bowl, add the citrus mix and toss really well.
3. Heat up a pan over medium-high heat, add pork steaks and the marinade, cook for 4 minutes on each side, introduce the pan in the oven and bake at 350 degrees F for 20 minutes.
4. Divide the steaks between plates, drizzle some of the cooking juices all over and serve with a side salad.
5. Enjoy!

Nutrition: Calories 270, Fat 7, Fiber 2, Carbs 8, Protein 20

763. Pork Chops with Nutmeg

Preparation time: 10 minutes
Cooking time: 40 minutes
Servings: 3
Ingredients:
- 8 ounces mushrooms, sliced
- ¼ cup coconut milk
- 1 teaspoon garlic powder
- 1 yellow onion, chopped
- 3 pork chops, boneless
- 2 teaspoons nutmeg, ground

- 1 tablespoon balsamic vinegar
- ½ cup olive oil

Directions:
1. Heat up a pan with the oil over medium heat, add mushrooms and onions, stir and cook for 5 minutes.
2. Add pork chops, nutmeg and garlic powder and cook for 5 minutes more.
3. Add vinegar and coconut milk, toss, introduce in the oven and bake at 350 degrees F and bake for 30 minutes.
4. Divide between plates and serve.
5. Enjoy!

Nutrition: Calories 260, Fat 10, Fiber 6, Carbs 8, Protein 22

764. Italian Parmesan Pork

Preparation time: 10 minutes
Cooking time: 30 minutes
Servings: 6
Ingredients:
- 2 tablespoons parsley, chopped
- 1 pound pork cutlets, thinly sliced
- 1 tablespoon olive oil
- ¼ cup yellow onion, chopped
- 3 garlic cloves, minced
- 2 tablespoons parmesan, grated
- 15 ounces canned tomatoes, no-salt-added and chopped
- 1/3 cup low sodium chicken stock
- Black pepper to the taste
- 1 teaspoon Italian seasoning

Directions:
1. Heat up a pan with the oil over medium-high heat, add pork cutlets, season with Italian seasoning and black pepper and cook for 4 minutes on each side.
2. Add onion, garlic, tomatoes, stock and top with parmesan, introduce the pan in the oven and bake at 350 degrees F for 20 minutes.
3. Sprinkle parsley on top, divide everything between plates and serve.
4. Enjoy!

Nutrition: Calories 280, Fat 17, Fiber 5, Carbs 12, Protein 34

765. Pork Roast with Cranberry

Preparation time: 10 minutes
Cooking time: 1 hour and 30 minutes
Servings: 4
Ingredients:
- 1 tablespoon coconut flour
- Black pepper to the taste
- 1 and ½ pounds pork loin roast
- ½ teaspoon ginger, grated
- ½ cup cranberries
- 2 garlic cloves, minced
- Juice of ½ lemon
- ½ cup low-sodium veggie stock

Directions:
1. Put the stock in a small pan, heat it up over medium-high heat, add black pepper, ginger, garlic, cranberries, lemon juice and the flour, whisk well and cook for 10 minutes.

2. Put the roast in a pan, add the cranberry sauce on top, introduce in the oven and bake at 375 degrees F for 1 hour and 20 minutes.
3. Slice the roast, divide it and the sauce between plates and serve.
4. Enjoy!

Nutrition: Calories 330, Fat 13, Fiber 2, Carbs 13, Protein 25

766. Pork Patties

Preparation time: 10 minutes
Cooking time: 35 minutes
Servings: 6
Ingredients:
- ½ cup coconut flour
- 2 tablespoons olive oil
- 2 egg, whisked
- Black pepper to the taste
- 1 and ½ pounds pork, ground
- 10 ounces low sodium veggie stock
- ¼ cup tomato sauce, no-salt-added
- ½ teaspoon mustard powder

Directions:
1. Put the flour in a bowl and the egg in another one.
2. Mix the pork with black pepper and a pinch of paprika, shape medium patties out of this mix, dip them in the egg and then dredge in flour.
3. Heat up a pan with the oil over medium-high heat, add the patties and cook them for 5 minutes on each side.
4. In a bowl, combine the stock with tomato sauce and mustard powder and whisk.
5. Add this over the patties, cook for 10 minutes over medium heat, divide everything between plates and serve.
6. Enjoy!

Nutrition: Calories 332, Fat 18, Fiber 4, Carbs 11, Protein 25

767. Pork, Water Chestnuts and Cabbage Salad

Preparation time: 10 minutes
Cooking time: 0 minutes
Servings: 10
Ingredients:
- 1 green cabbage head, shredded
- 1 and ½ cups brown rice, already cooked
- 2 cups pork roast, already cooked and shredded
- 10 ounces peas
- 8 ounces water chestnuts, drained and sliced
- ½ cup low-fat sour cream
- ½ cup avocado mayonnaise
- A pinch of black pepper

Directions:
1. In a bowl, combine the cabbage with the rice, shredded meat, peas, chestnuts, sour cream, mayo and black pepper, toss and serve cold.
2. Enjoy!

Nutrition: Calories 310, Fat 5, Fiber 4, Carbs 11, Protein 17

768. Pork and Zucchini Stew

Preparation time: 10 minutes
Cooking time: 1 hour
Servings: 4
Ingredients:

- 1 pound ground pork, cubed
- Black pepper to the taste
- ¼ teaspoon sweet paprika
- 1 tablespoon olive oil
- 1 and ½ cups low-sodium veggie stock
- 3 cups zucchinis, cubed
- 1 yellow onion, chopped
- ½ cup low-sodium tomato sauce
- 1 tablespoon parsley, chopped

Directions:

1. Heat up a pot with the oil over medium-high heat, add the pork, black pepper and paprika, stir and brown for 5 minutes.
2. Add stock, onion and tomato sauce, toss, bring to a simmer, reduce heat to medium and cook for 40 minutes.
3. Add the zucchinis and the parsley, toss, cook for 15 minutes more, divide into bowls and serve.
4. Enjoy!

Nutrition: Calories 270, Fat 7, Fiber 9, Carbs 12, Protein 17

769. Pork Roast, Leeks and Carrots

Preparation time: 10 minutes
Cooking time: 1 hour and 10 minutes
Servings: 4
Ingredients:

- 2 pounds pork roast, trimmed
- 4 carrots, chopped
- 4 leeks, chopped
- 1 teaspoon black peppercorns
- 2 yellow onions, cut into wedges
- 1 tablespoon parsley, chopped
- 1 cup low-sodium veggie stock
- 1 teaspoon mustard
- Black pepper to the taste

Directions:

1. Put the pork in a roasting pan, add carrots, leeks, peppercorns, onions, stock, mustard and black pepper, toss, cover the pan and bake in the oven at 375 degrees F for 1 hour and 10 minutes.
2. Slice the meat, divide it between plates, sprinkle parsley on top and serve with the carrots and leeks mix on the side.
3. Enjoy!

Nutrition: Calories 260, Fat 5, Fiber 7, Carbs 12, Protein 20

770. Easy Veal Chops

Preparation time: 10 minutes
Cooking time: 20 minutes
Servings: 4
Ingredients:

- 3 tablespoons whole wheat flour
- Black pepper to the taste
- 2 eggs
- 1 tablespoon milk
- 1 and ½ cups whole wheat breadcrumbs
- Zest of 1 lemon, grated
- 4 veal rib chops
- 3 tablespoons olive oil

Directions:

1. Put whole wheat flour in a bowl.
2. In another bowl, mix eggs with milk and whisk.
3. In a third bowl, mix the breadcrumbs with lemon zest.
4. Season veal chops with black pepper, dredge them in flour, dip in the egg mix and then in breadcrumbs.
5. Heat up a pan with the oil over medium-high heat, add veal chops, cook for 2 minutes on each side and transfer to a baking sheet, introduce them in the oven at 350 degrees F, bake for 15 minutes, divide between plates and serve with a side salad.
6. Enjoy!

Nutrition: Calories 270, Fat 6, Fiber 7, Carbs 10, Protein 16

771. Pork with Apple Sauce

Preparation time: 10 minutes
Cooking time: 1 hour and 30 minutes
Servings: 6
Ingredients:

- 1 tablespoon lemon juice
- 2 cups low-sodium veggie stock
- 17 ounces apples, cored and cut into wedges
- 2 pounds pork belly, trimmed and scored
- 1 teaspoons sweet paprika
- Black pepper to the taste
- A drizzle of olive oil

Directions:

1. In your blender, mix the stock with apples and lemon juice and pulse very well.
2. Put pork belly in a roasting pan, add apple sauce, also add the oil, paprika and black pepper, toss well, introduce in the oven and bake at 380 degrees F for 1 hour and 30 minutes.
3. Slice the pork belly, divide it between plates, drizzle the sauce all over and serve.
4. Enjoy!

Nutrition: Calories 356, Fat 14, Fiber 4, Carbs 10, Protein 27

772. Pork with Mushrooms Bowls

Preparation time: 10 minutes
Cooking time: 23 minutes
Servings: 6
Ingredients:

- Juice of 1 lime
- 1 and ½ pounds pork steak, cut into strips
- ½ teaspoon chili powder
- Black pepper to the taste
- 1 teaspoon sweet paprika
- ½ teaspoon oregano, dried

- 2 tablespoons olive oil
- 2 red bell peppers, chopped
- 1 yellow onion, sliced
- 5 ounces mushrooms, chopped
- 1 garlic clove, minced
- 2 green onions, chopped
- 1 jalapeno, chopped
- 1 cup low-sodium veggie stock
- ¼ cup parsley, chopped

Directions:
1. In a bowl, mix lime juice with black pepper, chili powder, paprika, oregano and meat strips and toss well.
2. Heat up a pan with the oil over medium-high heat, add the meat, and cook for 4 minutes on each side and transfer to a plate.
3. Heat up the same pan over medium heat, add bell peppers, mushrooms, garlic and onions, stir and cook for 5 minutes.
4. Add stock, green onion, lime juice, jalapeno, return the meat, stir and cook for 10 minutes more.
5. Divide everything between plates and serve with parsley on top.
6. Enjoy!

Nutrition: Calories 250, Fat 12, Fiber 3, Carbs 7, Protein 14

773. Pork and salsa

Preparation time: 10 minutes
Cooking time: 15 minutes
Servings: 4
Ingredients:
- 8 ounces canned pineapple, crushed
- 1 tablespoon olive oil
- 1 pound pork, ground
- 1 teaspoon chili powder
- 1 teaspoon garlic powder
- 1 teaspoon cumin, ground
- Black pepper to the taste
- 1 mango, chopped
- Juice of 1 lime
- 2 avocados, pitted, peeled and chopped
- ¼ cup cilantro, chopped

Directions:
1. Heat up a pan with the oil over medium heat, add pork meat stir and brown for 5 minutes.
2. Add garlic, cumin, chili powder, pineapple and pepper, stir and cook for 10 minutes.
3. In a bowl, mix mango with avocados, lime juice, cilantro and pepper and stir.
4. Divide the pork and pineapple mix between plates, top with the mango salsa and serve.
5. Enjoy!

Nutrition: Calories 270, Fat 6, Fiber 7, Carbs 12, Protein 22

774. Pork Stew with Shallots

Preparation time: 10 minutes
Cooking time: 15 minutes
Servings: 4
Ingredients:

- 2 shallots, chopped
- 2 tablespoons olive oil
- 4 garlic cloves, minced
- 1 pound pork, ground
- 1 eggplant, cubed
- 14 ounces canned tomatoes, no-salt-added and chopped
- Black pepper to the taste
- ½ cup basil, chopped
- 2 tablespoons low-sodium tomato paste
- ¾ cup coconut cream

Directions:
1. Heat up a pan with half of the oil over medium heat, add garlic and shallots, stir and cook for 5 minutes.
2. Add pork, stir and brown for 4 minutes.
3. Heat up another pan with the rest of the oil over medium heat, add eggplant, stir, cook for 5 minutes and add over the meat.
4. Also add tomatoes, pepper, basil, tomato paste and coconut cream, stir, cook for 1 minute, divide into bowls and serve.
5. Enjoy!

Nutrition: Calories 261, Fat 11, Fiber 1, Carbs 8, Protein 22

775. Pork Chops with Thyme and Apples

Preparation time: 10 minutes
Cooking time: 35 minutes
Servings: 4
Ingredients:
- 1 and ½ cups red onion, cut into wedges
- 2 and ½ teaspoons olive oil
- 2 cups apple, cored and cut into wedges
- Black pepper to the taste
- 2 teaspoons thyme, chopped
- 4 medium pork loin chops, bone-in
- 1 teaspoon cider vinegar
- ½ cup low-sodium chicken stock

Directions:
1. Heat up a pan with 1 teaspoon oil over medium-high heat, add the onions, stir and cook them for 2 minutes.
2. Add apples, stock, vinegar, black pepper and the thyme, toss introduce the pan in the oven at 400 degrees F and bake for 15 minutes.
3. Heat up another pan with the rest of the oil over medium-high heat, add pork, season with pepper and cook for 5 minutes on each side.
4. Add the apples and thyme mix, toss, everything, cook for 5 minutes more, divide between plates and serve.

Nutrition: Calories 240, Fat 7, Fiber 2, Carbs 10, Protein 17

776. Pork and Roasted Tomatoes Mix

Preparation time: 10 minutes
Cooking time: 15 minutes
Servings: 6
Ingredients:
- 1 pound pork meat, ground

- 2 cups zucchinis, chopped
- ½ cup yellow onion, chopped
- Black pepper to the taste
- 15 ounces canned roasted tomatoes, no-salt-added and chopped
- ¾ cup low-fat cheddar cheese, shredded

Directions:
1. Heat up a pan over medium-high heat, add pork, onion, black pepper and zucchini, stir and cook for 7 minutes.
2. Add roasted tomatoes, stir, bring to a boil, cook over medium heat for 8 minutes, divide into bowls, sprinkle cheddar on top and serve.
3. Enjoy!

Nutrition: Calories 270, Fat 5, Fiber 3, Carbs 10, Protein 12

777. Balsamic Chili Roast

Preparation time: 10 minutes
Cooking time: 4 hours
Servings: 6

Ingredients:
- 4 pound pork roast
- 6 garlic cloves, minced
- 1 yellow onion, chopped
- ½ cup balsamic vinegar
- 1 cup low-sodium chicken stock
- 2 tablespoons coconut aminos
- Black pepper to the taste
- A pinch of red chili pepper flakes

Directions:
1. Put the roast in a baking dish, add garlic, onion, vinegar, stock, aminos, black pepper and chili flakes, and cover, introduce in the oven and cook at 325 degrees F for 4 hours.
2. Slice, divide between plates and serve with a side salad.
3. Enjoy!

Nutrition: Calories 265, Fat 7, Fiber 6, Carbs 15, Protein 32

778. Spiced Winter Pork Roast

Preparation time: 10 minutes
Cooking time: 3 hours and 20 minutes
Servings: 6

Ingredients:
- 2 and ½ pounds pork roast
- Black pepper to the taste
- 1 teaspoon chili powder
- ½ teaspoon onion powder
- ¼ teaspoon cumin, ground
- 1 teaspoon cocoa powder

Directions:
1. In a roasting pan, combine the roast with black pepper, chili powder, onion powder, cumin and cocoa, rub, cover the pan, introduce in the oven and bake at 325 degrees F for 3 hours and 20 minutes.
2. Slice, divide between plates and serve with a side salad.
3. Enjoy!

Nutrition: Calories 288, Fat 5, Fiber 6, Carbs 12, Protein 23

779. Creamy Smoky Pork Chops

Preparation time: 10 minutes
Cooking time: 20 minutes
Servings: 4

Ingredients:
- 2 tablespoons olive oil
- 4 pork chops
- 1 tablespoon chili powder
- Black pepper to the taste
- 1 teaspoon sweet paprika
- 1 garlic clove, minced
- 1 cup coconut milk
- 1 teaspoon liquid smoke
- ¼ cup cilantro, chopped
- Juice of 1 lemon

Directions:
1. In a bowl, mix pork chops with pepper, chili powder, paprika and garlic and rub well.
2. Heat up a pan with the oil over medium-high heat, add pork chops and cook for 5 minutes on each side.
3. In a blender, mix coconut milk with liquid smoke, lemon juice and cilantro, blend well, pour over the chops, cook for 10 minutes more, divide everything between plates and serve.
4. Enjoy!

Nutrition: Calories 240, Fat 8, Fiber 6, Carbs 10, Protein 22

780. Pork with Dates Sauce

Preparation time: 10 minutes
Cooking time: 40 minutes
Servings: 6

Ingredients:
- 1 and ½ pounds pork tenderloin
- 2 tablespoons water
- 1/3 cup dates, pitted
- ¼ teaspoon onion powder
- ¼ teaspoon smoked paprika
- 2 tablespoons mustard
- ¼ cup coconut aminos
- Black pepper to the taste

Directions:
1. In your food processor, mix dates with water, coconut aminos, mustard, paprika, pepper and onion powder and blend well.
2. Put pork tenderloin in a roasting pan, add the dates sauce, toss to coat very well, introduce everything in the oven at 400 degrees F, bake for 40 minutes, slice the meat, divide it and the sauce between plates and serve.
3. Enjoy!

Nutrition: Calories 240, Fat 8, Fiber 4, Carbs 13, Protein 24

781. Pork Chops and Apples

Preparation time: 10 minutes
Cooking time: 1 hour
Servings: 4

Ingredients:
- 1 and ½ cups low-sodium chicken stock
- Black pepper to the taste
- 4 pork chops
- 1 yellow onion, chopped
- 1 tablespoon olive oil
- 2 garlic cloves, minced
- 3 apples, cored and sliced
- 1 tablespoon thyme, chopped

Directions:
1. Heat up a pan with the oil over medium-high heat, add pork chops, season with black pepper and cook for 5 minutes on each side.
2. Add onion, garlic, apples, thyme and stock, toss, introduce in the oven and bake at 350 degrees F for 50 minutes.
3. Divide everything between plates and serve.
4. Enjoy!

Nutrition: Calories 340, Fat 12, Fiber 9, Carbs 14, Protein 27

782. Spiced Beef

Preparation Time: 10 minutes
Cooking Time: 80 minutes
Servings: 2
Ingredients:
- 1-pound beef sirloin
- 1 tablespoon five-spice seasoning
- 1 bay leaf
- 2 cups of water
- 1 teaspoon peppercorn

Directions:
1. Rub the meat with five-spice seasoning and put in the saucepan.
2. Add nay leaf, water, and peppercorns.
3. Close the lid and simmer it for 80 minutes on the medium heat.
4. Chop the cooked meat and sprinkle it with hot spiced water from the saucepan.

Nutrition: 213 calories, 34.5g protein, 0.5g carbohydrates, 7.1g fat, 0.2g fiber, 101mg cholesterol, 116mg sodium, 466mg potassium.

783. Tomato Beef

Preparation Time: 10 minutes
Cooking Time: 17 minutes
Servings: 2
Ingredients:
- 2 chuck shoulder steaks
- ¼ cup tomato sauce
- 1 tablespoon olive oil

Directions:
1. Brush the steaks with tomato sauce and olive oil and transfer in the preheated to 390F grill.
2. Grill the meat for 9 minutes.
3. Then flip it on another side and cook for 8 minutes more.

Nutrition: 247 calories, 21.4g protein, 1.7g carbohydrates, 17.1g fat, 0.5g fiber, 70mg cholesterol, 231mg sodium, 101mg potassium.

784. Hoisin Pork

Preparation Time: 10 minutes
Cooking Time: 14 minutes
Servings: 2
Ingredients:
- 1-pound pork loin steaks
- 2 tablespoons hoisin sauce
- 1 tablespoon apple cider vinegar
- 1 teaspoon olive oil

Directions:
1. Rub the pork steaks with hoisin sauce, apple cider vinegar, and olive oil.
2. Then preheat the grill to 395F.
3. Put the pork steak in the grill and cook them for 7 minutes per side.

Nutrition: 263 calories, 39.3g protein, 3.6g carbohydrates, 10.1g fat, 0.2g fiber, 0mg cholesterol, 130mg sodium, 12mg potassium.

785. Sage Beef Loin

Preparation Time: 10 minutes
Cooking Time: 18 minutes
Servings: 2
Ingredients:
- 10 oz. beef loin, strips
- 1 garlic clove, diced
- 2 tablespoons margarine
- 1 teaspoon dried sage

Directions:
1. Toss margarine in the skillet.
2. Add garlic and dried sage and roast them for 2 minutes on low heat.
3. Add beef loin strips and roast them for 15 minutes on medium heat. Stir the meat occasionally.

Nutrition: 363 calories, 38.2g protein, 0.8g carbohydrates, 23.2g fat, 0.2g fiber, 101mg cholesterol, 211mg sodium, 497mg potassium.

786. Beef Chili

Preparation Time: 10 minutes
Cooking Time: 30 minutes
Servings: 2
Ingredients:
- 1 cup lean lean ground beef
- 1 onion, diced
- 1 tablespoon olive oil
- 1 cup crushed tomatoes
- ½ cup red kidney beans, cooked
- ½ cup of water
- 1 teaspoon chili seasonings

Directions:
1. Heat up olive oil in the saucepan and add lean ground beef.
2. Cook it for 7 minutes over the medium heat.
3. Then add chili seasonings and diced onion. Stir the ingredients and cook them for 10 minutes.
4. After this, add water, crushed tomatoes, red kidney beans, and stir the chili well.
5. Close the lid and simmer the meal for 13 minutes.

Nutrition: 220 calories, 18.3g protein, 22g carbohydrates, 6.7g fat, 6.1g fiber, 34mg cholesterol, 177mg sodium, 530mg potassium.

787. Ground Pork and Kale Soup

Preparation time: 10 minutes
Cooking time: 30 minutes
Servings: 4
Ingredients:
- 1 pound pork, ground
- 3 carrots, chopped
- 4 potatoes, chopped
- 1 yellow onion, chopped
- ½ bunch kale, chopped
- 4 garlic cloves, minced
- 2 cups squash, cooked and pureed
- 2 quarts low-sodium veggie stock
- Black pepper to the taste
- 3 teaspoons Italian seasoning

Directions:
1. Heat up a pot over medium-high heat, add pork, stir, and brown for 5 minutes and transfer to a bowl.
2. Heat up the pot again over medium heat, add potatoes, onion, carrots, kale, garlic and pepper, stir and cook for 10 minutes.
3. Return beef, also add stock, squash puree and Italian seasoning, stir, simmer over medium heat for 15 minutes, ladle into bowls and serve.
4. Enjoy!

Nutrition: Calories 270, Fat 12, Fiber 6, Carbs 12, Protein 23

788. Peaches and Kale Steak Salad

Preparation time: 10 minutes
Cooking time: 12 minutes
Servings: 2
Ingredients:
- 2 peaches, chopped
- 3 handfuls kale, chopped
- 8 ounces pork steak, cut into strips
- 1 tablespoon avocado oil
- A drizzle of olive oil
- 1 tablespoon balsamic vinegar

Directions:
1. Heat up a pan with the avocado oil over medium-high heat, add steak strips, cook them for 6 minutes on each side and transfer to a salad bowl.
2. Add peaches, kale, olive oil and vinegar, toss and serve.
3. Enjoy!

Nutrition: Calories 240, Fat 5, Fiber 4, Carbs 8, Protein 15

789. Garlic Pork Meatballs

Preparation Time: 10 minutes
Cooking Time: 28 minutes
Servings: 2

Ingredients:
- 2 pork medallions
- 1 teaspoon minced garlic
- ¼ cup of coconut milk
- 1 tablespoon olive oil
- 1 teaspoon cayenne pepper

Directions:
1. Sprinkle each pork medallion with cayenne pepper.
2. Heat up olive oil in the skillet and add meat.
3. Roast the pork medallions for 3 minutes from each side.
4. After this, add coconut milk and minced garlic. Close the lid and simmer the meat for 20 minutes on low heat.

Nutrition: 284 calories, 25.9g protein, 2.6g carbohydrates, 18.8g fat, 0.9g fiber, 70mg cholesterol, 60mg sodium, 103mg potassium.

790. Fajita Pork Strips

Preparation Time: 10 minutes
Cooking Time: 35 minutes
Servings: 2
Ingredients:
- 16 oz. pork sirloin
- 1 tablespoon Fajita seasonings
- 1 tablespoon canola oil

Directions:
1. Cut the pork sirloin into the strips and sprinkle with fajita seasonings and canola oil.
2. Then transfer the meat in the baking tray in one layer.
3. Bake it for 35 minutes at 365F. Stir the meat every 10 minutes during cooking.

Nutrition: 184 calories, 18.5g protein, 1.3g carbohydrates, 10.8g fat, 0g fiber, 64mg cholesterol, 157mg sodium, 0mg potassium.

791. Pepper Pork Tenderloins

Preparation Time: 15 minutes
Cooking Time: 60 minutes
Servings: 2
Ingredients:
- 8 oz. pork tenderloin
- 1 tablespoon mustard
- 1 teaspoon ground black pepper
- 2 tablespoons olive oil

Directions:
1. Rub the meat with mustard and sprinkle with ground black pepper.
2. Then brush it with olive oil and wrap in the foil.
3. Bake the meat for 60 minutes at 375F.
4. Then discard the foil and slice the tenderloin into servings.

Nutrition: 311 calories, 31.2g protein, 2.6g carbohydrates, 19.6g fat, 1.1g fiber, 83mg cholesterol, 65mg sodium, 529mg potassium.

792. Pork and Veggies Mix

Preparation time: 15 minutes
Cooking time: 1 hour
Servings: 6
Ingredients:

- 4 eggplants, cut into halves lengthwise
- 4 ounces olive oil
- 2 yellow onions, chopped
- 4 ounces pork meat, ground
- 2 green bell peppers, chopped
- 1 pound tomatoes, chopped
- 4 tomato slices
- 2 tablespoons low-sodium tomato paste
- ½ cup parsley, chopped
- 4 garlic cloves, minced
- ½ cup hot water
- Black pepper to the taste

Directions:
1. Heat up a pan with the olive oil over medium-high heat, add eggplant halves, cook for 5 minutes and transfer to a plate.
2. Heat up the same pan over medium-high heat, add onion, stir and cook for 3 minutes.
3. Add bell peppers, pork, tomato paste, pepper, parsley and chopped tomatoes, stir and cook for 7 minutes.
4. Arrange the eggplant halves in a baking tray, divide garlic in each, spoon meat filling and top with a tomato slice.
5. Pour the water over them, cover tray with foil, bake in the oven at 350 degrees F for 40 minutes, divide between plates and serve.
6. Enjoy!

Nutrition: Calories 253, Fat 3, Fiber 2, Carbs 12, Protein 14

793. Pork Chili

Preparation time: 10 minutes
Cooking time: 1 hour and 10 minutes
Servings: 6
Ingredients:
- 1 green bell pepper, chopped
- 1 pound pork, cubed
- 1 yellow onion, chopped
- 4 carrots, chopped
- Black pepper to the taste
- 26 ounces canned tomatoes, no-salt-added and chopped
- 1 teaspoon onion powder
- 1 tablespoon parsley, chopped
- 4 teaspoons chili powder
- 1 teaspoon garlic powder
- 1 teaspoon sweet paprika

Directions:
1. Heat up a pot over medium-high heat, add the meat and brown for 5 minutes.
2. Add bell pepper, carrots, onions, tomatoes, black pepper, onion powder, chili powder, paprika and garlic powder, and toss, bring to a simmer, reduce heat to medium, cover the pot and cook for 1 hour and 5 minutes.
3. Add parsley, toss, divide into bowls and serve.
4. Enjoy!

Nutrition: Calories 284, Fat 6, Fiber 6, Carbs 12, Protein 24

794. Pork and Sweet Potatoes with Chili

Preparation time: 10 minutes
Cooking time: 1 hour and 20 minutes
Servings: 8
Ingredients:
- 2 pounds sweet potatoes, chopped
- A drizzle of olive oil
- 1 yellow onion, chopped
- 2 pounds pork meat, ground
- 1 tablespoon chili powder
- Black pepper to the taste
- 1 teaspoon cumin, ground
- ½ teaspoon garlic powder
- ½ teaspoon oregano, chopped
- ½ teaspoon cinnamon powder
- 1 cup low-sodium veggie stock
- ½ cup cilantro, chopped

Directions:
1. Heat up the a pan with the oil over medium-high heat, add sweet potatoes and onion, stir, cook for 15 minutes and transfer to a bowl.
2. Heat up the pan again over medium-high heat, add pork, stir and brown for 5 minutes.
3. Add black pepper, cumin, garlic powder, oregano, chili powder, and cinnamon, stock, return potatoes and onion, stir and cook for 1 hour over medium heat.
4. Add the cilantro, toss, divide into bowls and serve.
5. Enjoy!

Nutrition: Calories 320, Fat 7, Fiber 6, Carbs 12, Protein 22

795. Pork and Pumpkin Chili

Preparation time: 10 minutes
Cooking time: 1 hour and 30 minutes
Servings: 6
Ingredients:
- 1 green bell pepper, chopped
- 2 cups yellow onion, chopped
- 1 tablespoon olive oil
- 6 garlic cloves, minced
- 28 ounces canned tomatoes, no-salt-added and chopped
- 1 and ½ pounds pork, ground
- 6 ounces low-sodium tomato paste
- 14 ounces pumpkin puree
- 1 cup low-sodium chicken stock
- 2 and ½ teaspoons oregano, dried
- 1 and ½ teaspoon cinnamon, ground
- 1 and ½ tablespoon chili powder
- Black pepper to the taste

Directions:
1. Heat up a pot with the oil over medium-high heat, add bell peppers and onion, stir and cook for 7 minutes.
2. Add garlic and the pork, toss and cook for 10 minutes.
3. Add tomatoes, tomato paste, pumpkin puree, stock, oregano, cinnamon, chili powder and pepper, stir, cover, cook over medium heat for 1 hour and 10 minutes, divide into bowls and serve.
4. Enjoy!

Nutrition: Calories 289, Fat 12, Fiber 8, Carbs 12, Protein 20

796. Spiced Pork Soup

Preparation time: 10 minutes
Cooking time: 1 hour and 30 minutes
Servings: 6
Ingredients:
- 3 carrots, chopped
- 1 pound pork meat, cubed
- 1 tomato, chopped
- 3 mushrooms, sliced
- 6 star anise
- 4 bay leaves
- 5 ginger slices
- 2 tablespoons Sichuan peppercorns
- 1 an ½ tablespoons fennel powder
- 1 teaspoon coriander, ground
- 1 tablespoon cumin powder
- ¼ teaspoon five spice powder
- Black pepper to the taste
- A bunch of scallions, chopped
- 8 cups water
- 1/3 cup coconut aminos

Directions:
1. Put the water in a pot and heat up over medium heat.
2. Add carrots, pork, tomato, mushrooms, star anise, bay leaves, ginger, peppercorns, fennel, coriander, cumin, five spice, black pepper, aminos and scallions, stir, bring to a boil and cook for 1 hour and 30 minutes.
3. Discard star anise, ginger, bay leaves and peppercorns, ladle the soup into bowls and serve.
4. Enjoy!

Nutrition: Calories 250, Fat 2, Fiber 7, Carbs 14, Protein 14

797. Tarragon Pork Steak with Tomatoes

Preparation time: 10 minutes
Cooking time: 22 minutes
Servings: 4
Ingredients:
- 4 medium pork steaks
- Black pepper to the taste
- 1 tablespoon olive oil
- 8 cherry tomatoes, halved
- A handful tarragon, chopped

Directions:
1. Heat up a pan with the oil over medium-high heat, add steaks, season with black pepper, cook them for 6 minutes on each side and divide between plates.
2. Heat up the same pan over medium heat, add the tomatoes and the tarragon, cook for 10 minutes, divide next to the pork and serve.
3. Enjoy!

Nutrition: Calories 263, Fat 4, Fiber 6, Carbs 12, Protein 16

798. Pork Meatballs

Preparation time: 10 minutes
Cooking time: 10 minutes
Servings: 4
Ingredients:
- 1 pound pork, ground
- 1/3 cup cilantro, chopped
- 1 cup red onion, chopped
- 4 garlic cloves, minced
- 1 tablespoon ginger, grated
- 1 Thai chili, chopped
- 2 tablespoons olive oil

Directions:
1. In a bowl, combine the meat with cilantro, onion, garlic, ginger and chili, stir well and shape medium meatballs out of this mix.
2. Heat up a pan with the oil over medium-high heat, add the meatballs, cook them for 5 minutes on each side, divide them between plates and serve with a side salad.
3. Enjoy!

Nutrition: Calories 220, Fat 4, Fiber 2, Carbs 8, Protein 14

799. Pork with Scallions and Peanuts

Preparation time: 10 minutes
Cooking time: 16 minutes
Servings: 4
Ingredients:
- 2 tablespoons lime juice
- 2 tablespoons coconut aminos
- 1 and ½ tablespoons brown sugar
- 5 garlic cloves, minced
- 3 tablespoons olive oil
- Black pepper to the taste
- 1 yellow onion, cut into wedges
- 1 and ½ pound pork tenderloin, cubed
- 3 tablespoons peanuts, chopped
- 2 scallions, chopped

Directions:
1. In a bowl, mix lime juice with aminos and sugar and stir very well.
2. In another bowl, mix garlic with 1 and ½ teaspoon oil and some black pepper and stir.
3. Heat up a pan with the rest of the oil over medium-high heat, add meat, and cook for 3 minutes on each side and transfer to a bowl.
4. Heat up the same pan over medium-high heat, add onion, stir and cook for 3 minutes.
5. Add the garlic mix, return the pork, also add the aminos mix, toss, cook for 6 minutes, divide between plates, sprinkle scallions and peanuts on top and serve.
6. Enjoy!

Nutrition: Calories 273, Fat 4, Fiber 5, Carbs 12, Protein 18

800. Mediterranean Lamb Mix

Preparation time: 10 minutes

Cooking time: 10 minutes
Servings: 4
Ingredients:
- 1 garlic clove, minced
- 2 red chilies, chopped
- 1 cucumber, sliced
- 2 tablespoons balsamic vinegar
- 1 carrot, sliced
- 1 radish, sliced
- ½ cup mint leaves, chopped
- ½ cup coriander leaves, chopped
- Black pepper to the taste
- 2 tablespoons olive oil
- 3 ounces bean sprouts
- 2 lamb fillets

Directions:
1. Put the chilies in a pan, add garlic and vinegar, bring to a boil, stir well and take off heat.
2. In a bowl, mix cucumber with radish, carrot, coriander, mint and sprouts.
3. Heat up your kitchen grill over medium-high heat, brush lamb fillets with the oil, season them with pepper, cook for 3 minutes on each side, slice the meat, add over the veggies, also add the vinegar mix, toss and serve.
4. Enjoy!

Nutrition: Calories 231, Fat 3, Fiber 5, Carbs 7, Protein 17

VEGETABLES

801. Loaded Baked Sweet Potatoes

Preparation time: 15 minutes
Cooking time: 20 minutes
Servings: 4
Ingredients:
6. 4 sweet potatoes
7. ½ cup nonfat or low-fat plain Greek yogurt
8. Freshly ground black pepper
9. 1 teaspoon olive oil
10. 1 red bell pepper, cored and diced
11. ½ red onion, diced
12. 1 teaspoon ground cumin
13. 1 (15-ounce) can chickpeas, drained and rinsed

Directions:
- Prick the potatoes using a fork and cook on your microwave's potato setting until potatoes are soft and cooked through, about 8 to 10 minutes for 4 potatoes. If you don't have a microwave, bake at 400°F for about 45 minutes.
- Combine the yogurt and black pepper in a small bowl and mix well. Heat the oil in a medium pot over medium heat. Add bell pepper, onion, cumin, and additional black pepper to taste.
- Add the chickpeas, stir to combine, and heat through about 5 minutes. Slice the potatoes lengthwise down the middle and top each half with a portion of the bean mixture followed by 1 to 2 tablespoons of the yogurt. Serve immediately.

Nutrition: Calories: 264 Fat: 2g Sodium: 124mg Carbohydrate: 51g Protein: 11g

802. White Beans with Spinach and Pan-Roasted Tomatoes

Preparation time: 15 minutes
Cooking time: 10 minutes
Servings: 2
Ingredients:

6. 1 tablespoon olive oil
7. 4 small plum tomatoes, halved lengthwise
8. 10 ounces frozen spinach, defrosted and squeezed of excess water
9. 2 garlic cloves, thinly sliced
10. 2 tablespoons water
11. ¼ teaspoon freshly ground black pepper
12. 1 can white beans, drained
13. Juice of 1 lemon

Directions:
- Heat-up the oil in a large skillet over medium-high heat. Put the tomatoes, cut-side down, and cook within 3 to 5 minutes; turn and cook within 1 minute more. Transfer to a plate.
- Reduce heat to medium and add the spinach, garlic, water, and pepper to the skillet. Cook, tossing until the spinach is heated through, 2 to 3 minutes.
- Return the tomatoes to the skillet, put the white beans and lemon juice, and toss until heated through 1 to 2 minutes.

Nutrition: Calories: 293 Fat: 9g Sodium: 267mg Carbohydrate: 43g Protein: 15g

803. Black-Eyed Peas and Greens Power Salad

Preparation time: 15 minutes
Cooking time: 6 minutes Servings: 2
Ingredients:
7. 1 tablespoon olive oil
8. 3 cups purple cabbage, chopped
9. 5 cups baby spinach
10. 1 cup shredded carrots
11. 1 can black-eyed peas, drained
12. Juice of ½ lemon
13. Salt
14. Freshly ground black pepper

Directions:
- In a medium pan, add the oil and cabbage and sauté for 1 to 2 minutes on medium heat. Add in your spinach, cover for 3 to 4 minutes on medium heat, until greens are wilted. Remove from the heat and add to a large bowl.

- Add in the carrots, black-eyed peas, and a splash of lemon juice. Season with salt and pepper, if desired. Toss and serve.

Nutrition: Calories: 320 Fat: 9g Sodium: 351mg Potassium: 544mg Carbohydrate: 49g Protein: 16g

804. Butternut-Squash Macaroni and Cheese

Preparation time: 15 minutes
Cooking time: 20 minutes
Servings: 2
Ingredients:
8. 1 cup whole-wheat ziti macaroni
9. 2 cups peeled and cubed butternut squash
10. 1 cup nonfat or low-fat milk, divided
11. Freshly ground black pepper
12. 1 teaspoon Dijon mustard
13. 1 tablespoon olive oil
14. ¼ cup shredded low-fat cheddar cheese

Directions:
- Cook the pasta al dente. Put the butternut squash plus ½ cup milk in a medium saucepan and place over medium-high heat. Season with black pepper. Bring it to a simmer. Lower the heat, then cook until fork-tender, 8 to 10 minutes.
- To a blender, add squash and Dijon mustard. Purée until smooth. Meanwhile, place a large sauté pan over medium heat and add olive oil. Add the squash purée and the remaining ½ cup of milk. Simmer within 5 minutes. Add the cheese and stir to combine.
- Add the pasta to the sauté pan and stir to combine. Serve immediately.

Nutrition: Calories: 373 Fat: 10g Sodium: 193mg Carbohydrate: 59g Protein: 14g

805. Pasta with Tomatoes and Peas

Preparation time: 15 minutes
Cooking time: 15 minutes
Servings: 2
Ingredients:
1. ½ cup whole-grain pasta of choice
2. 8 cups water, plus ¼ for finishing
3. 1 cup frozen peas
4. 1 tablespoon olive oil
5. 1 cup cherry tomatoes, halved
6. ¼ teaspoon freshly ground black pepper
7. 1 teaspoon dried basil
8. ¼ cup grated Parmesan cheese (low-sodium)

Directions:
- Cook the pasta al dente. Add the water to the same pot you used to cook the pasta, and when it's boiling, add the peas. Cook within 5 minutes. Drain and set aside.
- Heat-up the oil in a large skillet over medium heat. Add the cherry tomatoes, put a lid on the skillet and let the tomatoes soften for about 5 minutes, stirring a few times.
- Season with black pepper and basil. Toss in the pasta, peas, and ¼ cup of water, stir and remove from the heat. Serve topped with Parmesan.

Nutrition: Calories: 266 Fat: 12g Sodium: 320mg Carbohydrate: 30g Protein: 13g

806. Quinoa Bowl

Preparation Time: 15 minutes
Cooking Time: 15 minutes
Servings: 4
Ingredients:
- 1 cup quinoa
- 2 cups of water
- 1 cup tomatoes, diced
- 1 cup sweet pepper, diced
- ½ cup of rice, cooked
- 1 tablespoon lemon juice
- ½ teaspoon lemon zest, grated
- 1 tablespoon olive oil

Directions:
1. Mix up water and quinoa and cook it for 15 minutes. Then remove it from the heat and leave to rest for 10 minutes.
2. Transfer the cooked quinoa in the big bowl.
3. Add tomatoes, sweet pepper, rice, lemon juice, lemon zest, and olive oil.
4. Stir the mixture well and transfer in the serving bowls.

Nutrition: Calories 290; Protein 8.4g; Carbohydrates 49.9g; Fat 6.4g; Fiber 4.3g; Cholesterol 0mg; Sodium 11mg; Potassium 435mg

807. Vegan Meatloaf

Preparation Time: 10 minutes
Cooking Time: 30 minutes
Servings: 6
Ingredients:
- 1 cup chickpeas, cooked
- 1 onion, diced
- 1 tablespoon ground flax seeds
- ½ teaspoon chili flakes
- 1 tablespoon coconut oil
- ½ cup carrot, diced
- ½ cup celery stalk, chopped
- 1 tablespoon tomato paste

Directions:
1. Heat up coconut oil in the saucepan.
2. Add carrot, onion, and celery stalk. Cook the vegetables for 8 minutes or until they are soft.
3. Then add chickpeas, chili flakes, and ground flax seeds.
4. Blend the mixture until smooth with the help of the immersion blender.
5. Then line the loaf mold with baking paper and transfer the blended mixture inside.
6. Flatten it well and spread with tomato paste.
7. Bake the meatloaf in the preheated to 365F oven for 20 minutes.

Nutrition: Calories 162; Protein 7.1g; Carbohydrates 23.9g; Fat 4.7g; Fiber 7g; Cholesterol 0mg; Sodium 25mg; Potassium 407mg

808. Red Beans and Rice

Preparation time: 15 minutes
Cooking time: 45 minutes
Servings: 2
Ingredients:

- ½ cup dry brown rice
- 1 cup water, plus ¼ cup
- 1 can red beans, drained
- 1 tablespoon ground cumin
- Juice of 1 lime
- 4 handfuls of fresh spinach
- Optional toppings: avocado, chopped tomatoes, Greek yogurt, onions

Directions:

1. Mix rice plus water in a pot and bring to a boil. Cover and reduce heat to a low simmer. Cook within 30 to 40 minutes or according to package directions.
2. Meanwhile, add the beans, ¼ cup of water, cumin, and lime juice to a medium skillet. Simmer within 5 to 7 minutes.
3. Once the liquid is mostly gone, remove from the heat and add the spinach. Cover and let spinach wilt slightly, 2 to 3 minutes. Mix in with the beans. Serve beans with rice. Add toppings, if using.

Nutrition: Calories: 232 Fat: 2g Sodium: 210mg Carbohydrate: 41g Protein: 13g

809. Hearty Lentil Soup

Preparation time: 15 minutes
Cooking time: 30 minutes
Servings: 4
Ingredients:

- 1 tablespoon olive oil
- 2 carrots, peeled and chopped
- 2 celery stalks, diced
- 1 onion, chopped
- 1 teaspoon dried thyme
- ½ teaspoon garlic powder
- Freshly ground black pepper
- 1 (28-ounce) can no-salt diced tomatoes, drained
- 1 cup dry lentils
- 5 cups of water
- Salt

Directions:

1. Heat-up the oil in a large Dutch oven or pot over medium heat. Once the oil is simmering, add the carrot, celery, and onion. Cook, often stirring within 5 minutes.
2. Add the thyme, garlic powder, and black pepper. Cook within 30 seconds. Pour in the drained diced tomatoes and cook for a few more minutes, often stirring to enhance their flavor.
3. Put the lentils, water, plus a pinch of salt. Raise the heat and bring to a boil, then partially cover the pot and reduce heat to maintain a gentle simmer.
4. Cook within 30 minutes, or until lentils are tender but still hold their shape. Ladle into serving bowls and serve with a fresh green salad and whole-grain bread.

Nutrition: Calories: 168 Fat: 4g Sodium: 130mg Carbohydrate: 35g Protein: 10g

810. Black-Bean Soup

Preparation time: 15 minutes
Cooking time: 20 minutes
Servings: 4
Ingredients:

- 1 yellow onion
- 1 tablespoon olive oil
- 2 cans black beans, drained
- 1 cup diced fresh tomatoes
- 5 cups low-sodium vegetable broth
- ¼ teaspoon freshly ground black pepper
- ¼ cup chopped fresh cilantro

Directions:

1. Cook or sauté the onion in the olive oil within 4 to 5 minutes in a large saucepan over medium heat. Put the black beans, tomatoes, vegetable broth, and black pepper. Boil, then adjust heat to simmer within 15 minutes.
2. Remove, then working in batches, ladle the soup into a blender and process until somewhat smooth. Put it back to the pot, add the cilantro, and heat until warmed through. Serve immediately.

Nutrition: Calories: 234 Fat: 5g Sodium: 363mg Carbohydrate: 37g Protein: 11g

811. Paella

Preparation Time: 10 minutes
Cooking Time: 25 minutes
Servings: 6
Ingredients:

- 1 teaspoon dried saffron
- 1 cup short-grain rice
- 1 tablespoon olive oil
- 2 cups of water
- 1 teaspoon chili flakes
- 6 oz. artichoke hearts, chopped
- ½ cup green peas
- 1 onion, sliced
- 1 cup bell pepper, sliced

Directions:

9. Pour water in the saucepan. Add rice and cook it for 15 minutes.
10. Meanwhile, heat up olive oil in the skillet.
11. Add dried saffron, chili flakes, onion, and bell pepper.
12. Roast the vegetables for 5 minutes.
13. Add them to the cooked rice.
14. Then add artichoke hearts and green peas. Stir the paella well and cook it for 10 minutes over the low heat.

Nutrition: Calories 170; Protein 4.2g; Carbohydrates 32.7g; Fat 2.7g; Fiber 3.2g; Cholesterol 0mg; Sodium 33mg; Potassium 237mg

812. Mushroom Cakes

Preparation Time: 15 minutes
Cooking Time: 10 minutes
Servings: 4
Ingredients:

- 2 cups mushrooms, chopped
- 3 garlic cloves, chopped

- 1 tablespoon dried dill
- 1 egg, beaten
- ¼ cup of rice, cooked
- 1 tablespoon sesame oil
- 1 teaspoon chili powder

Directions:
1. Grind the mushrooms in the food processor.
2. Add garlic, dill, egg, rice, and chili powder.
3. Blend the mixture for 10 seconds.
4. After this, heat up sesame oil for 1 minute.
5. Make the medium size mushroom cakes and put in the hot sesame oil.
6. Cook the mushroom cakes for 5 minutes per side on the medium heat.

Nutrition: Calories 103; Protein 3.7g; Carbohydrates 12g; Fat 4.8g; Fiber 0.9g; Cholesterol 41mg; Sodium 27mg; Potassium 187mg

813. Glazed Eggplant Rings

Preparation Time: 10 minutes
Cooking Time: 10 minutes
Servings: 4
Ingredients:
- 3 eggplants, sliced
- 1 tablespoon liquid honey
- 1 teaspoon minced ginger
- 2 tablespoons lemon juice
- 3 tablespoons avocado oil
- ½ teaspoon ground coriander
- 3 tablespoons water

Directions:
1. Rub the eggplants with ground coriander.
2. Then heat up the avocado oil in the skillet for 1 minute.
3. When the oil is hot, add the sliced eggplant and arrange it in one layer.
4. Cook the vegetables for 1 minute per side.
5. Transfer the eggplant in the bowl.
6. Then add minced ginger, liquid honey, lemon juice, and water in the skillet.
7. Bring it to boil and add cooked eggplants.
8. Coat the vegetables in the sweet liquid well and cook for 2 minutes more.

Nutrition: Calories 136; Protein 4.3g; Carbohydrates 29.6g; Fat 2.2g; Fiber 15.1g; Cholesterol 0mg; Sodium 11mg; Potassium 993mg

814. Sweet Potato Balls

Preparation Time: 15 minutes
Cooking Time: 10 minutes
Servings: 4
Ingredients:
- 1 cup sweet potato, mashed, cooked
- 1 tablespoon fresh cilantro, chopped
- 1 egg, beaten
- 3 tablespoons ground oatmeal
- 1 teaspoon ground paprika
- ½ teaspoon ground turmeric
- 2 tablespoons coconut oil

Directions:

1. In the bowl mix up mashed sweet potato, fresh cilantro, egg, ground oatmeal, paprika, and turmeric.
2. Stir the mixture until smooth and make the small balls.
3. Heat up the coconut oil in the saucepan.
4. When the coconut oil is hot, add the sweet potato balls.
5. Cook them until golden brown.

Nutrition: Calories 133; Protein 2.8g; Carbohydrates 13.1g; Fat 8.2g; Fiber 2.2g; Cholesterol 41mg; Sodium 44mg; Potassium 283mg

815. Chickpea Curry

Preparation Time: 10 minutes
Cooking Time: 10 minutes
Servings: 4
Ingredients:
- 1 ½ cup chickpeas, boiled
- 1 teaspoon curry powder
- ½ teaspoon garam masala
- 1 cup spinach, chopped
- 1 teaspoon coconut oil
- ¼ cup of soy milk
- 1 tablespoon tomato paste
- ½ cup of water

Directions:
1. Heat up coconut oil in the saucepan.
2. Add curry powder, garam masala, tomato paste, and soy milk.
3. Whisk the mixture until smooth and bring it to boil.
4. Add water, spinach, and chickpeas.
5. Stir the meal and close the lid.
6. Cook it for 5 minutes over the medium heat.

Nutrition: Calories 298; Protein 15.4g; Carbohydrates 47.8g; Fat 6.1g; Fiber 13.6g; Cholesterol 0mg; Sodium 37mg; Potassium 765mg

816. Tofu Turkey

Preparation Time: 15 minutes
Cooking Time: 75 minutes
Servings: 6
Ingredients:
- 1 onion, diced
- 1 cup mushrooms, chopped
- 1 bell pepper, chopped
- 12 oz. firm tofu, crumbled
- 1 teaspoon dried rosemary
- 1 tablespoon avocado oil
- ½ cup marinara sauce
- 1 teaspoon miso paste

Directions:
1. Sauté onion, mushrooms, bell pepper, rosemary, miso paste, and avocado oil in the saucepan until the ingredients are cooked (appx.10-15 minutes).
2. Then put ½ part of tofu in the round baking pan. Press well and make the medium whole in the center.
3. Put the mushroom mixture in the tofu whole and top it with marinara sauce.
4. Add remaining tofu and press it well. Cover the meal with foil.
5. Bake the tofu turkey for 60 minutes at 395F.

Nutrition: Calories 80; Protein 5.9g; Carbohydrates 7.9g; Fat 3.4; Fiber 2.1g; Cholesterol 0mg; Sodium 130mg Potassium 262mg

817. Cauliflower Tots

Preparation Time: 15 minutes
Cooking Time: 20 minutes
Servings: 4
Ingredients:
- 1 cup cauliflower, shredded
- 3 oz. vegan Parmesan, grated
- 1/3 cup flax seeds meal
- 1 egg, beaten
- 1 teaspoon Italian seasonings
- 1 teaspoon olive oil

Directions:
1. In the bowl mix up shredded cauliflower, vegan Parmesan, flax seeds meal, egg, and Italian seasonings.
2. Knead the cauliflower mixture. Add water if needed.
3. After this, make the cauliflower tots from the mixture.
4. Line the baking tray with baking paper and place the cauliflower tots inside.
5. Sprinkle them with the olive oil and transfer in the preheated to 375F oven.
6. Bake the meal for 15-20 minutes or until golden brown.

Nutrition: Calories 109; Protein 6.1g; Carbohydrates 6.3g; Fat 6.6g; Fiber 3.7g; Cholesterol 42mg Sodium 72mg Potassium 158mg

818. Aromatic Whole Grain Spaghetti

Preparation Time: 5 minutes
Cooking Time: 10 minutes
Servings: 2
Ingredients:
- 1 teaspoon dried basil
- ¼ cup of soy milk
- 6 oz. whole-grain spaghetti
- 2 cups of water
- 1 teaspoon ground nutmeg

Directions:
1. Bring the water to boil, add spaghetti and cook them for 8-10 minutes.
2. Meanwhile, bring the soy milk to boil.
3. Drain the cooked spaghetti and mix them up with soy milk, ground nutmeg, and dried basil.
4. Stir the meal well.

Nutrition: Calories 128; Protein 5.6g; Carbohydrates 25g; Fat 1.4g; Fiber 4.3g; Cholesterol 0mg; Sodium 25mg; Potassium 81mg

819. Chunky Tomatoes

Preparation Time: 5 minutes
Cooking Time: 15 minutes
Servings: 3
Ingredients:
- 2 cups plum tomatoes, roughly chopped
- ½ cup onion, diced

- ½ teaspoon garlic, diced
- 1 teaspoon Italian seasonings
- 1 teaspoon canola oil
- 1 chili pepper, chopped

Directions:
1. Heat up canola oil in the saucepan.
2. Add chili pepper and onion. Cook the vegetables for 5 minutes. Stir them from time to time.
3. After this, add tomatoes, garlic, and Italian seasonings.
4. Close the lid and sauté the meal for 10 minutes.

Nutrition: Calories 550; Protein 1.7g; Carbohydrates 8.4g; Fat 2.3g; Fiber 1.8g; Cholesterol 1mg; Sodium 17mg; Potassium 279mg

820. Baked Falafel

Preparation Time: 10 minutes
Cooking Time: 25 minutes
Servings: 6
Ingredients:
- 2 cups chickpeas, cooked
- 1 yellow onion, diced
- 3 tablespoons olive oil
- 1 cup fresh parsley, chopped
- 1 teaspoon ground cumin
- ½ teaspoon coriander
- 2 garlic cloves, diced

Directions:
1. Put all ingredients in the food processor and blend until smooth.
2. Preheat the oven to 375F.
3. Then line the baking tray with the baking paper.
4. Make the balls from the chickpeas mixture and press them gently in the shape of the falafel.
5. Put the falafel in the tray and bake in the oven for 25 minutes.

Nutrition: Calories 316; Protein 13.5g; Carbohydrates 43.3g; Fat 11.2g; Fiber 12.4g; Cholesterol 0mg; Sodium 23mg; Potassium 676mg

821. Stuffed Portobello

Preparation Time: 10 minutes
Cooking Time: 20 minutes
Servings: 2
Ingredients:
- 4 Portobello mushroom caps
- ½ zucchini, grated
- 1 tomato, diced
- 1 teaspoon olive oil
- ½ teaspoon dried parsley
- ¼ teaspoon minced garlic

Directions:
1. In the mixing bowl, mix up diced tomato, grated zucchini, dried parsley, and minced garlic.
2. Then fill the mushroom caps with zucchini mixture and transfer in the lined with baking paper tray.
3. Bake the vegetables for 20 minutes or until they are soft.

Nutrition: 24 calories, 1.2g protein, 2.9g carbohydrates, 1.3g fat, 0.9g fiber, 0mg cholesterol, 5mg sodium, 238mg potassium.

822. Chile Relents

Preparation Time: 10 minutes
Cooking Time: 30 minutes
Servings: 2
Ingredients:

- 2 chili peppers
- 2 oz. vegan Mozzarella cheese, shredded
- 2 oz. tomato puree
- 1 tablespoon coconut oil
- 2 tablespoons whole-grain wheat flour
- 1 tablespoon potato starch
- ¼ cup of water
- ½ teaspoon chili flakes

Directions:
1. Bake the chili peppers for 15 minutes in the preheated to 375F oven.
2. Meanwhile, pour tomato puree in the saucepan.
3. Add chili flakes and bring the mixture to boil. Remove it from the heat.
4. After this, mix up potato starch, flour, and water.
5. When the chili peppers are cooked, make the cuts in them and remove the seeds.
6. Then fill the peppers with shredded cheese and secure the cuts with toothpicks.
7. Heat up coconut oil in the skillet.
8. Dip the chili peppers in the flour mixture and roast in the coconut oil until they are golden brown.
9. Sprinkle the cooked chilies with tomato puree mixture.

Nutrition: 187 calories, 4.2g protein, 16g carbohydrates, 12g fat, 3.7g fiber, 0mg cholesterol, 122mg sodium, 41mg potassium.

823. Carrot Cakes

Preparation Time: 10 minutes
Cooking Time: 10 minutes
Servings: 4
Ingredients:

- 1 cup carrot, grated
- 1 tablespoon semolina
- 1 egg, beaten
- 1 teaspoon Italian seasonings
- 1 tablespoon sesame oil

Directions:
7. In the mixing bowl, mix up grated carrot, semolina, egg, and Italian seasonings.
8. Heat up sesame oil in the skillet.
9. Make the carrot cakes with the help of 2 spoons and put in the skillet.
10. Roast the cakes for 4 minutes per side.

Nutrition: Calories 70; Protein 1.9g; Carbohydrates 4.8g; Fat 4.9g; Fiber 0.8g; Cholesterol 42mg; Sodium 35mg Potassium 108mg

824. Vegan Chili

Preparation Time: 10 minutes
Cooking Time: 25 minutes
Servings: 4
Ingredients:

- ½ cup bulgur
- 1 cup tomatoes, chopped
- 1 chili pepper, chopped
- 1 cup red kidney beans, cooked
- 2 cups low-sodium chicken broth
- 1 teaspoon tomato paste
- ½ cup celery stalk, chopped

Directions:
6. Put all ingredients in the big saucepan and stir well.
7. Close the lid and simmer the chili for 25 minutes over the medium-low heat.

Nutrition: Calories 234; Protein 14.1g; Carbohydrates 44.4g; Fat 0.9g; Fiber 1g; Cholesterol 0mg Sodium 57mg; Potassium 52mg

825. Spinach Casserole

Preparation Time: 5 minutes
Cooking Time: 30 minutes
Servings: 3
Ingredients:

- 2 cups spinach, chopped
- 4 oz. artichoke hearts, chopped
- ¼ cup low-fat yogurt
- 1 teaspoon Italian seasonings
- 2 oz. vegan mozzarella, shredded

Directions:
8. Mix up all ingredients in the casserole mold and cover it with foil.
9. Then transfer it in the preheated to 365F oven and bake it for 30 minutes.

Nutrition: Calories 102; Protein 3.7g; Carbohydrates 11g; Fat 4.9g; Fiber 2.5g; Cholesterol 2mg;Sodium 206mg Potassium 300mg

826. Mac Stuffed Sweet Potatoes

Preparation Time: 20 minutes
Cooking Time: 25 minutes
Servings: 2
Ingredients:

- 1 sweet potato
- ¼ cup whole-grain penne pasta
- 1 teaspoon tomato paste
- 1 teaspoon olive oil
- ¼ teaspoon minced garlic
- 1 tablespoon soy milk

Directions:
1. Cut the sweet potato in half and pierce it 3-4 times with the help of the fork.
2. Sprinkle the sweet potato halves with olive oil and bake in the preheated to 375F oven for 25-30 minutes or until the vegetables are tender.
3. Meanwhile, mix up penne pasta, tomato paste, minced garlic, and soy milk.
4. When the sweet potatoes are cooked, scoop out the vegetable meat and mix it up with a penne pasta mixture.
5. Fill the sweet potatoes with the pasta mixture.

Nutrition: 105 calories, 2.7g protein, 17.8g carbohydrates, 2.8g fat, 3g fiber,0mg cholesterol, 28mg sodium, 308mg potassium.

827. Tofu Tikka Masala

Preparation Time: 10 minutes
Cooking Time: 25 minutes
Servings: 2
Ingredients:
- 8 oz. tofu, chopped
- ½ cup of soy milk
- 1 teaspoon garam masala
- 1 teaspoon olive oil
- 1 teaspoon ground paprika
- ½ cup tomatoes, chopped
- ½ onion, diced

Directions:
1. Heat up olive oil in the saucepan.
2. Add diced onion and cook it until light brown.
3. Then add tomatoes, ground paprika, and garam masala. Bring the mixture to boil.
4. Add soy milk and stir well. Simmer it for 5 minutes.
5. Then add chopped tofu and cook the meal for 3 minutes.
6. Leave the cooked meal for 10 minutes to rest.

Nutrition: 155 calories, 12.2g protein, 20.7g carbohydrates, 8.4g fat, 2.9g fiber, 0mg cholesterol, 51mg sodium, 412mg potassium.

828. Tofu Parmigiana

Preparation Time: 15 minutes
Cooking Time: 8 minutes
Servings: 2
Ingredients:
- 6 oz. firm tofu, roughly sliced
- 1 teaspoon coconut oil
- 1 teaspoon tomato sauce
- ½ teaspoon Italian seasonings

Directions:
1. In the mixing bowl, mix up, tomato sauce, and Italian seasonings.
2. Then brush the sliced tofu with the tomato mixture well and leave for 10 minutes to marinate.
3. Heat up coconut oil.
4. Then put the sliced tofu in the hot oil and roast it for 3 minutes per side or until tofu is golden brown.

Nutrition: 83 calories, 7g protein, 1.7g carbohydrates, 6.2g fat, 0.8 fiber, 1mg cholesterol, 24mg sodium, 135mg potassium.

829. Mushroom Stroganoff

Preparation Time: 10 minutes
Cooking Time: 20 minutes
Servings: 2
Ingredients:
- 2 cups mushrooms, sliced
- 1 teaspoon whole-grain wheat flour
- 1 tablespoon coconut oil
- 1 onion, chopped
- 1 teaspoon dried thyme
- 1 garlic clove, diced
- 1 teaspoon ground black pepper
- ½ cup of soy milk

Directions:
1. Heat up coconut oil in the saucepan.
2. Add mushrooms and onion and cook them for 10 minutes. Stir the vegetables from time to time.
3. After this, sprinkle them with ground black pepper, thyme, and garlic.
4. Add soy milk and bring the mixture to boil.
5. Then add flour and stir it well until homogenous.
6. Cook the mushroom stroganoff until it thickens.

Nutrition: 70 calories, 2.6g protein, 6.9g carbohydrates, 4.1g fat, 1.5g fiber, 0mg cholesterol, 19mg sodium, 202mg potassium.

830. Eggplant Croquettes

Preparation Time: 15 minutes
Cooking Time: 5 minutes
Servings: 2
Ingredients:
- 1 eggplant, peeled, boiled
- 2 potatoes, mashed
- 2 tablespoons almond meal
- 1 teaspoon chili pepper
- 1 tablespoon coconut oil
- 1 tablespoon olive oil
- ¼ teaspoon ground nutmeg

Directions:
1. Blend the eggplant until smooth.
2. Then mix it up with mashed potato, chili pepper, coconut oil, and ground nutmeg.
3. Make the croquettes from the eggplant mixture.
4. Heat up olive oil in the skillet.
5. Put the croquettes in the hot oil and cook them for 2 minutes per side or until they are light brown.

Nutrition: 180 calories, 3.6g protein, 24.3g carbohydrates, 8.8g fat, 7.1g fiber, 0mg cholesterol, 9mg sodium, 721mg potassium.

831. Baked Eggs in Avocado

Preparation time: 15 minutes
Cooking time: 15 minutes
Servings: 2
Ingredients:
- 2 avocados
- Juice of 2 limes
- Freshly ground black pepper
- 4 eggs
- 2 (8-inch) whole-wheat or corn tortillas, warmed
- Optional for serving: halved cherry tomatoes and chopped cilantro

Directions:
1. Adjust the oven rack to the middle position and preheat the oven to 450°F. Scrape out the center of halved avocado using a spoon about 1½ tablespoons.
2. Press lime juice over the avocados and season with black pepper to taste, and then place it on a baking sheet. Crack an egg into the avocado.
3. Bake within 10 to 15 minutes. Remove from oven and garnish with optional cilantro and cherry tomatoes and serve with warm tortillas.

Nutrition: Calories: 534 Fat: 39g Sodium: 462mg Potassium: 1,095mg Carbohydrate: 30g Fiber: 20g Sugars: 3g Protein: 23g

832. Vegetarian Lasagna

Preparation Time: 10 minutes
Cooking Time: 30 minutes
Servings: 6
Ingredients:

- 1 cup carrot, diced
- ½ cup bell pepper, diced
- 1 cup spinach, chopped
- 1 tablespoon olive oil
- 1 teaspoon chili powder
- 1 cup tomatoes, chopped
- 4 oz. low-fat cottage cheese
- 1 eggplant, sliced
- 1 cup low-sodium chicken broth

Directions:
1. Put carrot, bell pepper, and spinach in the saucepan.
2. Add olive oil and chili powder and stir the vegetables well. Cook them for 5 minutes.
3. After this, make the layer of sliced eggplants in the casserole mold and top it with vegetable mixture.
4. Add tomatoes and cottage cheese.
5. Bake the lasagna for 30 minutes at 375F.

Nutrition: Calories 77; Protein 4.4g; Carbohydrates 9.5g; Fat 3g; Fiber 3.9g; Cholesterol 2mg; Sodium 113mg; Potassium 377mg

833. Lentil Quiche

Preparation Time: 15 minutes
Cooking Time: 35 minutes
Servings: 2
Ingredients:

- 1 cup green lentils, boiled
- ½ cup carrot, grated
- 1 onion, diced
- 1 tablespoon olive oil
- ¼ cup flax seeds meal
- 1 teaspoon ground black pepper
- ¼ cup of soy milk

Directions:
1. Cook the onion with olive oil in the skillet until light brown.
2. Then mix up cooked onion, lentils, and carrot.
3. Add flax seeds meal, ground black pepper, and soy milk. Stir the mixture until homogenous.
4. After this, transfer it in the baking pan and flatten ell.
5. Bake the quiche for 35 minutes at 375F.

Nutrition: 351 calories, 17.1g protein, 41.6g carbohydrates, 13.1g fat, 23.3g fiber, 0mg cholesterol, 29mg sodium, 567mg potassium

834. Corn Patties

Preparation Time: 15 minutes
Cooking Time: 10 minutes
Servings: 1
Ingredients:

- ½ cup chickpeas, cooked
- 1 cup corn kernels, cooked
- 1 tablespoon fresh parsley, chopped
- 1 teaspoon chili powder

- ½ teaspoon ground coriander
- 1 tablespoon tomato paste
- 1 tablespoon almond meal
- 1 tablespoon olive oil

Directions:
1. Mash the cooked chickpeas and combine them with corn kernels, parsley, chili powder, ground coriander, tomato paste, and almond meal.
2. Stir the mixture until homogenous.
3. Make the small patties.
4. After this, heat up olive oil in the skillet.
5. Put the prepared patties in the hot oil and cook them for 3 minutes per side or until they are golden brown.
6. Dry the cooked patties with the help of the paper towel if needed.

Nutrition: 168 calories, 6.7g protein, 23.9g carbohydrates, 6.3g fat, 6g fiber, 0mg cholesterol, 23mg sodium, 392mg potassium.

835. Tofu Stir Fry

Preparation Time: 15 minutes
Cooking Time: 10 minutes
Servings: 2
Ingredients:

- 9 oz. firm tofu, cubed
- 3 tablespoons low-sodium soy sauce
- 1 teaspoon sesame seeds
- 1 tablespoon sesame oil
- 1 cup spinach, chopped
- ¼ cup of water

Directions:
1. In the mixing bowl mix up soy sauce, and sesame oil.
2. Dip the tofu cubes in the soy sauce mixture and leave for 10 minutes to marinate.
3. Heat up a skillet and put the tofu cubes inside. Roast them for 1.5 minutes from each side.
4. Then add water, remaining soy sauce mixture, and chopped spinach.
5. Close the lid and cook the meal for 5 minutes more.

Nutrition: 118 calories, 8.5g protein, 3.1g carbohydrates, 8.6g fat, 1.1g fiber, 0mg cholesterol, 406mg sodium, 193mg potassium.

836. Greek Flatbread with Spinach, Tomatoes & Feta

Preparation time: 15 minutes
Cooking time: 9 minutes
Servings: 2
Ingredients:

- 2 cups fresh baby spinach, coarsely chopped
- 2 teaspoons olive oil
- 2 slices Naan, or another flatbread
- ¼ cup sliced black olives
- 2 plum tomatoes, thinly sliced
- 1 teaspoon salt-free Italian seasoning blend
- ¼ cup crumbled feta

Directions:
1. Preheat the oven to 400°F. Heat 3 tablespoons of water in a small skillet over medium heat. Add the spinach,

cover, and steam until wilted, about 2 minutes. Drain off any excess water, then put aside.
2. Drizzle the oil evenly onto both flatbreads. Top each evenly with the spinach, olives, tomatoes, seasoning, and feta. Bake the flatbreads within 5 to 7 minutes, or until lightly browned. Cut each into four pieces and serve hot.

Nutrition: Calories: 411 Fat: 15g Carbohydrates: 53g Fiber: 7g Protein: 15g Sodium: 621mg Potassium: 522mg

837. Mushroom Risotto with Peas

Preparation time: 15 minutes
Cooking time: 20 minutes
Servings: 2
Ingredients:
- 2 cups low-sodium vegetable or chicken broth
- 1 teaspoon olive oil
- 8 ounces baby portobello mushrooms, thinly sliced
- ½ cup frozen peas
- 1 teaspoon butter
- 1 cup Arborio rice
- 1 tablespoon grated Parmesan cheese

Directions:
1. Pour the broth into a microwave-proof glass measuring cup. Microwave on high for 1½ minutes or until hot. Warm-up oil over medium heat in a large saucepan. Add the mushrooms and stir for 1 minute. Cover and cook until soft, about 3 more minutes. Stir in the peas and reduce the heat to low.
2. Put the mushroom batter to the saucepan's sides and add the butter to the middle, heating until melted. Put the rice in the saucepan and stir for 1 to 2 minutes to lightly toast. Add the hot broth, ½ cup at a time, and stir gently.
3. As the broth is cooked into the rice, continue adding more broth, ½ cup at a time, stirring after each addition, until all broth is added. Once all of the liquid is absorbed (this should take 15 minutes), remove from the heat. Serve immediately, topped with Parmesan cheese.

Nutrition: Calories: 430 Fat: 6g Carbohydrates: 83g Fiber: 5g Protein: 10g Sodium: 78mg Potassium: 558mg

838. Loaded Tofu Burrito with Black Beans

Preparation time: 15 minutes
Cooking time: 20 minutes
Servings: 2
Ingredients:
- 4 ounces extra-firm tofu, pressed and cut into 2-inch cubes
- 2 teaspoons mesquite salt-free seasoning, divided
- 2 teaspoons canola oil
- 1 cup thinly sliced bell peppers
- ½ cup diced onions
- 2/3 cup of black beans, drained
- 2 (10-inch) whole-wheat tortillas
- 1 tablespoon sriracha
- Nonfat Greek yogurt, for serving

Directions:

1. Put the tofu and 1 teaspoon of seasoning in a medium zip-top plastic freezer bag and toss until the tofu is well coated.
2. Heat-up the oil in a medium skillet over medium-high heat. Put the tofu in the skillet. Don't stir; allow the tofu to brown before turning. When lightly browned, about 6 minutes, transfer the tofu from the skillet to a small bowl and set aside.
3. Put the peppers plus onions in the skillet and sauté until tender, about 5 minutes. Lower the heat to medium-low, then put the beans and the remaining seasoning. Cook within 5 minutes.
4. For the burritos, lay each tortilla flat on a work surface. Place half of the tofu in the center of each tortilla, top with half of the pepper-bean mixture, and drizzle with the sriracha.
5. Fold the bottom portion of each tortilla up and over the tofu mixture. Then fold each side into the middle, tuck in, and tightly roll it up toward the open end. Serve with a dollop of yogurt.

Nutrition: Calories: 327 Fat: 12g Carbohydrates: 41g Fiber: 11g Protein: 16g Sodium: 282mg

839. Southwest Tofu Scramble

Preparation time: 15 minutes
Cooking time: 15 minutes
Servings: 1
Ingredients:
- ½ tablespoon olive oil
- ½ red onion, chopped
- 2 cups chopped spinach
- 8 ounces firm tofu, drained well
- 1 teaspoon ground cumin
- ½ teaspoon garlic powder
- Optional for serving: sliced avocado or sliced tomatoes

Directions:
1. Heat-up the olive oil in a medium skillet over medium heat. Put the onion and cook within 5 minutes. Add the spinach and cover to steam for 2 minutes.
2. Using a spatula, move the veggies to one side of the pan. Crumble the tofu into the open area in the pan, breaking it up with a fork. Add the cumin and garlic to the crumbled tofu and mix well. Sauté for 5 to 7 minutes until the tofu is slightly browned.
3. Serve immediately with whole-grain bread, fruit, or beans. Top with optional sliced avocado and tomato, if using.

Nutrition: Calories: 267 Fat: 17g Sodium: 75mg Carbohydrate: 13g Protein: 23g

840. Black-Bean and Vegetable Burrito

Preparation time: 15 minutes
Cooking time: 15 minutes
Servings: 4
Ingredients:
- ½ tablespoon olive oil
- 2 red or green bell peppers, chopped

- 1 zucchini or summer squash, diced
- ½ teaspoon chili powder
- 1 teaspoon cumin
- Freshly ground black pepper
- 2cans black beans drained and rinsed
- 1 cup cherry tomatoes, halved
- 4 (8-inch) whole-wheat tortillas
- Optional for serving: spinach, sliced avocado, chopped scallions, or hot sauce

Directions:
1. Heat-up the oil in a large sauté pan over medium heat. Add the bell peppers and sauté until crisp-tender, about 4 minutes. Add the zucchini, chili powder, cumin, and black pepper to taste, and continue to sauté until the vegetables are tender, about 5 minutes.
2. Add the black beans and cherry tomatoes and cook within 5 minutes. Divide between 4 burritos and serve topped with optional ingredients as desired. Enjoy immediately.

Nutrition: Calories: 311 Fat: 6g Sodium: 499mg Carbohydrate: 52g Protein: 19g

841. Tomato & Olive Orecchiette with Basil Pesto

Preparation time: 15 minutes
Cooking time: 25 minutes
Servings: 6
Ingredients:
- 12 ounces orecchiette pasta
- 2 tablespoons olive oil
- 1-pint cherry tomatoes, quartered
- ½ cup Basil Pesto or store-bought pesto
- ¼ cup Kalamata olives, sliced
- 1 tablespoon dried oregano leaves
- ¼ teaspoon kosher or sea salt
- ½ teaspoon freshly cracked black pepper
- ¼ teaspoon crushed red pepper flakes
- 2 tablespoons freshly grated Parmesan cheese

Directions:
1. Boil a large pot of water. Cook the orecchiette, drain and transfer the pasta to a large nonstick skillet.
2. Put the skillet over medium-low heat, then heat the olive oil. Stir in the cherry tomatoes, pesto, olives, oregano, salt, black pepper, and crushed red pepper flakes. Cook within 8 to 10 minutes, until heated throughout. Serve the pasta with the freshly grated Parmesan cheese.

Nutrition: Calories: 332 Fat: 13g Sodium: 389mg Carbohydrate: 44g Protein: 9g

842. Italian Stuffed Portobello Mushroom Burgers

Preparation time: 15 minutes
Cooking time: 25 minutes
Servings: 4
Ingredients:

- 1 tablespoon olive oil
- 4 large portobello mushrooms, washed and dried
- ½ yellow onion, peeled and diced
- 4 garlic cloves, peeled and minced
- 1 can cannellini beans, drained
- ½ cup fresh basil leaves, torn
- ½ cup panko bread crumbs
- 1/8 teaspoon kosher or sea salt
- ¼ teaspoon ground black pepper
- 1 cup lower-sodium marinara, divided
- ½ cup shredded mozzarella cheese
- 4 whole-wheat buns, toasted
- 1 cup fresh arugula

Directions:
1. Heat-up the olive oil in a large skillet to medium-high heat. Sear the mushrooms for 4 to 5 minutes per side, until slightly soft. Place on a baking sheet. Preheat the oven to a low broil.
2. Put the onion in the skillet and cook for 4 to 5 minutes, until slightly soft. Mix in the garlic then cooks within 30 to 60 seconds. Move the onions plus garlic to a bowl. Add the cannellini beans and smash with the back of a fork to form a chunky paste. Stir in the basil, bread crumbs, salt, and black pepper and half of the marinara. Cook for 5 minutes.
3. Remove the bean mixture from the stove and divide among the mushroom caps. Spoon the remaining marinara over the stuffed mushrooms and top each with the mozzarella cheese. Broil within 3 to 4 minutes, until the cheese is melted and bubbly. Transfer the burgers to the toasted whole-wheat buns and top with the arugula.

Nutrition: Calories: 407 Fat: 9g Sodium: 575mg Carbohydrate: 63g Protein: 25g

843. Gnocchi with Tomato Basil Sauce

Preparation time: 15 minutes
Cooking time: 25 minutes
Servings: 6
Ingredients:
- 2 tablespoons olive oil
- ½ yellow onion, peeled and diced
- 3 cloves garlic, peeled and minced
- 1 (32-ounce) can no-salt-added crushed San Marzano tomatoes
- ¼ cup fresh basil leaves
- 2 teaspoons Italian seasoning
- ½ teaspoon kosher or sea salt
- 1 teaspoon granulated sugar
- ½ teaspoon ground black pepper
- 1/8 teaspoon crushed red pepper flakes
- 1 tablespoon heavy cream (optional)
- 12 ounces gnocchi
- ¼ cup freshly grated Parmesan cheese

Directions:
1. Heat-up the olive oil in a Dutch oven or stockpot over medium heat. Add the onion and sauté for 5 to 6 minutes, until soft. Stir in the garlic and stir until fragrant, 30 to 60 seconds. Then stir in the tomatoes, basil, Italian

seasoning, salt, sugar, black pepper, and crushed red pepper flakes.
2. Bring to a simmer for 15 minutes. Stir in the heavy cream, if desired. For a smooth, puréed sauce, use an immersion blender or transfer sauce to a blender and purée until smooth. Taste and adjust the seasoning, if necessary.
3. While the sauce simmers, cook the gnocchi according to the package instructions, remove with a slotted spoon, and transfer to 6 bowls. Pour the sauce over the gnocchi and top with the Parmesan cheese.

Nutrition: Calories: 287 Fat: 7g Sodium: 527mg Carbohydrate: 41g Protein: 10g

844. Creamy Pumpkin Pasta

Preparation time: 15 minutes
Cooking time: 30 minutes
Servings: 6
Ingredients:
- 1-pound whole-grain linguine
- 1 tablespoon olive oil
- 3 garlic cloves, peeled and minced
- 2 tablespoons chopped fresh sage
- 1½ cups pumpkin purée
- 1 cup unsalted vegetable stock
- ½ cup low-fat evaporated milk
- ¾ teaspoon kosher or sea salt
- ½ teaspoon ground black pepper
- ½ teaspoon ground nutmeg
- ¼ teaspoon ground cayenne pepper
- ½ cup freshly grated Parmesan cheese, divided

Directions:
1. Cook the whole-grain linguine in a large pot of boiled water. Reserve ½ cup of pasta water and drain the rest. Set the pasta aside.
2. Warm-up olive oil over medium heat in a large skillet. Add the garlic and sage and sauté for 1 to 2 minutes, until soft and fragrant. Whisk in the pumpkin purée, stock, milk, and reserved pasta water and simmer for 4 to 5 minutes, until thickened.
3. Whisk in the salt, black pepper, nutmeg, and cayenne pepper and half of the Parmesan cheese. Stir in the cooked whole-grain linguine. Evenly divide the pasta among 6 bowls and top with the remaining Parmesan cheese.

Nutrition: Calories: 381 Fat: 8g Sodium: 175mg Carbohydrate: 63g Protein: 15g

845. Quinoa-Stuffed Peppers

Preparation time: 15 minutes
Cooking time: 35 minutes
Servings: 2
Ingredients:
- 2 large green bell peppers, halved
- 1½ teaspoons olive oil, divided
- ½ cup quinoa
- ½ cup minced onion
- 1 garlic clove, pressed or minced
- 1 cup chopped portobello mushrooms
- 3 tablespoons grated Parmesan cheese, divided

- 4 ounces tomato sauce

Directions:
1. Preheat the oven to 400°F. Put the pepper halves on your prepared baking sheet. Brush the insides of peppers with ½ teaspoon olive oil and bake for 10 minutes.
2. Remove the baking sheet, then set aside. While the peppers bake, cook the quinoa in a large saucepan over medium heat according to the package directions and set aside.
3. Warm-up the rest of the oil in a medium-size skillet over medium heat. Add the onion and sauté until it's translucent about 3 minutes. Put the garlic and cook within 1 minute.
4. Put the mushrooms in the skillet, adjust the heat to medium-low, cover, and cook within 5 to 6 minutes. Uncover, and if there's still liquid in the pan, reduce the heat and cook until the liquid evaporates.
5. Add the mushroom mixture, 1 tablespoon of Parmesan, and the tomato sauce to the quinoa and gently stir to combine. Carefully spoon the quinoa mixture into each pepper half and sprinkle with the remaining Parmesan. Return the peppers to the oven, bake for 10 to 15 more minutes until tender, and serve.

Nutrition: Calories: 292 Fat: 9g Carbohydrates: 45g Fiber: 8g Protein: 12g Sodium: 154mg Potassium: 929mg

846. Sweet Potato Cakes with Classic Guacamole

Preparation time: 15 minutes
Cooking time: 20 minutes
Servings: 4
Ingredients:
- For the guacamole:
- 2 ripe avocados, peeled and pitted
- ½ jalapeño, seeded and finely minced
- ¼ red onion, peeled and finely diced
- ¼ cup fresh cilantro leaves, chopped
- Zest and juice of 1 lime
- ¼ teaspoon kosher or sea salt
- For the cakes:
- 3 sweet potatoes, cooked and peeled
- ½ cup cooked black beans
- 1 large egg
- ½ cup panko bread crumbs
- 1 teaspoon ground cumin
- 1 teaspoon chili powder
- ½ teaspoon kosher or sea salt
- ¼ teaspoon ground black pepper
- 2 tablespoons canola oil

Directions:
1. Mash the avocado, then stir in the jalapeño, red onion, cilantro, lime zest and juice, and salt in a bowl. Taste and adjust the seasoning, if necessary.
2. Put the cooked sweet potatoes plus black beans in a bowl and mash until a paste form. Stir in the egg, bread crumbs, cumin, chili powder, salt, and black pepper until combined.
3. Warm-up canola oil in a large skillet at medium heat. Form the sweet potato mixture into 4 patties, place them in the hot skillet, and cook within 3 to 4 minutes per side,

until browned and crispy. Serve the sweet potato cakes with guacamole on top.

Nutrition: Calories: 369 Fat: 22g Sodium: 521mg Carbohydrate: 38g Protein: 8g

847. Chickpea Cauliflower Tikka Masala

Preparation time: 15 minutes
Cooking time: 40 minutes
Servings: 6
Ingredients:
- 2 tablespoons olive oil
- 1 yellow onion, peeled and diced
- 4 garlic cloves, peeled and minced
- 1-inch piece fresh ginger, peeled and minced
- 2 tablespoons Garam Masala
- 1 teaspoon kosher or sea salt
- ½ teaspoon ground black pepper
- ¼ teaspoon ground cayenne pepper
- ½ small head cauliflower, small florets
- 2 (15-ounce) cans no-salt-added chickpeas, rinsed and drained
- 1 (15-ounce) can no-salt-added petite diced tomatoes, drained
- 1½ cups unsalted vegetable broth
- ½ (15-ounce) can coconut milk
- Zest and juice of 1 lime
- ½ cup fresh cilantro leaves, chopped, divided
- 1½ cups cooked Fluffy Brown Rice, divided

Directions:
1. Warm-up olive oil over medium heat, then put the onion and sauté within 4 to 5 minutes in a large Dutch oven or stockpot. Stir in the garlic, ginger, garam masala, salt, black pepper, and cayenne pepper and toast for 30 to 60 seconds, until fragrant.
2. Stir in the cauliflower florets, chickpeas, diced tomatoes, and vegetable broth and increase to medium-high. Simmer within 15 minutes, until the cauliflower is fork-tender.
3. Remove, then stir in the coconut milk, lime juice, lime zest, and half of the cilantro. Taste and adjust the seasoning, if necessary. Serve over the rice and the remaining chopped cilantro.

Nutrition: Calories: 323 Fat: 12g Sodium: 444mg Carbohydrate: 44g Protein: 11g

848. Eggplant Parmesan Stacks

Preparation time: 15 minutes
Cooking time: 20 minutes
Servings: 4
Ingredients:
- 1 large eggplant, cut into thick slices
- 2 tablespoons olive oil, divided
- ¼ teaspoon kosher or sea salt
- ¼ teaspoon ground black pepper
- 1 cup panko bread crumbs
- ¼ cup freshly grated Parmesan cheese
- 5 to 6 garlic cloves, minced
- ½ pound fresh mozzarella, sliced
- 1½ cups lower-sodium marinara
- ½ cup fresh basil leaves, torn

Directions:
1. Preheat the oven to 425°F. Coat the eggplant slices in 1 tablespoon olive oil and sprinkle with the salt and black pepper. Put on a large baking sheet, then roast for 10 to 12 minutes, until soft with crispy edges. Remove the eggplant and set the oven to a low broil.
2. In a bowl, stir the remaining tablespoon of olive oil, bread crumbs, Parmesan cheese, and garlic. Remove the cooled eggplant from the baking sheet and clean it.
3. Create layers on the same baking sheet by stacking a roasted eggplant slice with a slice of mozzarella, a tablespoon of marinara, and a tablespoon of the bread crumb mixture, repeating with 2 layers of each ingredient. Cook under the broiler within 3 to 4 minutes until the cheese is melted and bubbly.

Nutrition: Calories: 377 Fat: 22g Sodium: 509mg Carbohydrate: 29g Protein: 16g

849. Roasted Vegetable Enchiladas

Preparation time: 15 minutes
Cooking time: 45 minutes
Servings: 8
Ingredients:
- 2 zucchinis, diced
- 1 red bell pepper, seeded and sliced
- 1 red onion, peeled and sliced
- 2 ears corn
- 2 tablespoons canola oil
- 1 can no-salt-added black beans, drained
- 1½ tablespoons chili powder
- 2 teaspoon ground cumin
- 1/8 teaspoon kosher or sea salt
- ½ teaspoon ground black pepper
- 8 (8-inch) whole-wheat tortillas
- 1 cup Enchilada Sauce or store-bought enchilada sauce
- ½ cup shredded Mexican-style cheese
- ½ cup plain nonfat Greek yogurt
- ½ cup cilantro leaves, chopped

Directions:
1. Preheat oven to 400°F. Place the zucchini, red bell pepper, and red onion on a baking sheet. Place the ears of corn separately on the same baking sheet. Drizzle all with the canola oil and toss to coat. Roast for 10 to 12 minutes, until the vegetables are tender. Remove and reduce the temperature to 375°F.
2. Cut the corn from the cob. Transfer the corn kernels, zucchini, red bell pepper, and onion to a bowl and stir in the black beans, chili powder, cumin, salt, and black pepper until combined.
3. Oiled a 9-by-13-inch baking dish with cooking spray. Line up the tortillas in the greased baking dish. Evenly distribute the vegetable bean filling into each tortilla. Pour half of the enchilada sauce and sprinkle half of the shredded cheese on top of the filling.

4. Roll each tortilla into enchilada shape and place them seam-side down. Pour the remaining enchilada sauce and sprinkle the remaining cheese over the enchiladas. Bake for 25 minutes until the cheese is melted and bubbly. Serve the enchiladas with Greek yogurt and chopped cilantro.

Nutrition: Calories: 335 Fat: 15g Sodium: 557mg Carbohydrate: 42g Protein: 13g

850. Lentil Avocado Tacos

Preparation time: 15 minutes
Cooking time: 35 minutes
Servings: 6
Ingredients:
- 1 tablespoon canola oil
- ½ yellow onion, peeled and diced
- 2-3 garlic cloves, minced
- 1½ cups dried lentils
- ½ teaspoon kosher or sea salt
- 3 to 3½ cups unsalted vegetable or chicken stock
- 2½ tablespoons Taco Seasoning or store-bought low-sodium taco seasoning
- 16 (6-inch) corn tortillas, toasted
- 2 ripe avocados, peeled and sliced

Directions:
1. Heat-up the canola oil in a large skillet or Dutch oven over medium heat. Cook the onion within 4 to 5 minutes, until soft. Mix in the garlic and cook within 30 seconds until fragrant. Then add the lentils, salt, and stock. Bring to a simmer for 25 to 35 minutes, adding additional stock if needed.
2. When there's only a small amount of liquid left in the pan, and the lentils are al dente, stir in the taco seasoning and let simmer for 1 to 2 minutes. Taste and adjust the seasoning, if necessary. Spoon the lentil mixture into tortillas and serve with the avocado slices.

Nutrition: Calories: 400 Fat: 14g Sodium: 336mg Carbohydrate: 64g Fiber: 15g Protein: 16g

851. Stuffed Eggplant Shells

Preparation time: 10 minutes
Cooking time: 25 minutes
Servings: 2
Ingredients:
- 1 medium eggplant
- 1 cup of water
- 1 tablespoon olive oil
- 4 oz. cooked white beans
- 1/4 cup onion, chopped
- 1/2 cup red, green, or yellow bell peppers, chopped
- 1 cup canned unsalted tomatoes
- 1/4 cup tomatoes liquid
- 1/4 cup celery, chopped
- 1 cup fresh mushrooms, sliced
- 3/4 cup whole-wheat breadcrumbs
- Freshly ground black pepper, to taste

Directions:

1. Prepare the oven to 350 degrees F to preheat. Grease a baking dish with cooking spray and set it aside. Trim and cut the eggplant into half, lengthwise. Scoop out the pulp using a spoon and leave the shell about ¼ inch thick.
2. Place the shells in the baking dish with their cut side up. Add water to the bottom of the dish. Dice the eggplant pulp into cubes and set them aside. Add oil to an iron skillet and heat it over medium heat. Stir in onions, peppers, chopped eggplant, tomatoes, celery, mushrooms, and tomato juice.
3. Cook for 10 minutes on simmering heat, then stirs in beans, black pepper, and breadcrumbs. Divide this mixture into the eggplant shells. Cover the shells with a foil sheet and bake for 15 minutes. Serve warm.

Nutrition: Calories 334; Fat 10 g; Sodium 142 mg; Carbs 35 g; Protein 26 g

852. Southwestern Vegetables Tacos

Preparation time: 10 minutes
Cooking time: 20 minutes
Servings: 4
Ingredients:
- 1 tablespoon olive oil
- 1 cup red onion, chopped
- 1 cup yellow summer squash, diced
- 1 cup green zucchini, diced
- 3 large garlic cloves, minced
- 4 medium tomatoes, seeded and chopped
- 1 jalapeno chili, seeded and chopped
- 1 cup fresh corn kernels
- 1 cup canned pinto, rinsed and drained
- 1/2 cup fresh cilantro, chopped
- 8 corn tortillas
- 1/2 cup smoke-flavored salsa

Directions:
1. Add olive oil to a saucepan, then heat it over medium heat. Stir in onion and sauté until soft. Add zucchini and summer squash. Cook for 5 minutes.
2. Stir in corn kernels, jalapeno, garlic, beans, and tomatoes. Cook for another 5 minutes. Stir in cilantro, then remove the pan from the heat.
3. Warm each tortilla in a dry nonstick skillet for 20 secs per side. Place the tortilla on the serving plate. Spoon the vegetable mixture in each tortilla. Top the mixture with salsa. Serve.

Nutrition: Calories 310; Fat 6 g; Sodium 97 mg; Carbs 54 g; Protein 10g

853. Tofu & Green Bean Stir-Fry

Preparation time: 15 minutes
Cooking time: 20 minutes
Servings: 4
Ingredients:
- 1 (14-ounce) package extra-firm tofu
- 2 tablespoons canola oil
- 1-pound green beans, chopped

- 2 carrots, peeled and thinly sliced
- ½ cup Stir-Fry Sauce or store-bought lower-sodium stir-fry sauce
- 2 cups Fluffy Brown Rice
- 2 scallions, thinly sliced
- 2 tablespoons sesame seeds

Directions:
1. Put the tofu on your plate lined with a kitchen towel, put separate kitchen towel over the tofu, and place a heavy pot on top, changing towels every time they become soaked. Let sit within 15 minutes to remove the moisture. Cut the tofu into 1-inch cubes.
2. Heat the canola oil in a large wok or skillet to medium-high heat. Add the tofu cubes and cook, flipping every 1 to 2 minutes, so all sides become browned. Remove from the skillet and place the green beans and carrots in the hot oil. Stir-fry for 4 to 5 minutes, occasionally tossing, until crisp and slightly tender.
3. While the vegetables are cooking, prepare the Stir-Fry Sauce (if using homemade). Place the tofu back in the skillet. Put the sauce over the tofu and vegetables and let simmer for 2 to 3 minutes. Serve over rice, then top with scallions and sesame seeds.

Nutrition: Calories: 380 Fat: 15g Sodium: 440mg Potassium: 454mg Carbohydrate: 45g Protein: 16g

854. Peanut Vegetable Pad Thai

Preparation time: 15 minutes
Cooking time: 20 minutes
Servings: 6
Ingredients:
- 8 ounces brown rice noodles
- 1/3 cup natural peanut butter
- 3 tablespoons unsalted vegetable broth
- 1 tablespoon low-sodium soy sauce
- 2 tablespoons of rice wine vinegar
- 1 tablespoon honey
- 2 teaspoons sesame oil
- 1 teaspoon sriracha (optional)
- 1 tablespoon canola oil
- 1 red bell pepper, thinly sliced
- 1 zucchini, cut into matchsticks
- 2 large carrots, cut into matchsticks
- 3 large eggs, beaten
- ¾ teaspoon kosher or sea salt
- ½ cup unsalted peanuts, chopped
- ½ cup cilantro leaves, chopped

Directions:
1. Boil a large pot of water. Cook the rice noodles as stated in package directions. Mix the peanut butter, vegetable broth, soy sauce, rice wine vinegar, honey, sesame oil, and sriracha in a bowl. Set aside.
2. Warm-up canola oil over medium heat in a large nonstick skillet. Add the red bell pepper, zucchini, and carrots, and sauté for 2 to 3 minutes, until slightly soft. Stir in the eggs and fold with a spatula until scrambled. Add the cooked rice noodles, sauce, and salt. Toss to combine. Spoon into bowls and evenly top with the peanuts and cilantro.

Nutrition: Calories: 393 Fat: 19g Sodium: 561mg Carbohydrate: 45g Protein: 13g

855. Spicy Tofu Burrito Bowls with Cilantro Avocado Sauce

Preparation time: 15 minutes
Cooking time: 15 minutes
Servings: 4
Ingredients:
- For the sauce:
- ¼ cup plain nonfat Greek yogurt
- ½ cup fresh cilantro leaves
- ½ ripe avocado, peeled
- Zest and juice of 1 lime
- 2 garlic cloves, peeled
- ¼ teaspoon kosher or sea salt
- 2 tablespoons water
- For the burrito bowls:
- 1 (14-ounce) package extra-firm tofu
- 1 tablespoon canola oil
- 1 yellow or orange bell pepper, diced
- 2 tablespoons Taco Seasoning
- ¼ teaspoon kosher or sea salt
- 2 cups Fluffy Brown Rice
- 1 (15-ounce) can black beans, drained

Directions:
1. Place all the sauce ingredients in the bowl of a food processor or blender and purée until smooth. Taste and adjust the seasoning, if necessary. Refrigerate until ready for use.
2. Put the tofu on your plate lined with a kitchen towel. Put another kitchen towel over the tofu and place a heavy pot on top, changing towels if they become soaked. Let it stand within 15 minutes to remove the moisture. Cut the tofu into 1-inch cubes.
3. Warm-up canola oil in a large skillet over medium heat. Add the tofu and bell pepper and sauté, breaking up the tofu into smaller pieces for 4 to 5 minutes. Stir in the taco seasoning, salt, and ¼ cup of water. Evenly divide the rice and black beans among 4 bowls. Top with the tofu/bell pepper mixture and top with the cilantro avocado sauce.

Nutrition: Calories: 383 Fat: 13g Sodium: 438mg Carbohydrate: 48g Protein: 21g

856. Vegetable Cheese Calzone

Preparation time: 15 minutes
Cooking time: 20 minutes
Servings: 4
Ingredients:
- 3 asparagus stalks, cut into pieces
- 1/2 cup spinach, chopped
- 1/2 cup broccoli, chopped
- 1/2 cup sliced
- 2 tablespoons garlic, minced
- 2 teaspoons olive oil, divided
- 1/2 lb. frozen whole-wheat bread dough, thawed

- 1 medium tomato, sliced
- 1/2 cup mozzarella, shredded
- 2/3 cup pizza sauce

Directions:
1. Prepare the oven to 400 degrees F to preheat. Grease a baking sheet with cooking oil and set it aside. Toss asparagus with mushrooms, garlic, broccoli, and spinach in a bowl. Stir in 1 teaspoon olive oil and mix well. Heat a greased skillet on medium heat.
2. Stir in vegetable mixture and sauté for 5 minutes. Set these vegetables aside. Cut the bread dough into quarters.
3. Spread each bread quarter on a floured surface into an oval. Add sautéed vegetables, 2 tbsp. cheese, and tomato slice to half of each oval.
4. Wet the edges of each oval and fold the dough over the vegetable filling. Pinch and press the two edges.
5. Place these calzones on the baking sheet. Brush each calzone with foil and bake for 10 minutes. Heat pizza sauce in a saucepan for a minute. Serve the calzone with pizza sauce.

Nutritional: Calories 198; Fat 8 g; Sodium 124 mg; Carbs 36 g; Protein 12 g

857. Mixed Vegetarian Chili

Preparation time: 10 minutes
Cooking time: 36 minutes
Servings: 4

Ingredients:
- 1 tablespoon olive oil
- 14 oz. canned black beans, rinsed and drained
- ½ cup yellow Onion, chopped
- 12 oz. extra-firm tofu, cut into pieces
- 14 oz. canned kidney beans, rinsed and drained
- 2 cans (14 oz.) diced tomatoes
- 3 tablespoons chili powder
- 1 tablespoon oregano
- 1 tablespoon chopped cilantro (fresh coriander)

Directions:
1. Take a soup pot and heat olive oil in it over medium heat. Add onions and sauté for 6 minutes until soft. Add tomatoes, beans, chili powder, oregano, and beans. Boil it first, then reduce the heat to a simmer. Cook for 30 minutes, then add cilantro. Serve warm.

Nutrition: Calories 314; Fat 6 g; Sodium 119 mg; Carbs 46g; Protein 19 g

858. Zucchini Pepper Kebabs

Preparation time: 15 minutes
Cooking time: 40 minutes
Servings: 2

Ingredients:
- 1 small zucchini, sliced into 8 pieces
- 1 red onion, cut into 4 wedges
- 1 green bell pepper, cut into 4 chunks
- 8 cherry tomatoes
- 8 button mushrooms
- 1 red bell pepper, cut into 4 chunks
- 1/2 cup Italian dressing, fat-free

- 1/2 cup brown rice
- 1 cup of water
- 4 wooden skewers, soaked and drained

Directions:
1. Toss tomatoes with zucchini, onion, peppers, and mushrooms in a bowl. Stir in Italian dressing and mix well to coat the vegetables. Marinate them for 10 minutes. Boil water with rice in a saucepan, then reduce the heat to a simmer.
2. Cover the rice and cook for 30 minutes until rice is done. Meanwhile, prepare the grill and preheat it on medium heat. Grease the grilling rack with cooking spray and place it 4 inches above the heat.
3. Thread 2 mushrooms, 2 tomatoes, and 2 zucchini slices along with 1 onions wedge, 1 green and red pepper slice on each skewer. Grill these kebabs for 5 minutes per side. Serve warm with boiled rice.

Nutrition: Calories 335; Fat 8.2 g; Sodium 516 mg; Carbs 67 g; Protein 8.8 g

859. Asparagus Cheese Vermicelli

Preparation time: 10 minutes
Cooking time: 15 minutes
Servings: 4

Ingredients:
- 2 teaspoons olive oil, divided
- 6 asparagus spears, cut into pieces
- 4 oz. dried whole-grain vermicelli
- 1 medium tomato, chopped
- 1 tablespoon garlic, minced
- 2 tablespoons fresh basil, chopped
- 4 tablespoons Parmesan, freshly grated, divided
- 1/8 teaspoon black pepper, ground

Directions:
1. Add 1 tsp. oil to a skillet and heat it. Stir in asparagus and sauté until golden brown.
2. Cut the sautéed asparagus into 1-inch pieces. Fill a sauce pot with water up to ¾ full. After boiling the water, add pasta and cook for 10 minutes until it is all done.
3. Drain and rinse the pasta under tap water. Add pasta to a large bowl, then toss in olive oil, tomato, garlic, asparagus, basil, garlic, and parmesan. Serve with black pepper on top.

Nutrition: Calories 325; Fat 8 g; Sodium 350 mg; Carbs 48 g; Protein 7.3 g

860. Corn Stuffed Peppers

Preparation time: 10 minutes
Cooking time: 35 minutes
Servings: 4

Ingredients:
- 4 red or green bell peppers
- 1 tablespoon olive oil
- ¼ cup onion, chopped
- 1 green bell pepper, chopped
- 2 1/2 cups fresh corn kernels
- 1/8 teaspoon chili powder

- 2 tablespoons chopped fresh parsley
- 3 egg whites
- 1/2 cup skim milk
- 1/2 cup water

Directions:

1. Prepare the oven to 350 F to preheat. Layer a baking dish with cooking spray. Cut the bell peppers from the top and remove their seeds from inside. Put the peppers in your prepared baking dish with their cut side up.
2. Add oil to a skillet, then heat it on medium flame. Stir in onion, corn, and green pepper. Sauté for 5 minutes. Add cilantro and chili powder. Switch the heat to low. Mix milk plus egg whites in a bowl. Pour this mixture into the skillet and cook for 5 minutes while stirring.
3. Divide this mixture into each pepper. Add some water to the baking dish. Cover the stuffed peppers with an aluminum sheet. Bake for 15 minutes, then serves warm.

Nutrition: Calories 197; Fat 5 g; Sodium 749 mg; Carbs 29 g; Protein 9 g

861. Chunky Black-Bean Dip

Preparation time: 5 minutes
Cooking time: 1 minute
Servings: 2

Ingredients:

- 1 (15-ounce) can black beans, drained, with liquid reserved
- ½-can of chipotle peppers in adobo sauce
- ¼ cup plain Greek yogurt
- Freshly ground black pepper

Directions:

1. Combine beans, peppers, and yogurt in a food processor or blender and process until smooth. Add some of the bean liquid, 1 tablespoon at a time, for a thinner consistency. Season to taste with black pepper. Serve.

Nutrition: Calories: 70g; Fat: 1g; Sodium: 159mg; Carbohydrate: 11g; Protein: 5g

862. Classic Hummus

Preparation time: 5 minutes
Cooking time: 0 minutes
Servings: 6–8

Ingredients:

- 1 (15-ounce) can chickpeas, drained and rinsed
- 3 tablespoons sesame tahini
- 2 tablespoons olive oil
- 3 garlic cloves, chopped
- Juice of 1 lemon
- Salt
- Freshly ground black pepper

Directions:

1. Mix all the ingredients until smooth but thick in a food processor or blender. Add water if necessary to produce a smoother hummus. Store covered for up to 5 days.

Nutrition: Calories: 147g; Fat: 10g; Sodium: 64mg; Carbohydrate: 11g; Protein: 6g.

863. Crispy Potato Skins

Preparation time: 2 minutes
Cooking time: 19 minutes
Servings: 2

Ingredients:

- 2 russet potatoes
- Cooking spray
- 1 teaspoon dried rosemary
- 1/8 teaspoon freshly ground black pepper

Directions:

1. Preheat the oven to 375°f. Prick or pierce the potatoes all over using a fork. Put on a plate. Cook on full power in the microwave within 5 minutes. Flip over, and cook again within 3 to 4 minutes more, or until soft.
2. Carefully—the potatoes will be very hot—scoop out the pulp of the potatoes, leaving a 1/8 inch of potato pulp attached to the skin. Set aside.
3. Spray the inside of each potato with cooking spray. Press in the rosemary and pepper. Place the skins on a baking sheet and bake in a preheated oven for 5 to 10 minutes until slightly browned and crispy. Serve immediately.

Nutrition: Calories 114; Fat: 0g; Sodium: 0mg; Carbohydrate: 27g; Protein: 3g

864. Roasted Chickpeas

Preparation time: 5 minutes
Cooking time: 30 minutes
Servings: 2

Ingredients:

- 1 (15-ounce can) chickpeas, drained and rinsed
- ½ teaspoon olive oil
- 2 teaspoons of your favorite herbs or spice blend
- ¼ teaspoon salt

Directions:

1. Preheat the oven to 400°f.
2. Wrap a rimmed baking sheet with paper towels, place the chickpeas on it in an even layer, and blot with more paper towels until most of the liquid is absorbed.
3. In a medium bowl, gently toss the chickpeas and olive oil until combined. Sprinkle the mixture with the herbs and salt and toss again.
4. Place the chickpeas back on the baking sheet and spread in an even layer. Bake for 30 to 40 minutes, until crunchy and golden brown. Stir halfway through. Serve.

Nutrition: Calories: 175g; Fat: 3g; Sodium: 474mg; Carbohydrate: 29g; Protein: 11g

865. Carrot-Cake Smoothie

Preparation time 5 minutes
Cooking time: 0 minutes
Servings: 2

Ingredients:

- 1 frozen banana, peeled and diced
- 1 cup carrots, diced (peeled if preferred)
- 1 cup nonfat or low-fat milk
- ½ cup nonfat or low-fat vanilla Greek yogurt
- ½ cup ice

- ¼ cup diced pineapple, frozen
- ½ teaspoon ground cinnamon
- Pinch nutmeg
- Optional toppings: chopped walnuts, grated carrots

Directions:
1. Process all of the fixings to a blender. Serve immediately with optional toppings as desired.

Nutrition: Calories: 180g; Fat: 1g; Sodium: 114mg; Carbohydrate: 36g; Protein 10g

866. Southwestern Bean-And-Pepper Salad

Preparation time: 6 minutes
Cooking time: 0 minutes
Servings: 4
Ingredients:
- 1 can pinto beans, drained
- 2 bell peppers, cored and chopped
- 1 cup corn kernels
- Salt
- Freshly ground black pepper
- Juice of 2 limes
- 1 tablespoon olive oil
- 1 avocado, chopped

Directions:
1. Mix beans, peppers, corn, salt, plus pepper in a large bowl. Press fresh lime juice, then mix in olive oil. Let the salad stand in the fridge within 30 minutes. Add avocado just before serving.

Nutrition: Calories: 245; Fat: 11g; Sodium: 97mg; Carbohydrate: 32g; Protein: 8g

867. Cauliflower Mashed Potatoes

Preparation time: 10 minutes
Cooking time: 10 minutes
Servings: 4
Ingredients:
- 16 cups water (enough to cover cauliflower)
- 1 head cauliflower (about 3 pounds), trimmed and cut into florets
- 4 garlic cloves
- 1 tablespoon olive oil
- ¼ teaspoon salt
- 1/8 teaspoon freshly ground black pepper
- 2 teaspoons dried parsley

Directions:
1. Boil a large pot of water, then the cauliflower and garlic. Cook within 10 minutes, then strain. Move it back to the hot pan, and let it stand within 2 to 3 minutes with the lid on.
2. Put the cauliflower plus garlic in a food processor or blender. Add the olive oil, salt, pepper, and purée until smooth. Taste and adjust the salt and pepper.
3. Remove, then put the parsley, and mix until combined. Garnish with additional olive oil, if desired. Serve immediately.

Nutrition: Calories: 87g; Fat: 4g; Sodium: 210mg; Carbohydrate: 12g; Protein: 4g

868. Roasted Brussels sprouts

Preparation time: 5 minutes
Cooking time: 20 minutes
Servings: 4
Ingredients:
- 1½ pounds Brussels sprouts, trimmed and halved
- 2 tablespoons olive oil
- ¼ teaspoon salt
- ½ teaspoon freshly ground black pepper

Directions:
1. Preheat the oven to 400°f. Combine the Brussels sprouts and olive oil in a large mixing bowl and toss until they are evenly coated.
2. Turn the Brussels sprouts out onto a large baking sheet and flip them over, so they are cut-side down with the flat part touching the baking sheet. Sprinkle with salt and pepper.
3. Bake within 20 to 30 minutes or until the Brussels sprouts are lightly charred and crisp on the outside and toasted on the bottom. The outer leaves will be extra dark, too. Serve immediately.

Nutrition: Calories: 134; Fat: 8g; Sodium: 189mg; Carbohydrate: 15g; Protein: 6g

869. Broccoli with Garlic and Lemon

Preparation time: 2 minutes
Cooking time: 4 minutes
Servings: 4
Ingredients:
- 1 cup of water
- 4 cups broccoli florets
- 1 teaspoon olive oil
- 1 tablespoon minced garlic
- 1 teaspoon lemon zest
- Salt
- Freshly ground black pepper

Directions:
1. Put the broccoli in the boiling water in a small saucepan and cook within 2 to 3 minutes. The broccoli should retain its bright-green color. Drain the water from the broccoli.
2. Put the olive oil in a small sauté pan over medium-high heat. Add the garlic and sauté for 30 seconds. Put the broccoli, lemon zest, salt, plus pepper. Combine well and serve.

Nutrition: Calories: 38g; Fat: 1g; Sodium: 24mg; Carbohydrate: 5g; Protein: 3g

870. Brown Rice Pilaf

Preparation time: 5 minutes
Cooking time: 10 minutes
Servings: 4

Ingredients:

- 1 cup low-sodium vegetable broth
- ½ tablespoon olive oil
- 1 clove garlic, minced
- 1 scallion, thinly sliced
- 1 tablespoon minced onion flakes
- 1 cup instant brown rice
- 1/8 teaspoon freshly ground black pepper

Directions:

1. Mix the vegetable broth, olive oil, garlic, scallion, and minced onion flakes in a saucepan and boil. Put rice, then boil it again, adjust the heat and simmer within 10 minutes. Remove and let stand within 5 minutes. Fluff with a fork and season with black pepper.

Nutrition: Calories: 100g; Fat: 2g; Sodium: 35mg; Carbohydrate: 19g; Protein: 2g

871. Pasta with Tomatoes and Peas

Preparation time: 15 minutes
Cooking time: 15 minutes
Servings: 2
Ingredients:

- ½ cup whole-grain pasta of choice
- 8 cups water, plus ¼ for finishing
- 1 cup frozen peas
- 1 tablespoon olive oil
- 1 cup cherry tomatoes, halved
- ¼ teaspoon freshly ground black pepper
- 1 teaspoon dried basil
- ¼ cup grated Parmesan cheese (low-sodium)

Directions:

1. Cook the pasta al dente. Add the water to the same pot you used to cook the pasta, and when it's boiling, add the peas. Cook within 5 minutes. Drain and set aside.
2. Heat-up the oil in a large skillet over medium heat. Add the cherry tomatoes, put a lid on the skillet and let the tomatoes soften for about 5 minutes, stirring a few times.
3. Season with black pepper and basil. Toss in the pasta, peas, and ¼ cup of water, stir and remove from the heat. Serve topped with Parmesan.

Nutrition: Calories: 266; Fat: 12g; Sodium: 320mg; Carbohydrate: 30g; Protein: 13g

872. Healthy Vegetable Fried Rice

Preparation time: 15 minutes
Cooking time: 10 minutes
Servings: 4
Ingredients:

- For the sauce:
- 1/3 cup garlic vinegar
- 1½ tablespoons dark molasses
- 1 teaspoon onion powder
- For the fried rice:
- 1 teaspoon olive oil
- 2 lightly beaten whole eggs + 4 egg whites

- 1 cup of frozen mixed vegetables
- 1 cup frozen edamame
- 2 cups cooked brown rice

Directions:

1. Prepare the sauce by combining the garlic vinegar, molasses, and onion powder in a glass jar. Shake well.
2. Heat-up oil in a large wok or skillet over medium-high heat. Add eggs and egg whites, let cook until the eggs set, for about 1 minute.
3. Break up eggs with a spatula or spoon into small pieces. Add frozen mixed vegetables and frozen edamame. Cook for 4 minutes, stirring frequently.
4. Add the brown rice and sauce to the vegetable-and-egg mixture. Cook for 5 minutes or until heated through. Serve immediately.

Nutrition: Calories: 210; Fat: 6g; Sodium: 113mg; Carbohydrate: 28g; Protein: 13g

873. Portobello-Mushroom Cheeseburgers

Preparation time: 15 minutes
Cooking time: 10 minutes
Servings: 4
Ingredients:

- 4 portobello mushrooms, caps removed and brushed clean
- 1 tablespoon olive oil
- ½ teaspoon freshly ground black pepper
- 1 tablespoon red wine vinegar
- 4 slices reduced-fat Swiss cheese, sliced thin
- 4 whole-wheat 100-calorie sandwich thins
- ½ avocado, sliced thin

Directions:

1. Heat-up a skillet or grill pan over medium-high heat. Clean the mushrooms and remove the stems. Brush each cap with olive oil and sprinkle with black pepper. Place in skillet cap-side up and cook for about 4 minutes. Flip and cook for another 4 minutes.
2. Sprinkle with the red wine vinegar and flip. Add the cheese and cook for 2 more minutes. For optimal melting, place a lid loosely over the pan. Meanwhile, toast the sandwich thins. Create your burgers by topping each with sliced avocado. Enjoy immediately.

Nutrition: Calories: 245; Fat: 12g; Sodium: 266mg; Carbohydrate: 28g; Protein: 14g

874. And-Rosemary Omelet

Preparation time: 15 minutes
Cooking time: 15 minutes
Servings: 2
Ingredients:

- ½ tablespoon olive oil
- 4 eggs
- ¼ cup grated Parmesan cheese
- 1 (15-ounce) can chickpeas, drained and rinsed
- 2 cups packed baby spinach
- 1 cup button mushrooms, chopped

- 2 sprigs rosemary, leaves picked (or 2 teaspoons dried rosemary)
- Salt
- Freshly ground black pepper

Directions:
1. Warm oven to 400 F and puts a baking tray on the middle shelf. Line an 8-inch spring form pan with baking paper and grease generously with olive oil. If you don't have a spring form pan, grease an oven-safe skillet (or cast-iron skillet) with olive oil.
2. Lightly whisk the eggs and Parmesan. Place chickpeas in the prepared pan. Layer the spinach and mushrooms on top of the beans. Pour the egg mixture on top and scatter the rosemary. Season to taste with salt and pepper.
3. Place the pan on the preheated tray and bake until golden and puffy and the center feels firm and springy about 15 minutes. Remove from the oven, slice, and serve immediately.

Nutrition: Calories: 418; Fat: 19g; Sodium: 595mg; Carbohydrate: 33g; Protein: 30g

875. Chilled Cucumber-And-Avocado Soup with Dill

Preparation time: 15 minutes
Cooking time: 30 minutes
Servings: 4

Ingredients:
- 2 English cucumbers, peeled and diced, plus ¼ cup reserved for garnish
- 1 avocado, peeled, pitted, and chopped, plus ¼ cup reserved for garnish
- 1½ cups nonfat or low-fat plain Greek yogurt
- ½ cup of cold water
- 1/3 cup loosely packed dill, plus sprigs for garnish
- 1 tablespoon freshly squeezed lemon juice
- ¼ teaspoon freshly ground black pepper
- ¼ teaspoon salt
- 1 clove garlic

Directions:
1. Purée ingredients in a blender until smooth. If you prefer a thinner soup, add more water until you reach the desired consistency. Divide soup among 4 bowls. Cover with plastic wrap and refrigerate within 30 minutes. Garnish with cucumber, avocado, and dill sprigs, if desired.

Nutrition: Calories: 142; Fat: 7g; Sodium: 193mg; Carbohydrate: 12g; Protein: 11g

876. Black-Bean Soup

Preparation time: 15 minutes
Cooking time: 20 minutes
Servings: 4

Ingredients:
- 1 yellow onion
- 1 tablespoon olive oil
- 2 cans black beans, drained
- 1 cup diced fresh tomatoes
- 5 cups low-sodium vegetable broth

- ¼ teaspoon freshly ground black pepper
- ¼ cup chopped fresh cilantro

Directions:
1. Cook or sauté the onion in the olive oil within 4 to 5 minutes in a large saucepan over medium heat. Put the black beans, tomatoes, vegetable broth, and black pepper. Boil, then adjust heat to simmer within 15 minutes.
2. Remove, then working in batches, ladle the soup into a blender and process until somewhat smooth. Put it back to the pot, add the cilantro, and heat until warmed through. Serve immediately.

Nutrition: Calories: 234; Fat: 5g; Sodium: 363mg; Carbohydrate: 37g; Protein: 11g

877. Loaded Baked Sweet Potatoes

Preparation time: 15 minutes
Cooking time: 20 minutes
Servings: 4

Ingredients:
- 4 sweet potatoes
- ½ cup nonfat or low-fat plain Greek yogurt
- Freshly ground black pepper
- 1 teaspoon olive oil
- 1 red bell pepper, cored and diced
- ½ red onion, diced
- 1 teaspoon ground cumin
- 1 (15-ounce) can chickpeas, drained and rinsed

Directions:
1. Prick the potatoes using a fork and cook on your microwave's potato setting until potatoes are soft and cooked through, about 8 to 10 minutes for 4 potatoes. If you don't have a microwave, bake at 400°F for about 45 minutes.
2. Combine the yogurt and black pepper in a small bowl and mix well. Heat the oil in a medium pot over medium heat. Add bell pepper, onion, cumin, and additional black pepper to taste.
3. Add the chickpeas, stir to combine, and heat through about 5 minutes. Slice the potatoes lengthwise down the middle and top each half with a portion of the bean mixture followed by 1 to 2 tablespoons of the yogurt. Serve immediately.

Nutrition: Calories: 264; Fat: 2g; Sodium: 124mg; Carbohydrate: 51g; Protein: 11g

878. White Beans with Spinach and Pan-Roasted Tomatoes

Preparation time: 15 minutes
Cooking time: 10 minutes
Servings: 2

Ingredients:
- 1 tablespoon olive oil
- 4 small plum tomatoes, halved lengthwise
- 10 ounces frozen spinach, defrosted and squeezed of excess water

- 2 garlic cloves, thinly sliced
- 2 tablespoons water
- ¼ teaspoon freshly ground black pepper
- 1 can white beans, drained
- Juice of 1 lemon

Directions:
1. Heat-up the oil in a large skillet over medium-high heat. Put the tomatoes, cut-side down, and cook within 3 to 5 minutes; turn and cook within 1 minute more. Transfer to a plate.
2. Reduce heat to medium and add the spinach, garlic, water, and pepper to the skillet. Cook, tossing until the spinach is heated through, 2 to 3 minutes.
3. Return the tomatoes to the skillet, put the white beans and lemon juice, and toss until heated through 1 to 2 minutes.

Nutrition: Calories: 293; Fat: 9g; Sodium: 267mg; Carbohydrate: 43g; Protein: 15g

879. Black-Eyed Peas and Greens Power Salad

Preparation time: 15 minutes
Cooking time: 6 minutes
Servings: 2
Ingredients:
- 1 tablespoon olive oil
- 3 cups purple cabbage, chopped
- 5 cups baby spinach
- 1 cup shredded carrots
- 1 can black-eyed peas, drained
- Juice of ½ lemon
- Salt
- Freshly ground black pepper

Directions:
1. In a medium pan, add the oil and cabbage and sauté for 1 to 2 minutes on medium heat. Add in your spinach, cover for 3 to 4 minutes on medium heat, until greens are wilted. Remove from the heat and add to a large bowl.
2. Add in the carrots, black-eyed peas, and a splash of lemon juice. Season with salt and pepper, if desired. Toss and serve.

Nutrition: Calories: 320; Fat: 9g; Sodium: 351mg; Potassium: 544mg; Carbohydrate: 49g; Protein: 16g

880. Butternut-Squash Macaroni and Cheese

Preparation time: 15 minutes
Cooking time: 20 minutes
Servings: 2
Ingredients:
- 1 cup whole-wheat ziti macaroni
- 2 cups peeled and cubed butternut squash
- 1 cup nonfat or low-fat milk, divided
- Freshly ground black pepper
- 1 teaspoon Dijon mustard
- 1 tablespoon olive oil
- ¼ cup shredded low-fat cheddar cheese

Directions:
1. Cook the pasta al dente. Put the butternut squash plus ½ cup milk in a medium saucepan and place over medium-high heat. Season with black pepper. Bring it to a simmer. Lower the heat, then cook until fork-tender, 8 to 10 minutes.
2. To a blender, add squash and Dijon mustard. Purée until smooth. Meanwhile, place a large sauté pan over medium heat and add olive oil. Add the squash purée and the remaining ½ cup of milk. Simmer within 5 minutes. Add the cheese and stir to combine.
3. Add the pasta to the sauté pan and stir to combine. Serve immediately.

Nutrition: Calories: 373; Fat: 10g; Sodium: 193mg; Carbohydrate: 59g; Protein: 14g

881. Southwest Tofu Scramble

Preparation time: 15 minutes
Cooking time: 15 minutes
Servings: 1
Ingredients:
- ½ tablespoon olive oil
- ½ red onion, chopped
- 2 cups chopped spinach
- 8 ounces firm tofu, drained well
- 1 teaspoon ground cumin
- ½ teaspoon garlic powder
- Optional for serving: sliced avocado or sliced tomatoes

Directions:
1. Heat-up the olive oil in a medium skillet over medium heat. Put the onion and cook within 5 minutes. Add the spinach and cover to steam for 2 minutes.
2. Using a spatula, move the veggies to one side of the pan. Crumble the tofu into the open area in the pan, breaking it up with a fork. Add the cumin and garlic to the crumbled tofu and mix well. Sauté for 5 to 7 minutes until the tofu is slightly browned.
3. Serve immediately with whole-grain bread, fruit, or beans. Top with optional sliced avocado and tomato, if using.

Nutrition: Calories: 267; Fat: 17g; Sodium: 75mg; Carbohydrate: 13g; Protein: 23g

882. Black-Bean and Vegetable Burrito

Preparation time: 15 minutes
Cooking time: 15 minutes
Servings: 4
Ingredients:
- ½ tablespoon olive oil
- 2 red or green bell peppers, chopped
- 1 zucchini or summer squash, diced
- ½ teaspoon chili powder
- 1 teaspoon cumin
- Freshly ground black pepper
- 2cans black beans drained and rinsed
- 1 cup cherry tomatoes, halved
- 4 (8-inch) whole-wheat tortillas

- Optional for serving: spinach, sliced avocado, chopped scallions, or hot sauce

Directions:
1. Heat-up the oil in a large sauté pan over medium heat. Add the bell peppers and sauté until crisp-tender, about 4 minutes. Add the zucchini, chili powder, cumin, and black pepper to taste, and continue to sauté until the vegetables are tender, about 5 minutes.
2. Add the black beans and cherry tomatoes and cook within 5 minutes. Divide between 4 burritos and serve topped with optional ingredients as desired. Enjoy immediately.

Nutrition: Calories: 311; Fat: 6g; Sodium: 499mg; Carbohydrate: 52g; Protein: 19g

883. Baked Eggs in Avocado

Preparation time: 15 minutes
Cooking time: 15 minutes
Servings: 2
Ingredients:
- 2 avocados
- Juice of 2 limes
- Freshly ground black pepper
- 4 eggs
- 2 (8-inch) whole-wheat or corn tortillas, warmed
- Optional for serving: halved cherry tomatoes and chopped cilantro

Directions:
1. Adjust the oven rack to the middle position and preheat the oven to 450°F. Scrape out the center of halved avocado using a spoon about 1½ tablespoons.
2. Press lime juice over the avocados and season with black pepper to taste, and then place it on a baking sheet. Crack an egg into the avocado.
3. Bake within 10 to 15 minutes. Remove from oven and garnish with optional cilantro and cherry tomatoes and serve with warm tortillas.

Nutrition: Calories: 534; Fat: 39g; Sodium: 462mg; Potassium: 1,095mg; Carbohydrate: 30g; Fiber: 20g; Sugars: 3g; Protein: 23g

884. Red Beans and Rice

Preparation time: 15 minutes
Cooking time: 45 minutes
Servings: 2
Ingredients:
- ½ cup dry brown rice
- 1 cup water, plus ¼ cup
- 1 can red beans, drained
- 1 tablespoon ground cumin
- Juice of 1 lime
- 4 handfuls of fresh spinach
- Optional toppings: avocado, chopped tomatoes, Greek yogurt, onions

Directions:
1. Mix rice plus water in a pot and bring to a boil. Cover and reduce heat to a low simmer. Cook within 30 to 40 minutes or according to package directions.

2. Meanwhile, add the beans, ¼ cup of water, cumin, and lime juice to a medium skillet. Simmer within 5 to 7 minutes.
3. Once the liquid is mostly gone, remove from the heat and add the spinach. Cover and let spinach wilt slightly, 2 to 3 minutes. Mix in with the beans. Serve beans with rice. Add toppings, if using.

Nutrition: Calories: 232; Fat: 2g; Sodium: 210mg; Carbohydrate: 41g; Protein: 13g

885. Hearty Lentil Soup

Preparation time: 15 minutes
Cooking time: 30 minutes
Servings: 4
Ingredients:
- 1 tablespoon olive oil
- 2 carrots, peeled and chopped
- 2 celery stalks, diced
- 1 onion, chopped
- 1 teaspoon dried thyme
- ½ teaspoon garlic powder
- Freshly ground black pepper
- 1 (28-ounce) can no-salt diced tomatoes, drained
- 1 cup dry lentils
- 5 cups of water
- Salt

Directions:
1. Heat-up the oil in a large Dutch oven or pot over medium heat. Once the oil is simmering, add the carrot, celery, and onion. Cook, often stirring within 5 minutes.
2. Add the thyme, garlic powder, and black pepper. Cook within 30 seconds. Pour in the drained diced tomatoes and cook for a few more minutes, often stirring to enhance their flavor.
3. Put the lentils, water, plus a pinch of salt. Raise the heat and bring to a boil, then partially cover the pot and reduce heat to maintain a gentle simmer.
4. Cook within 30 minutes, or until lentils are tender but still hold their shape. Ladle into serving bowls and serve with a fresh green salad and whole-grain bread.

Nutrition: Calories: 168; Fat: 4g; Sodium: 130mg; Carbohydrate: 35g; Protein: 10g

886. Brown Rice Casserole with Cottage Cheese

Preparation time: 15 minutes
Cooking time: 45 minutes
Servings: 3
Ingredients:
- Nonstick cooking spray
- 1 cup quick-cooking brown rice
- 1 teaspoon olive oil
- ½ cup diced sweet onion
- 1 (10-ounce) bag of fresh spinach
- 1½ cups low-fat cottage cheese
- 1 tablespoon grated Parmesan cheese
- ¼ cup sunflower seed kernels

Directions:

1. Preheat the oven to 375°F. Spray a small 1½-quart casserole dish with cooking spray. Cook the rice, as stated in the package directions. Set aside.
2. Warm-up oil in a large nonstick skillet over medium-low heat. Add the onion and sauté for 3 to 4 minutes. Add the spinach and cover the skillet, cooking for 1 to 2 minutes until the spinach wilts. Remove the skillet from the heat.
3. In a medium bowl, mix the rice, spinach mixture, and cottage cheese. Transfer the mixture to the prepared casserole dish. Top with the Parmesan cheese and sunflower seeds, bake for 25 minutes until lightly browned, and serve.

Nutrition: Calories: 334; Fat: 9g; Carbohydrates: 47g; Fiber: 5g; Protein: 19g; Sodium: 425mg; Potassium: 553mg

887. Quinoa-Stuffed Peppers

Preparation time: 15 minutes
Cooking time: 35 minutes
Servings: 2
Ingredients:
- 2 large green bell peppers, halved
- 1½ teaspoons olive oil, divided
- ½ cup quinoa
- ½ cup minced onion
- 1 garlic clove, pressed or minced
- 1 cup chopped portobello mushrooms
- 3 tablespoons grated Parmesan cheese, divided
- 4 ounces tomato sauce

Directions:
1. Preheat the oven to 400°F. Put the pepper halves on your prepared baking sheet. Brush the insides of peppers with ½ teaspoon olive oil and bake for 10 minutes.
2. Remove the baking sheet, then set aside. While the peppers bake, cook the quinoa in a large saucepan over medium heat according to the package directions and set aside.
3. Warm-up the rest of the oil in a medium-size skillet over medium heat. Add the onion and sauté until it's translucent about 3 minutes. Put the garlic and cook within 1 minute.
4. Put the mushrooms in the skillet, adjust the heat to medium-low, cover, and cook within 5 to 6 minutes. Uncover, and if there's still liquid in the pan, reduce the heat and cook until the liquid evaporates.
5. Add the mushroom mixture, 1 tablespoon of Parmesan, and the tomato sauce to the quinoa and gently stir to combine. Carefully spoon the quinoa mixture into each pepper half and sprinkle with the remaining Parmesan. Return the peppers to the oven, bake for 10 to 15 more minutes until tender, and serve.

Nutrition: Calories: 292; Fat: 9g; Carbohydrates: 45g; Fiber: 8g; Protein: 12g; Sodium: 154mg; Potassium: 929mg

888. Greek Flatbread with Spinach, Tomatoes & Feta

Preparation time: 15 minutes
Cooking time: 9 minutes
Servings: 2

Ingredients:
- 2 cups fresh baby spinach, coarsely chopped
- 2 teaspoons olive oil
- 2 slices Naan, or another flatbread
- ¼ cup sliced black olives
- 2 plum tomatoes, thinly sliced
- 1 teaspoon salt-free Italian seasoning blend
- ¼ cup crumbled feta

Directions:
1. Preheat the oven to 400°F. Heat 3 tablespoons of water in a small skillet over medium heat. Add the spinach, cover, and steam until wilted, about 2 minutes. Drain off any excess water, then put aside.
2. Drizzle the oil evenly onto both flatbreads. Top each evenly with the spinach, olives, tomatoes, seasoning, and feta. Bake the flatbreads within 5 to 7 minutes, or until lightly browned. Cut each into four pieces and serve hot.

Nutrition: Calories: 411; Fat: 15g; Carbohydrates: 53g; Fiber: 7g; Protein: 15g; Sodium: 621mg; Potassium: 522mg

889. Mushroom Risotto with Peas

Preparation time: 15 minutes
Cooking time: 20 minutes
Servings: 2
Ingredients:
- 2 cups low-sodium vegetable or chicken broth
- 1 teaspoon olive oil
- 8 ounces baby portobello mushrooms, thinly sliced
- ½ cup frozen peas
- 1 teaspoon butter
- 1 cup Arborio rice
- 1 tablespoon grated Parmesan cheese

Directions:
1. Pour the broth into a microwave-proof glass measuring cup. Microwave on high for 1½ minutes or until hot. Warm-up oil over medium heat in a large saucepan. Add the mushrooms and stir for 1 minute. Cover and cook until soft, about 3 more minutes. Stir in the peas and reduce the heat to low.
2. Put the mushroom batter to the saucepan's sides and add the butter to the middle, heating until melted. Put the rice in the saucepan and stir for 1 to 2 minutes to lightly toast. Add the hot broth, ½ cup at a time, and stir gently.
3. As the broth is cooked into the rice, continue adding more broth, ½ cup at a time, stirring after each addition, until all broth is added. Once all of the liquid is absorbed (this should take 15 minutes), remove from the heat. Serve immediately, topped with Parmesan cheese.

Nutrition: Calories: 430; Fat: 6g; Carbohydrates: 83g; Fiber: 5g; Protein: 10g; Sodium: 78mg; Potassium: 558mg

890. Loaded Tofu Burrito with Black Beans

Preparation time: 15 minutes
Cooking time: 20 minutes
Servings: 2
Ingredients:

- 4 ounces extra-firm tofu, pressed and cut into 2-inch cubes
- 2 teaspoons mesquite salt-free seasoning, divided
- 2 teaspoons canola oil
- 1 cup thinly sliced bell peppers
- ½ cup diced onions
- 2/3 cup of black beans, drained
- 2 (10-inch) whole-wheat tortillas
- 1 tablespoon sriracha
- Nonfat Greek yogurt, for serving

Directions:
1. Put the tofu and 1 teaspoon of seasoning in a medium zip-top plastic freezer bag and toss until the tofu is well coated.
2. Heat-up the oil in a medium skillet over medium-high heat. Put the tofu in the skillet. Don't stir; allow the tofu to brown before turning. When lightly browned, about 6 minutes, transfer the tofu from the skillet to a small bowl and set aside.
3. Put the peppers plus onions in the skillet and sauté until tender, about 5 minutes. Lower the heat to medium-low, then put the beans and the remaining seasoning. Cook within 5 minutes.
4. For the burritos, lay each tortilla flat on a work surface. Place half of the tofu in the center of each tortilla, top with half of the pepper-bean mixture, and drizzle with the sriracha.
5. Fold the bottom portion of each tortilla up and over the tofu mixture. Then fold each side into the middle, tuck in, and tightly roll it up toward the open end. Serve with a dollop of yogurt.

Nutrition: Calories: 327; Fat: 12g; Carbohydrates: 41g; Fiber: 11g; Protein: 16g; Sodium: 282mg

891. Sweet Potato Rice with Spicy Peanut Sauce

Preparation time: 15 minutes
Cooking time: 25 minutes
Servings: 2
Ingredients:
- ½ cup basmati rice
- 2 teaspoons olive oil, divided
- 1 (8-ounce) can chickpeas, drained and rinsed
- 2 medium sweet potatoes, small cubes
- ¼ teaspoon ground cumin
- 1 cup of water
- 1/8 teaspoon salt
- 2 tablespoons chopped cilantro
- 3 tablespoons peanut butter
- 1 tablespoon sriracha
- 2 teaspoons reduced-sodium soy sauce
- ½ teaspoon garlic powder
- ¼ teaspoon ground ginger

Directions:
1. Heat-up 1 teaspoon of oil in a large nonstick skillet over medium-high heat. Add the chickpeas and heat for 3 minutes. Stir and cook until lightly browned. Transfer the chickpeas to a small bowl.
2. Put the rest of the1 teaspoon of oil to the skillet, then add the potatoes and cumin, distributing them evenly. Cook

the potatoes until they become lightly browned before turning them.
3. While the potatoes are cooking, boil the water with the salt in a large saucepan over medium-high heat. Put the rice in the boiling water, adjust the heat to low, cover, and simmer for 20 minutes.
4. When the potatoes have fully cooked, about 10 minutes in total, remove the skillet from the heat. Transfer the potatoes and chickpeas to the rice, folding all gently. Add the chopped cilantro.
5. In a small bowl, whisk the peanut butter, sriracha, soy sauce, garlic powder, and ginger until well blended. Divide the rice mixture between two serving bowls. Drizzle with the sauce and serve.

Nutrition: Calories: 667; Fat: 22g; Carbohydrates: 100g; Fiber: 14g; Protein: 20g; Sodium: 563mg; Potassium: 963mg

892. Vegetable Red Curry

Preparation time: 15 minutes
Cooking time: 25 minutes
Servings: 2
Ingredients:
- 2 teaspoons olive oil
- 1 cup sliced carrots
- ½ cup chopped onion
- 1 garlic clove, pressed or minced
- 2 bell peppers, seeded and thinly sliced
- 1 cup chopped cauliflower
- 2/3 cup light coconut milk
- ½ cup low-sodium vegetable broth
- 1 tablespoon tomato paste
- 1 teaspoon curry powder
- ½ teaspoon ground cumin
- ½ teaspoon ground coriander
- ¼ teaspoon turmeric
- 2 cups fresh baby spinach
- 1 cup quick-cooking brown rice

Directions:
1. Heat-up oil in a large nonstick skillet over medium heat. Add the carrots, onion, and garlic and cook for 2 to 3 minutes. Reduce the heat to medium-low, add the peppers and cauliflower to the skillet, cover, and cook within 5 minutes.
2. Add the coconut milk, broth, tomato paste, curry powder, cumin, coriander, and turmeric, stirring to combine. Simmer, covered (vent the lid slightly), for 10 to 15 minutes until the curry is slightly reduced and thickened.
3. Uncover, add the spinach, and stir for 2 minutes until it is wilted and mixed into the vegetables. Remove from the heat. Cook the rice as stated to the package instructions. Serve the curry over the rice.

Nutrition: Calories: 584; Fat: 16g; Carbohydrates: 101g; Fiber: 10g; Protein: 13g; Sodium: 102mg; Potassium: 1430mg

893. Black Bean Burgers

Preparation time: 15 minutes
Cooking time: 20 minutes
Servings: 4
Ingredients:

- ½ cup quick-cooking brown rice
- 2 teaspoons canola oil, divided
- ½ cup finely chopped carrots
- ¼ cup finely chopped onion
- 1 can black beans, drained
- 1 tablespoon salt-free mesquite seasoning blend
- 4 small, hard rolls

Directions:

1. Cook the rice as stated in the package directions and set aside. Heat-up 1 teaspoon of oil in a large nonstick skillet over medium heat. Add the carrots and onions and cook until the onions are translucent about 4 minutes. Adjust the heat to low, and cook again for 5 to 6 minutes, until the carrots are tender.
2. Add the beans and seasoning to the skillet and continue cooking for 2 to 3 more minutes. Pulse bean mixture in a food processor within 3 to 4 times or until the mixture is coarsely blended. Put the batter in a medium bowl and fold in the brown rice until well combined.
3. Divide the mixture evenly and form it into 4 patties with your hands. Heat the remaining oil in the skillet. Cook the patties within 4 to 5 minutes per side, turning once. Serve the burgers on the rolls with your choice of toppings.

Nutrition: Calories: 368; Fat: 6g; Carbohydrates: 66g; Fiber: 8g; Protein: 13g; Sodium: 322mg; Potassium: 413mg

894. Summer Barley Pilaf with Yogurt Dill Sauce

Preparation time: 15 minutes
Cooking time: 30 minutes
Servings: 3

Ingredients:

- 2 2/3 cups low-sodium vegetable broth
- 2 teaspoons avocado oil
- 1 small zucchini, diced
- 1/3 cup slivered almonds
- 2 scallions, sliced
- 1 cup barley
- ½ cup plain nonfat Greek yogurt
- 2 teaspoons grated lemon zest
- ¼ teaspoon dried dill

Directions:

1. Boil the broth in a large saucepan. Heat-up the oil in a skillet. Add the zucchini and sauté 3 to 4 minutes. Add the almonds and the white parts of the scallions and sauté for 2 minutes. Remove, and transfer it to a small bowl.
2. Add the barley to the skillet and sauté for 2 to 3 minutes to toast. Transfer the barley to the boiling broth and reduce the heat to low, cover, and simmer for 25 minutes or until tender. Remove, and let stand within 10 minutes or until the liquid is absorbed.
3. Simultaneously, mix the yogurt, lemon zest, and dill in a small bowl and set aside. Fluff the barley with a fork. Add the zucchini, almond, and onion mixture and mix gently. To serve, divide the pilaf between two bowls and drizzle the yogurt over each bowl.

Nutrition: Calories: 545; Fat: 15g; Carbohydrates: 87g; Fiber: 19g; Protein: 21g; Sodium: 37mg; Potassium: 694mg

895. Lentil Quinoa Gratin with Butternut Squash

Preparation time: 15 minutes
Cooking time: 1 hour & 15 minutes
Servings: 3

Ingredients:

- For the Lentils and Squash:
- Nonstick cooking spray
- 2 cups of water
- ½ cup dried green or red lentils, rinsed
- Pinch salt
- 1 teaspoon olive oil, divided
- ½ cup quinoa
- ¼ cup diced shallot
- 2 cups frozen cubed butternut squash
- ¼ cup low-fat milk
- 1 teaspoon chopped fresh rosemary
- Freshly ground black pepper
- For the Gratin Topping:
- ¼ cup panko bread crumbs
- 1 teaspoon olive oil
- 1/3 cup shredded Gruyere cheese

Directions:

5. Preheat the oven to 400°F. Spray a 1½-quart casserole dish or an 8-by-8-inch baking dish with cooking spray.
6. In a medium saucepan, stir the water, lentils, and salt and boil over medium-high heat. Lower the heat once the water is boiling, cover, and simmer for 20 to 25 minutes. Then drain and transfer the lentils to a large bowl and set aside.
7. In the same saucepan, heat-up ½ teaspoon of oil over medium heat. Add the quinoa and quickly stir for 1 minute to toast it lightly. Cook according to the package directions, about 20 minutes.
8. While the quinoa cooks, heat the remaining olive oil in a medium skillet over medium-low heat, add the shallots, and sauté them until they are translucent, about 3 minutes. Add the squash, milk, and rosemary and cook for 1 to 2 minutes.
9. Remove, then transfer to the lentil bowl. Add in the quinoa and gently toss all. Season with pepper to taste. Transfer the mixture to the casserole dish.
10. For the gratin topping, mix the panko bread crumbs with the olive oil in a small bowl. Put the bread crumbs over the casserole and top them with the cheese. Bake the casserole for 25 minutes and serve.

Nutrition: Calories: 576; Fat: 15g; Carbohydrates: 87g; Fiber: 12g; Protein: 28g; Sodium: 329mg; Potassium: 1176mg

896. Moroccan-Inspired Tagine with Chickpeas & Vegetables

Preparation time: 15 minutes
Cooking time: 45 minutes
Servings: 3

Ingredients:

- 2 teaspoons olive oil
- 1 cup chopped carrots

- ½ cup finely chopped onion
- 1 sweet potato, diced
- 1 cup low-sodium vegetable broth
- ¼ teaspoon ground cinnamon
- 1/8 teaspoon salt
- 1½ cups chopped bell peppers, any color
- 3 ripe plum tomatoes, chopped
- 1 tablespoon tomato paste
- 1 garlic clove, pressed or minced
- 1 (15-ounce) can chickpeas, drained and rinsed
- ½ cup chopped dried apricots
- 1 teaspoon curry powder
- ½ teaspoon paprika
- ½ teaspoon turmeric

Directions:
1. Warm-up oil over medium heat in a large Dutch oven or saucepan. Add the carrots and onion and cook until the onion is translucent about 4 minutes. Add the sweet potato, broth, cinnamon, and salt and cook for 5 to 6 minutes, until the broth is slightly reduced.
2. Add the peppers, tomatoes, tomato paste, and garlic. Stir and cook for another 5 minutes. Add the chickpeas, apricots, curry powder, paprika, and turmeric to the pot. Bring all to a boil, then reduce the heat to low, cover, simmer for about 30 minutes, and serve.

Nutrition: Calories: 469; Fat: 9g; Carbohydrates: 88g; Protein: 16g; Sodium: 256mg

897. Spaghetti Squash with Maple Glaze & Tofu Crumbles

Preparation time: 15 minutes
Cooking time: 22 minutes
Servings: 3
Ingredients:
- 2 ounces firm tofu, well-drained
- 1 small spaghetti squash, halved lengthwise
- 2½ teaspoons olive oil, divided
- 1/8 teaspoon salt
- ½ cup chopped onion
- 1 teaspoon dried rosemary
- ¼ cup dry white wine
- 2 tablespoons maple syrup
- ½ teaspoon garlic powder
- ¼ cup shredded Gruyere cheese

Directions:
1. Put the tofu in a large mesh colander and place over a large bowl to drain. Score the squash using a paring knife so the steam can vent while it cooks. Place the squash in a medium microwave-safe dish and microwave on high for 5 minutes. Remove the squash from the microwave and allow it to cool.
2. Cut the cooled squash in half on a cutting board. Remove the seeds, then put the squash halves into a 9-by-11-inch baking dish.
3. Drizzle the squash with half a teaspoon of olive oil and season it with the salt, then wrap it using wax paper and put it back in the microwave for 5 more minutes on high. Once it's cooked, scrape the squash strands with a fork into a small bowl and cover it to keep it warm.

4. While the squash is cooking, heat 1 teaspoon of oil in a large skillet over medium-high heat. Put the onion and sauté for within minutes. Add the rosemary and stir for 1 minute, until fragrant.
5. Put the rest of the oil in the same skillet. Crumble the tofu into the skillet, stir fry until lightly browned, about 4 minutes, and transfer it to a small bowl.
6. Add the wine, maple syrup, and garlic powder to the skillet and stir to combine. Cook for 2 minutes until slightly reduced and thickened. Remove from the heat. Evenly divide the squash between two plates, then top it with the tofu mixture. Drizzle the maple glaze over the top, then add the grated cheese.

Nutrition: Calories: 330; Fat: 15g; Carbohydrates: 36g; Fiber: 5g; Protein: 12g; Sodium: 326mg; Potassium: 474mg

898. Stuffed Tex-Mex Baked Potatoes

Preparation time: 15 minutes
Cooking time: 45 minutes
Servings: 2
Ingredients:
- 2 large Idaho potatoes
- ½ cup black beans, rinsed and drained
- ¼ cup store-bought salsa
- 1 avocado, diced
- 1 teaspoon freshly squeezed lime juice
- ½ cup nonfat plain Greek yogurt
- ¼ teaspoon reduced-sodium taco seasoning
- ¼ cup shredded sharp cheddar cheese

Directions:
1. Preheat the oven to 400°F. Scrub the potatoes, then slice an "X" into the top of each using a paring knife. Put the potatoes on the oven rack, then bake for 45 minutes until they are tender.
2. In a small bowl, stir the beans and salsa and set aside. In another small bowl, mix the avocado and lime juice and set aside. In a third small bowl, stir the yogurt and the taco seasoning until well blended.
3. When the potatoes are baked, carefully open them up. Top each potato with the bean and salsa mixture, avocado, seasoned yogurt, and cheddar cheese, evenly dividing each component, and serve.

Nutrition: Calories: 624; Fat: 21g; Carbohydrates: 91g; Fiber: 21g; Protein: 24g; Sodium: 366mg; Potassium: 2134mg

899. Lentil-Stuffed Zucchini Boats

Preparation time: 15 minutes
Cooking time: 45 minutes
Servings: 2
Ingredients:
- 2 medium zucchinis, halved lengthwise and seeded
- 2¼ cups water, divided
- 1 cup green or red lentils, dried & rinsed
- 2 teaspoons olive oil
- 1/3 cup diced onion
- 2 tablespoons tomato paste

- ½ teaspoon oregano
- ¼ teaspoon garlic powder
- Pinch salt
- ¼ cup grated part-skim mozzarella cheese

Directions:
1. Preheat the oven to 375°F. Line a baking sheet with parchment paper. Place the zucchini, hollow sides up, on the baking sheet, and set aside.
2. Boil 2 cups of water to a boil over high heat in a medium saucepan and add the lentils. Lower the heat, then simmer within 20 to 25 minutes. Drain and set aside.
3. Heat-up the olive oil in a medium skillet over medium-low heat. Sauté the onions until they are translucent, about 4 minutes. Lower the heat and add the cooked lentils, tomato paste, oregano, garlic powder, and salt.
4. Add the last quarter cup of water and simmer for 3 minutes, until the liquid reduces and forms a sauce. Remove from heat.
5. Stuff each zucchini half with the lentil mixture, dividing it evenly, and top with cheese, bake for 25 minutes and serve. The zucchini should be fork-tender, and the cheese should be melted.

Nutrition: Calories: 479; Fat: 9g; Carbohydrates: 74g; Fiber: 14g; Protein: 31g; Sodium: 206mg; Potassium: 1389mg

900. Baked Eggplant Parmesan

Preparation time: 15 minutes
Cooking time: 35 minutes
Servings: 4
Ingredients:

- 1 small to medium eggplant, cut into ¼-inch slices
- ½ teaspoon salt-free Italian seasoning blend
- 1 tablespoon olive oil
- ¼ cup diced onion
- ½ cup diced yellow or red bell pepper
- 2 garlic cloves, pressed or minced
- 1 (8-ounce) can tomato sauce
- 3 ounces fresh mozzarella, cut into 6 pieces
- 1 tablespoon grated Parmesan cheese, divided
- 5 to 6 fresh basil leaves, chopped

Directions:
1. Preheat an oven-style air fryer to 400°F.
2. Working in two batches, place the eggplant slices onto the air-fryer tray and sprinkle them with Italian seasoning. Bake for 7 minutes. Repeat with the remaining slices, then set them aside on a plate.
3. In a medium skillet, heat the oil over medium heat and sauté the onion and peppers until softened about 5 minutes. Add the garlic and sauté for 1 to 2 more minutes. Add the tomato sauce and stir to combine. Remove the sauce from the heat.
4. Spray a 9-by-6-inch casserole dish with cooking spray. Spread one-third of the sauce into the bottom of the dish. Layer eggplant slices onto the sauce. Sprinkle with half of the Parmesan cheese.
5. Continue layering the sauce and eggplant, ending with the sauce. Place the mozzarella pieces on the top. Sprinkle the remaining Parmesan evenly over the entire dish. Bake in the oven for 20 minutes. Garnish with fresh basil, cut into four servings, and serve.

Nutrition: Calories: 213; Fat: 12g; Carbohydrates: 20g; Fiber: 7g; Protein: 10g; Sodium: 222mg; Potassium: 763mg

SNACK AND DESSERTS

901. The Mean Green Smoothie

Preparation time: 5 minutes
Cooking time: 10 minutes
Serving: 2
Ingredients:

- 1 avocado
- 1 handful spinach, chopped
- Cucumber, 2 inch slices, peeled
- 1 lime, chopped
- Handful of grapes, chopped
- 5 dates, stoned and chopped
- 1 cup apple juice (fresh)

Directions:
1. Add all the listed ingredients to your blender.
2. Blend until smooth.
3. Add a few ice cubes and serve the smoothie.
4. Enjoy!

Nutrition: Calories: 200; Fat: 10g; Carbohydrates: 14g; Protein 2g

902. Mint Flavored Pear Smoothie

Preparation time: 5 minutes
Cooking time: 5 minutes
Serving: 2
Ingredients:

- ¼ honey dew
- 2 green pears, ripe
- ½ apple, juiced
- 1 cup ice cubes
- ½ cup fresh mint leaves

Directions:
1. Add the listed ingredients to your blender and blend until smooth.
2. Serve chilled!

Nutrition: Calories: 200; Fat: 10g; Carbohydrates: 14g; Protein 2g

903. Chilled Watermelon Smoothie

Preparation time: 5 minutes
Cooking time: 10 minutes
Serving: 2
Ingredients:
- 1 cup watermelon chunks
- ½ cup coconut water
- 1 ½ teaspoons lime juice
- 4 mint leaves
- 4 ice cubes

Directions:
1. Add the listed ingredients to your blender and blend until smooth.
2. Serve chilled!

Nutrition: Calories: 200; Fat: 10g; Carbohydrates: 14g; Protein 2g

904. Banana Ginger Medley

Preparation time: 5 minutes
Cooking time: 10 minutes
Serving: 2
Ingredients:
- 1 banana, sliced
- ¾ cup vanilla yogurt
- 1 tablespoon honey
- ½ teaspoon ginger, grated

Directions:
1. Add the listed ingredients to your blender and blend until smooth.
2. Serve chilled!

Nutrition: Calories: 200; Fat: 10g; Carbohydrates: 14g; Protein 2g

905. Banana and Almond Flax Glass

Preparation time: 5 minutes
Cooking time: 10 minutes
Serving: 2
Ingredients:
- 1 ripe frozen banana, diced
- 2/3 cup unsweetened almond milk
- 1/3 cup fat free plain Greek Yogurt
- 1 ½ tablespoons almond butter
- 1 tablespoon flaxseed meal
- 1 teaspoon honey
- 2-3 drops almond extract

Directions:
1. Add the listed ingredients to your blender and blend until smooth
2. Serve chilled!

Nutrition: Calories: 200; Fat: 10g; Carbohydrates: 14g; Protein 2g

906. Sensational Strawberry Medley

Preparation time: 5 minutes
Cooking time: 10 minutes
Serving: 2
Ingredients:
- 1-2 handful baby greens
- 3 medium kale leaves
- 5-8 mint leaves
- 1 inch piece ginger , peeled
- 1 avocado
- 1 cup strawberries
- 6-8 ounces coconut water + 6-8 ounces filtered water
- Fresh juice of one lime
- 1-2 teaspoon olive oil

Directions:
1. Add all the listed ingredients to your blender.
2. Blend until smooth.
3. Add a few ice cubes and serve the smoothie.
4. Enjoy!

Nutrition: Calories: 200; Fat: 10g; Carbohydrates: 14g; Protein 2g

907. Sweet Almond and Coconut Fat Bombs

Preparation time: 10 minutes
Cooking Time: /Freeze Time: 20 minutes
Serving: 6
Ingredients:
- ¼ cup melted coconut oil
- 9 ½ tablespoons almond butter
- 90 drops liquid stevia
- 3 tablespoons cocoa
- 9 tablespoons melted butter, salted

Directions:
1. Take a bowl and add all of the listed ingredients.
2. Mix them well.
3. Pour scant 2 tablespoons of the mixture into as many muffin molds as you like.
4. Chill for 20 minutes and pop them out.
5. Serve and enjoy!

Nutrition: Total Carbs: 2g; Fiber: 0g; Protein: 2.53g; Fat: 14g

908. Almond and Tomato Balls

Preparation time: 10 minutes
Cooking Time: Freeze Time: 20 minutes
Servings: 6
Ingredients:
- 1/3 cup pistachios, de-shelled
- 10 ounces cream cheese
- 1/3 cup sun dried tomatoes, diced

Directions:
1. Chop pistachios into small pieces.
2. Add cream cheese, tomatoes in a bowl and mix well.
3. Chill for 15-20 minutes and turn into balls.

4. Roll into pistachios.
5. Serve and enjoy!
Nutrition: Carb: 183; Fat: 18g; Carb: 5g; Protein: 5g

909. Avocado Tuna Bites

Preparation time: 10 minutes
Cooking Time: Nil
Serving: 4
Ingredients:
1/3 cup coconut oil
1 avocado, cut into cubes
10 ounces canned tuna, drained
¼ cup parmesan cheese, grated
¼ teaspoon garlic powder
1/4 teaspoon onion powder
1/3 cup almond flour
¼ teaspoon pepper
¼ cup low fat mayonnaise
Pepper as needed
Directions:
Take a bowl and add tuna, mayo, flour, parmesan, spices and mix well.
Fold in avocado and make 12 balls out of the mixture.
Melt coconut oil in pan and cook over medium heat, until all sides are golden.
Serve and enjoy!
Nutrition: Calories: 185; Fat: 18g; Carbohydrates: 1g; Protein: 5g

910. Mediterranean Pop Corn Bites

Preparation time: 5 minutes + 20 minutes chill time
Cooking Time: 2-3 minutes
Servings: 4
Ingredients:
- 3 cups Medjool dates, chopped
- 12 ounces brewed coffee
- 1 cup pecan, chopped
- ½ cup coconut, shredded
- ½ cup cocoa powder
Directions:
1. Soak dates in warm coffee for 5 minutes.
2. Remove dates from coffee and mash them, making a fine smooth mixture.
3. Stir in remaining ingredients (except cocoa powder) and form small balls out of the mixture.
4. Coat with cocoa powder, serve and enjoy!
Nutrition: Calories: 265; Fat: 12g; Carbohydrates: 43g; Protein 3g

911. Hearty Buttery Walnuts

Preparation time: 10 minutes
Cooking Time: Nil
Serving: 4
Ingredients:
- 4 walnut halves
- ½ tablespoon almond butter
Directions:

1. Spread butter over two walnut halves.
2. Top with other halves.
3. Serve and enjoy!
Nutrition: Calories: 90; Fat: 10g; Carbohydrates: 0g; Protein: 1g

912. Refreshing Watermelon Sorbet

Preparation time: 20 minutes + 20 hours chill time
Cooking Time: Nil
Serving: 4
Ingredients:
- 4 cups watermelon, seedless and chunked
- ¼ cup coconut sugar
- 2 tablespoons lime juice
Directions:
1. Add the listed ingredients to a blender and puree.
2. Transfer to a freezer container with a tight-fitting lid.
3. Freeze the mix for about 4-6 hours until you have gelatin-like consistency.
4. Puree the mix once again in batches and return to the container.
5. Chill overnight.
6. Allow the sorbet to stand for 5 minutes before serving and enjoy!
Nutrition: Calories: 91; Fat: 0g; Carbohydrates: 25g; Protein: 1g

913. Refreshing Mango and Pear Smoothie

Preparation time: 10 minutes
Cooking Time: Nil
Serving: 1
Ingredients:
- 1 ripe mango, cored and chopped
- ½ mango, peeled, pitted and chopped
- 1 cup kale, chopped
- ½ cup plain Greek yogurt
- 2 ice cubes
Directions:
1. Add pear, mango, yogurt, kale, and mango to a blender and puree.
2. Add ice and blend until you have a smooth texture.
3. Serve and enjoy!
Nutrition: Calories: 293; Fat: 8g; Carbohydrates: 53g; Protein: 8g

914. Epic Pineapple Juice

Preparation time: 10 minutes
Cooking Time: Nil
Serving: 4
Ingredients:
- 4 cups fresh pineapple, chopped
- 1 pinch sunflower seeds
- 1 ½ cups water
Directions:
1. Add the listed ingredients to your blender and blend well until you have a smoothie-like texture.

2. Chill and serve.
3. Enjoy!
Nutrition: Calories: 82; Fat: 0.2g; Carbohydrates: 21g; Protein: 21

915. Choco Lovers Strawberry Shake

Preparation time: 10 minutes
Serving: 1
Ingredients:
- ½ cup heavy cream, liquid
- 1 tablespoons cocoa powder
- 1 pack stevia
- ½ cup strawberry, sliced
- 1 tablespoon coconut flakes, unsweetened
- 1 ½ cups water

Directions:
1. Add listed ingredients to blender.
2. Blend until you have a smooth and creamy texture.
3. Serve chilled and enjoy!
Nutrition: Calories: 470; Fat: 46g; Carbohydrates: 15g; Protein: 4g

916. Healthy Coffee Smoothie

Preparation time: 10 minutes
Cooking time: 20 minutes
Serving: 1
Ingredients:
- 1 tablespoon chia seeds
- 2 cups strongly brewed coffee, chilled
- 1 ounce Macadamia Nuts
- 1-2 packets stevia, optional
- 1 tablespoon MCT oil

Directions:
1. Add all the listed ingredients to a blender.
2. Blend on high until smooth and creamy.
3. Enjoy your smoothie.
Nutrition: Calories: 395; Fat: 39g; Carbohydrates: 11g; Protein: 5.2g

917. Blackberry and Apple Smoothie

Preparation time: 5 minutes
Cooking time: 20 minutes
Serving: 2
Ingredients:
- 2 cups frozen blackberries
- ½ cup apple cider
- 1 apple, cubed
- 2/3 cup non-fat lemon yogurt

Directions:
1. Add the listed ingredients to your blender and blend until smooth.
2. Serve chilled!
Nutrition: Calories: 200; Fat: 10g; Carbohydrates: 14g; Protein 2g

918. Tasty Mediterranean Peanut Almond butter Popcorns

Preparation time: 5 minutes + 20 minutes chill time
Cooking Time: 2-3 minutes
Servings: 4
Ingredients:
- 3 cups Medjool dates, chopped
- 12 ounces brewed coffee
- 1 cup pecans, chopped
- ½ cup coconut, shredded
- ½ cup cocoa powder

Directions:
1. Soak dates in warm coffee for 5 minutes.
2. Remove dates from coffee and mash them, making a fine smooth mixture.
3. Stir in remaining ingredients (except cocoa powder) and form small balls out of the mixture.
4. Coat with cocoa powder, serve and enjoy!
Nutrition: Calories: 265; Fat: 12g; Carbohydrates: 43g; Protein 3g

919. Just a Minute worth Muffin

Preparation time: 5 minutes
Cooking Time: 1 minutes
Serving: 2
Ingredients:
- Coconut oil for grease
- 2 teaspoons coconut flour
- 1 pinch baking soda
- 1 pinch sunflower seeds
- 1 whole egg

Directions:
1. Grease ramekin dish with coconut oil and keep it on the side.
2. Add ingredients to a bowl and combine until no lumps.
3. Pour batter into ramekin.
4. Microwave for 1 minute on HIGH.
5. Slice in half and serve.
6. Enjoy!
Nutrition: Total Carbs: 5.4; Fiber: 2g; Protein: 7.3g

920. Hearty Almond Bread

Preparation time: 15 minutes
Cooking Time: 60 minutes
Serving: 8
Ingredients:
- 3 cups almond flour
- 1 teaspoon baking soda
- 2 teaspoons baking powder
- ¼ teaspoon sunflower seeds
- ¼ cup almond milk
- ½ cup + 2 tablespoons olive oil
- 3 whole eggs

Directions:

1. Preheat your oven to 300 degrees F.
2. Take a 9x5 inch loaf pan and grease, keep it on the side.
3. Add listed ingredients to a bowl and pour the batter into the loaf pan.
4. Bake for 60 minutes.
5. Once baked, remove from oven and let it cool.
6. Slice and serve!

Nutrition: Calories: 277; Fat: 21g; Carbohydrates: 7g; Protein: 10g

921. Mixed Berries Smoothie

Preparation time: 4 minutes
Cooking Time: 0 minutes
Serving: 2
Ingredients:
- ¼ cup frozen blueberries
- ¼ cup frozen blackberries
- 1 cup unsweetened almond milk
- 1 teaspoon vanilla bean extract
- 3 teaspoons flaxseeds
- 1 scoop chilled Greek yogurt
- Stevia as needed

Directions:
1. Mix everything in a blender and emulsify.
2. Pulse the mixture four time until you have your desired thickness.
3. Pour the mixture into a glass and enjoy!

Nutrition: Calories: 221; Fat: 9g; Protein: 21g; Carbohydrates: 10g

922. Satisfying Berry and Almond Smoothie

Preparation time: 10 minutes
Cooking Time: Nil
Serving: 4
Ingredients:
- 1 cup blueberries, frozen
- 1 whole banana
- ½ cup almond milk
- 1 tablespoon almond butter
- Water as needed

Directions:
1. Add the listed ingredients to your blender and blend well until you have a smoothie-like texture.
2. Chill and serve.
3. Enjoy!

Nutrition: Calories: 321; Fat: 11g; Carbohydrates: 55g; Protein: 5g

923. Decisive Lime and Strawberry Popsicle

Preparation time: 2 hours
Cooking Time: Nil
Serving: 4
Ingredients:
- 1 tablespoon lime juice, fresh
- ¼ cup strawberries, hulled and sliced
- ¼ cup coconut almond milk, unsweetened and full fat

- 2 teaspoons natural sweetener

Directions:
1. Blend the listed ingredients in a blender until smooth.
2. Pour mix into Popsicle molds and let them chill for 2 hours.
3. Serve and enjoy!

Nutrition: Calories: 166; Fat: 17g; Carbohydrates: 3g; Protein: 1g

924. Ravaging Blueberry Muffin

Preparation time: 10 minutes
Cooking Time: 30 minutes
Serving: 4
Ingredients:
- 1 cup almond flour
- Pinch of sunflower seeds
- 1/8 teaspoon baking soda
- 1 whole egg
- 2 tablespoons coconut oil, melted
- ½ cup coconut almond milk
- ¼ cup fresh blueberries

Directions:
1. Preheat your oven to 350 degrees F.
2. Line a muffin tin with paper muffin cups.
3. Add almond flour, sunflower seeds, baking soda to a bowl and mix, keep it on the side.
4. Take another bowl and add egg, coconut oil, coconut almond milk and mix.
5. Add mix to flour mix and gently combine until incorporated.
6. Mix in blueberries and fill the cupcakes tins with batter.
7. Bake for 20-25 minutes.
8. Enjoy!

Nutrition: Calories: 167; Fat: 15g; Carbohydrates: 2.1g; Protein: 5.2g

925. The Coconut Loaf

Preparation time: 15 minutes
Cooking Time: 40 minutes
Serving: 4
Ingredients:
- 1 ½ tablespoons coconut flour
- ¼ teaspoon baking powder
- 1/8 teaspoon sunflower seeds
- 1 tablespoons coconut oil, melted
- 1 whole egg

Directions:
1. Preheat your oven to 350 degrees F.
2. Add coconut flour, baking powder, sunflower seeds.
3. Add coconut oil, eggs and stir well until mixed.
4. Leave batter for several minutes.
5. Pour half batter onto baking pan.
6. Spread it to form a circle, repeat with remaining batter.
7. Bake in oven for 10 minutes.
8. Once you have a golden-brown texture, let it cool and serve.
9. Enjoy!

Nutrition: Calories: 297; Fat: 14g; Carbohydrates: 15g; Protein: 15g

926. Fresh Figs with Walnuts and Ricotta

Preparation time: 5 minutes
Cooking Time: 2-3 minutes
Servings: 4
Ingredients:
- 8 dried figs, halved
- ¼ cup ricotta cheese
- 16 walnuts, halved
- 1 tablespoon honey

Directions:
1. Take a skillet and place it over medium heat, add walnuts and toast for 2 minutes.
2. Top figs with cheese and walnuts.
3. Drizzle honey on top.
4. Enjoy!

Nutrition: Calories: 142; Fat: 8g; Carbohydrates: 10g; Protein: 4g

927. Authentic Medjool Date Truffles

Preparation time: 10-15 minutes
Cooking Time: Nil
Serving: 4
Ingredients:
- 2 tablespoons peanut oil
- ½ cup popcorn kernels
- 1/3 cup peanuts, chopped
- 1/3 cup peanut almond butter
- ¼ cup wildflower honey

Directions:
1. Take a pot and add popcorn kernels, peanut oil.
2. Place it over medium heat and shake the pot gently until all corn has popped.
3. Take a saucepan and add honey, gently simmer for 2-3 minutes.
4. Add peanut almond butter and stir.
5. Coat popcorn with the mixture and enjoy!

Nutrition: Calories: 430; Fat: 20g; Carbohydrates: 56g; Protein 9g

928. Fennel and Almond Bites

Preparation time: 10 minutes
Cooking Time: None Freeze Time: 3 hours
Servings: 12
Ingredients:
- 1 teaspoon vanilla extract
- ¼ cup almond milk
- ¼ cup cocoa powder
- ½ cup almond oil
- A pinch of sunflower seeds
- 1 teaspoon fennel seeds

Directions:
6. Take a bowl and mix the almond oil and almond milk.
7. Beat until smooth and glossy using electric beater.
8. Mix in the rest of the ingredients.
9. Take a piping bag and pour into a parchment paper lined baking sheet.

10. Freeze for 3 hours and store in the fridge.
Nutrition: Total Carbs: 1g; Fiber: 1g; Protein: 1g; Fat: 20g

929. Feisty Coconut Fudge

Preparation time: 20 minutes
Cooking Time: None Freeze Time: 2 hours
Servings: 12
Ingredients:
- ¼ cup coconut, shredded
- 2 cups coconut oil
- ½ cup coconut cream
- ¼ cup almonds, chopped
- 1 teaspoon almond extract
- A pinch of sunflower seeds
- Stevia to taste

Directions:
8. Take a large bowl and pour coconut cream and coconut oil into it.
9. Whisk using an electric beater.
10. Whisk until the mixture becomes smooth and glossy.
11. Add cocoa powder slowly and mix well.
12. Add in the rest of the ingredients.
13. Pour into a bread pan lined with parchment paper.
14. Freeze until set.
15. Cut them into squares and serve.

Nutrition: Total Carbs: 1g; Fiber: 1g; Protein: 0g; Fat: 20g

930. No Bake Cheesecake

Preparation time: 120 minutes
Cooking Time: Nil
Serving: 10
Ingredients:
- For Crust
- 2 tablespoons ground flaxseeds
- 2 tablespoons desiccated coconut
- 1 teaspoon cinnamon
- For Filling
- 4 ounces vegan cream cheese
- 1 cup cashews, soaked
- ½ cup frozen blueberries
- 2 tablespoons coconut oil
- 1 tablespoon lemon juice
- 1 teaspoon vanilla extract
- Liquid stevia

Directions:
6. Take a container and mix in the crust ingredients, mix well.
7. Flatten the mixture at the bottom to prepare the crust of your cheesecake.
8. Take a blender/ food processor and add the filling ingredients, blend until smooth.
9. Gently pour the batter on top of your crust and chill for 2 hours.
10. Serve and enjoy!

Nutrition: Calories: 182; Fat: 16g; Carbohydrates: 4g; Protein: 3g

931. Easy Chia Seed Pumpkin Pudding

Preparation time: 10-15 minutes/ overnight chill time
Cooking Time: Nil
Serving: 4
Ingredients:
- 1 cup maple syrup
- 2 teaspoons pumpkin spice
- 1 cup pumpkin puree
- 1 ¼ cup almond milk
- ½ cup chia seeds

Directions:
1. Add all of the ingredients to a bowl and gently stir.
2. Let it refrigerate overnight or at least 15 minutes.
3. Top with your desired ingredients, such as blueberries, almonds, etc.
4. Serve and enjoy!

Nutrition: Calories: 230; Fat: 10g; Carbohydrates: 22g; Protein: 11g

932. Lovely Blueberry Pudding

Preparation time: 20 minutes
Cooking Time: Nil
Serving: 4
Ingredients:
- 2 cups frozen blueberries
- 2 teaspoons lime zest, grated freshly
- 20 drops liquid stevia
- 2 small avocados, peeled, pitted and chopped
- ½ teaspoon fresh ginger, grated freshly
- 4 tablespoons fresh lime juice
- 10 tablespoons water

Directions:
1. Add all of the listed ingredients to a blender (except blueberries) and pulse the mixture well.
2. Transfer the mix into small serving bowls and chill the bowls.
3. Serve with a topping of blueberries.
4. Enjoy!

Nutrition: Calories: 166; Fat: 13g; Carbohydrates: 13g; Protein: 1.7g

933. Heart Warming Cinnamon Rice Pudding

Preparation time: 10 minutes
Cooking Time: 5 hours
Servings: 4
Ingredients:
- 6 ½ cups water
- 1 cup coconut sugar
- 2 cups white rice
- 2 cinnamon sticks
- ½ cup coconut, shredded

Directions:
1. Add water, rice, sugar, cinnamon and coconut to your Slow Cooker.

2. Gently stir.
3. Place lid and cook on HIGH for 5 hours.
4. Discard cinnamon.
5. Divide pudding between dessert dishes and enjoy!

Nutrition: Calories: 173; Fat: 4g; Carbohydrates: 9g; Protein: 4g

934. Pure Avocado Pudding

Preparation time: 3 hours
Cooking Time: Nil
Serving: 4
Ingredients:
- 1 cup almond milk
- 2 avocados, peeled and pitted
- ¾ cup cocoa powder
- 1 teaspoon vanilla extract
- 2 tablespoons stevia
- ¼ teaspoon cinnamon
- Walnuts, chopped for serving

Directions:
1. Add avocados to a blender and pulse well.
2. Add cocoa powder, almond milk, stevia, vanilla bean extract and pulse the mixture well.
3. Pour into serving bowls and top with walnuts.
4. Chill for 2-3 hours and serve!

Nutrition: Calories: 221; Fat: 8g; Carbohydrates: 7g; Protein: 3g

935. Sweet Almond and Coconut Fat Bombs

Preparation time: 10 minutes
Cooking Time: 20 minutes
Freeze Time: 20 minutes
Serving: 6
Ingredients:
- ¼ cup melted coconut oil
- 9 ½ tablespoons almond butter
- 90 drops liquid stevia
- 3 tablespoons cocoa
- 9 tablespoons melted almond butter, sunflower seeds

Directions:
1. Take a bowl and add all of the listed ingredients.
2. Mix them well.
3. Pour 2 tablespoons of the mixture into as many muffin molds as you like.
4. Chill for 20 minutes and pop them out.
5. Serve and enjoy!

Nutrition: Total Carbs: 2g; Fiber: 0g; Protein: 2.53g; Fat: 14g

936. Spicy Popper Mug Cake

Preparation time: 5 minutes
Cooking Time: 5 minutes
Serving: 2
Ingredients:
- 2 tablespoons almond flour
- 1 tablespoon flaxseed meal
- 1 tablespoon almond butter

- 1 tablespoon cream cheese
- 1 large egg
- 1 bacon, cooked and sliced
- ½ jalapeno pepper
- ½ teaspoon baking powder
- ¼ teaspoon sunflower seeds

Directions:
1. Take a frying pan and place it over medium heat.
2. Add slice of bacon and cook until it has a crispy texture.
3. Take a microwave proof container and mix all of the listed ingredients (including cooked bacon), clean the sides.
4. Microwave for 75 seconds, making to put your microwave to high power.
5. Take out the cup and tap it against a surface to take the cake out.
6. Garnish with a bit of jalapeno and serve!

Nutrition: Calories: 429; Fat: 38g; Carbohydrates: 6g; Protein: 16g

937. The Most Elegant Parsley Soufflé Ever

Preparation time: 5 minutes
Cooking Time: 6 minutes
Serving: 5
Ingredients:
- 2 whole eggs
- 1 fresh red chili pepper, chopped
- 2 tablespoons coconut cream
- 1 tablespoon fresh parsley, chopped
- Sunflower seeds to taste

Directions:
1. Preheat your oven to 390 degrees F.
2. Almond butter 2 soufflé dishes.
3. Add the ingredients to a blender and mix well.
4. Divide batter into soufflé dishes and bake for 6 minutes.
5. Serve and enjoy!

Nutrition: Calories: 108; Fat: 9g; Carbohydrates: 9g; Protein: 6g

938. Mesmerizing Avocado and Chocolate Pudding

Preparation time: 30 minutes
Cooking Time: Nil
Serving: 2
Ingredients:
- 1 avocado, chunked
- 1 tablespoon natural sweetener such as stevia
- 2 ounces cream cheese, at room temp
- ¼ teaspoon vanilla extract
- 4 tablespoons cocoa powder, unsweetened

Directions:
3. Blend listed ingredients in blender until smooth.
4. Divide the mix between dessert bowls, chill for 30 minutes.
5. Serve and enjoy!

Nutrition: Calories: 281; Fat: 27g; Carbohydrates: 12g; Protein: 8g

939. Hearty Pineapple Pudding

Preparation time: 10 minutes
Cooking Time: 5 hours
serving: 4
Ingredients:
- 1 teaspoon baking powder
- 1 cup coconut flour
- 3 tablespoons stevia
- 3 tablespoons avocado oil
- ½ cup coconut milk
- ½ cup pecans, chopped
- ½ cup pineapple, chopped
- ½ cup lemon zest, grated
- 1 cup pineapple juice, natural

Directions:
3. Grease Slow Cooker with oil.
4. Take a bowl and mix in flour, stevia, baking powder, oil, milk, pecans, pineapple, lemon zest, pineapple juice and stir well.
5. Pour the mix into the Slow Cooker.
6. Place lid and cook on LOW for 5 hours.
7. Divide between bowls and serve.
8. Enjoy!

Nutrition: Calories: 188; Fat: 3g; Carbohydrates: 14g; Protein: 5g

940. Healthy Berry Cobbler

Preparation time: 10 minutes
Cooking Time: 2 hours 30 minutes
Serving: 8
Ingredients:
- 1 ¼ cups almond flour
- 1 cup coconut sugar
- 1 teaspoon baking powder
- ½ teaspoon cinnamon powder
- 1 whole egg
- ¼ cup low-fat milk
- 2 tablespoons olive oil
- 2 cups raspberries
- 2 cups blueberries

Directions:
4. Take a bowl and add almond flour, coconut sugar, baking powder and cinnamon.
5. Stir well.
6. Take another bowl and add egg, milk, oil, raspberries, blueberries and stir.
7. Combine both of the mixtures.
8. Grease your Slow Cooker.
9. Pour the combined mixture into your Slow Cooker and cook on HIGH for 2 hours 30 minutes.
10. Divide between serving bowls and enjoy!

Nutrition: Calories: 250; Fat: 4g; Carbohydrates: 30g; Protein: 3g

941. Tasty Poached Apples

Preparation time: 10 minutes
Cooking Time: 2 hours 30 minutes

Serving: 8
Ingredients:
- 6 apples, cored, peeled and sliced
- 1 cup apple juice, natural
- 1 cup coconut sugar
- 1 tablespoon cinnamon powder

Directions:
4. Grease Slow Cooker with cooking spray.
5. Add apples, sugar, juice, cinnamon to your Slow Cooker.
6. Stir gently.
7. Place lid and cook on HIGH for 4 hours.
8. Serve cold and enjoy!

Nutrition: Calories: 180; Fat: 5g; Carbohydrates: 8g; Protein: 4g

942. Home Made Trail Mix for the Trip

Preparation time: 10 minutes
Cooking Time: 55 minutes
Serving: 4
Ingredients:
- ¼ cup raw cashews
- ¼ cup almonds
- ¼ cup walnuts
- 1 teaspoon cinnamon
- 2 tablespoons melted coconut oil
- Sunflower seeds as needed

Directions:
4. The side.
5. Combine nuts to large mixing bowl and add cinnamon and melted coconut oil.
6. Stir. Line baking sheet with parchment paper.
7. Preheat your oven to 275 degrees F.
8. Melt coconut oil and keep it on
9. Sprinkle sunflower seeds.
10. Place in oven and brown for 6 minutes.
11. Enjoy!

Nutrition: Calories: 363; Fat: 22g; Carbohydrates: 41g; Protein: 7g

943. Mini Teriyaki Turkey Sandwiches

Preparation time: 20 minutes
Cooking Time: 30 minutes
Servings: 20
Ingredients:
- 2 chicken breast halves
- 1 cup soy sauce, low-salt
- ¼ cup cider vinegar
- 3 minced garlic cloves
- 1 tablespoon fresh ginger root
- 2 tablespoons cornstarch
- 20 Hawaiian sweet rolls
- ½ teaspoon pepper
- 2 tablespoons melted butter

Directions:
1. Put turkey in pressure cooker and combine the first six ingredients over it.

2. Cook it on manual for 25 minutes, and when finished, natural pressure release.
3. Push sauté after removing the turkey, then mix cornstarch and water, stirring into cooking juices, and cook until sauce is thickened. Shred meat and stir to heat.
4. You can split the rolls, buttering each side, and bake till golden brown, adding the meat mixture to the top.

Nutrition: Calories: 252, Fat: 5g, Carbs: 25g, Net Carbs: 24g, Protein: 26g, Fiber: 1g

944. Elegant Cranberry Muffins

Preparation time: 10 minutes
Cooking Time: 20 minutes
Serving: 24 muffins
Ingredients:
- 2 cups almond flour
- 2 teaspoons baking soda
- ¼ cup avocado oil
- 1 whole egg
- ¾ cup almond milk
- ½ cup Erythritol
- ½ cup apple sauce
- Zest of 1 orange
- 2 teaspoons ground cinnamon
- 2 cup fresh cranberries

Directions:
1. Preheat your oven to 350 degrees F.
2. Line muffin tin with paper muffin cups and keep them on the side.
3. Add flour, baking soda and keep it on the side.
4. Take another bowl and whisk in remaining ingredients and add flour, mix well.
5. Pour batter into prepared muffin tin and bake for 20 minutes.
6. Once done, let it cool for 10 minutes.
7. Serve and enjoy!

Nutrition: Total Carbs: 7g; Fiber: 2g; Protein: 2.3g; Fat: 7g

945. Apple and Almond Muffins

Preparation time: 10 minutes
Cooking Time: 20 minutes
Serving: 6 muffins
Ingredients:
- 6 ounces ground almonds
- 1 teaspoon cinnamon
- ½ teaspoon baking powder
- 1 pinch sunflower seeds
- 1 whole egg
- 1 teaspoon apple cider vinegar
- 2 tablespoons Erythritol
- 1/3 cup apple sauce

Directions:
1. Preheat your oven to 350 degrees F.
2. Line muffin tin with paper muffin cups, keep them on the side.

3. Mix in almonds, cinnamon, baking powder, sunflower seeds and keep it on the side.
4. Take another bowl and beat in eggs, apple cider vinegar, apple sauce, Erythritol.
5. Add the mix to dry ingredients and mix well until you have a smooth batter.
6. Pour batter into tin and bake for 20 minutes.
7. Once done, let them cool.
8. Serve and enjoy!

Nutrition: Total Carbs: 10; Fiber: 4g; Protein: 13g; Fat: 17g

946. Stylish Chocolate Parfait

Preparation time: 2 hours
Cooking Time: Nil
Serving: 4
Ingredients:
- 2 tablespoons cocoa powder
- 1 cup almond milk
- 1 tablespoon chia seeds
- Pinch of sunflower seeds
- ½ teaspoon vanilla extract

Directions:
1. Take a bowl and add cocoa powder, almond milk, chia seeds, vanilla extract and stir.
2. Transfer to dessert glass and place in your fridge for 2 hours.
3. Serve and enjoy!

Nutrition: Calories: 130; Fat: 5g; Carbohydrates: 7g; Protein: 16g

947. Supreme Matcha Bomb

Preparation time: 100 minutes
Cooking Time: Nil
Serving: 10
Ingredients:
- 3/4 cup hemp seeds
- ½ cup coconut oil
- 2 tablespoons coconut almond butter
- 1 teaspoon Matcha powder
- 2 tablespoons vanilla bean extract
- ½ teaspoon mint extract
- Liquid stevia

Directions:
1. Take your blender/food processor and add hemp seeds, coconut oil, Matcha, vanilla extract and stevia.
2. Blend until you have a nice batter and divide into silicon molds.
3. Melt coconut almond butter and drizzle on top.
4. Let the cups chill and enjoy!

Nutrition: Calories: 200; Fat: 20g; Carbohydrates: 3g; Protein: 5g

948. Pork Beef Bean Nachos

Preparation time: 15 minutes
Cooking Time: 40 minutes
Servings: 10
Ingredients:
- 1 package beef jerky

- 4 cans black beans, drained and rinsed
- 6 bacon strips, crumbled
- 3 pounds pork spareribs
- 1 cup chopped onion
- 4 teaspoons minced garlic
- 4 cups divided beef broth
- optional toppings such as cheddar, sour cream, green onions, jalapeno slices
- 1 teaspoon crushed red pepper flakes
- Tortilla chips

Directions:
1. Pulse jerky in processor till ground, working in batches, put the ribs in the instant pot, topping with half jerky, two beans, and ½ cup onion, three pieces of bacon, 2 teaspoons garlic, 2 cups broth, and half teaspoon red pepper flakes. Cook on high for forty minutes.
2. Let it natural pressure release for 10 minutes, then quick release what's next, and do the same with the second batch.
3. Discard bones, and shred meat and then sauté it, and strain the mixture, and then discard juice and serve with chips and your desired toppings.

Nutrition: Calories: 469, Fat: 24g, Carbs: 27g Net Carbs: 20g, Protein: 33g, Fiber: 7g

949. Pressure Cooker Cranberry Hot Wings

Preparation time: 45 minutes
Cooking Time: 35 minutes
Servings: 4 dozen
Ingredients:
- 1 can jellied cranberry sauce
- ¼ cup Louisiana-style hot sauce
- 2 tablespoons honey
- 1 tablespoon Dijon mustard
- ½ cup sugar-free orange juice
- 2 tablespoons soy sauce
- 2 teaspoons garlic powder
- 1 minced garlic clove
- 1 teaspoon dried minced onion
- 5 pounds chicken wings
- 1 teaspoon salt
- 2 tablespoons cold water
- 4 teaspoons cornstarch

Directions:
1. Whisk the ingredients together but discard wing tips.
2. Put the wins in your instant pot, and then put cranberry mixture over top.
3. Lock lid, and then adjust pressure to high for 10 minutes.
4. You can from there, natural pressure release, and quick pressure.
5. Preheat broiler, skim fat, and from there, let it broil for 20-25 minutes.
6. When browned, brush with the glaze before serving

Nutrition: Calories: 71 per piece, Fat: 4g, Carbs: 5g, Net Carbs: 5g, Protein: 5g, Fiber: 0g

950. Bacon hot Dog Bites

Preparation time: 5 minutes
Cooking Time: 10 minutes
Servings: 12
Ingredients:
- 1 pack of hot dogs
- ½ bottle cocktail sauce
- 4 slices smoked bacon

Directions:
10. Cut up the meat, putting the dogs aside and cook bacon till done.
11. Separate the bacon from grease and put the hot dogs and bacon in pot, and then add the cocktail sauce until hated, and then cook on high pressure 5 minutes, quick release.
12. Turn off cooker and put in serving dish, it'll thicken over time.

Nutrition: Calories: 83, Fat: 10g, Carbs: 2g, Net Carbs: 2g, Protein: 10g, Fiber: 0g

951. Instant Pot cocktail Wieners

Preparation time: 2 minutes
Cooking Time: 1 minutes
Servings: 12
Ingredients:
- 1 package 12 cocktail wieners
- ¼ teaspoon brown sugar
- ½ cup chicken or veggie broth
- 1 jar jalapeno jelly
- ¼ cup chili sauce
- 1 diced jalapeno

Directions:
14. Put ½ cup of chicken broth into instant pot, then add wieners and rest of ingredients, still till everything is coated.
15. Cook on high pressure for a minute, and quick pressure then serve!

Nutrition: Calories: 92, Fat: 5g, Carbs: 6g, Net Carbs: 5g, Protein: 10g, Fiber: 1g

952. Pressure Cooker Braised Pulled Ham

Preparation time: 10 minutes
Cooking Time: 25 minutes
Servings: 16
Ingredients:
- 2 bottles beer, or nonalcoholic beer
- ½ teaspoon coarse ground pepper
- 1 cup Dijon mustard, divided
- 1 cooked bone-in ham
- 16 split pretzel hamburger buns
- 4 rosemary sprigs
- dill pickle slices

Directions:

11. Whisk the beer, pepper and mustard, and then add ham and rosemary, lock lid, and set pressure to high for 20 minutes, then natural pressure release.
12. Let it cool, discard rosemary, and skim the fat, and then let it boil for 5 minutes.
13. When ham is cool, shred with forks, discard bone, heat it again, and then put the ham on the pretzel buns, adding Dijon mustard at the end and the dill pickle slices.

Nutrition: Calories: 378, Fat: 9g, Carbs: 50g, Net Carbs: 2g, Protein: 25g, Fiber: 2g

953. Ginger and Cinnamon Pudding

Preparation time: 10 minutes
Cooking time: 1 hour
Servings: 4
Ingredients:
- ½ cup pumpkin puree
- 2 tablespoons maple syrup
- 1 and ½ cup coconut milk
- ½ cup chia seeds
- ¼ teaspoon ginger, grated
- ½ teaspoon cinnamon powder

Directions:
1. In your slow cooker, mix the milk with the pumpkin puree, maple syrup, chia, cinnamon and ginger, stir, cover, cook on High for 1 hour, divide into bowls and serve.

Nutrition: Calories 366, Fat 29.3g, Cholesterol 0mg, Sodium 20mg, Carbohydrate 24.8g, Fiber 11.5g, Sugars 10g, Protein 6.6g, Potassium 423mg

954. Honey Compote

Preparation time: 10 minutes
Cooking time: 2 hours
Servings: 6
Ingredients:
- 64 ounces red grapefruit juice
- 1 cup honey
- ½ cup mint, chopped
- 1 cup water
- 2 grapefruits, peeled and chopped

Directions:
1. In your slow cooker, mix grapefruit with water, honey, mint and grapefruit juice, stir, cover, cook on High for 2 hours, divide into bowls and serve cold.

Nutrition: Calories 364, Fat 0.1g, Cholesterol 0mg, Sodium 52mg, Carbohydrate 94.9g, Fiber 1.1g, Sugars 49.4g, Protein 0.7g, Potassium 124mg

955. Dark Cherry and Stevia Compote

Preparation time: 10 minutes
Cooking time: 2 hours

Servings: 6
Ingredients:
- 1-pound dark cherries, pitted and halved
- ¾ cup red grape juice
- ¼ cup maple syrup
- ½ cup dark cocoa powder
- 2 tablespoons stevia
- 2 cups water

Directions:
1. In your slow cooker, mix cocoa powder with grape juice, maple syrup, cherries, water and stevia, stir, cover, cook on High for 2 hours, divide into bowls and serve cold.

Nutrition: Calories 132, Fat 1.4g, Cholesterol 0mg, Sodium 179mg, Carbohydrate 37.9g, Fiber 7g, Sugars 23g, Protein 3.2g, Potassium 28mg

956. Vanilla Grapes Bowls

Preparation time: 10 minutes
Cooking time: 2 hours
Servings: 4
Ingredients:
- 1-pound green grapes
- 3 tablespoons coconut sugar
- 1 and ½ cups coconut cream
- 2 teaspoons vanilla extract

Directions:
1. In the slow cooker, combine the grapes with the cream and the other ingredients, put the lid on and cook on High for 2 hours.
2. Divide into bowls and serve.

Nutrition: Calories 360, Fat 21.9g, Cholesterol 0mg, Sodium 46mg, Carbohydrate 39g, Fiber 3g, Sugars 21.7g, Protein 3.5g, Potassium 456mg

957. Pears Mix

Preparation time: 10 minutes
Cooking time: 1 hour
Servings: 6
Ingredients:
- 1 quart water
- 5 star anise
- 2 tablespoons stevia
- ½ pound pears, cored and cut into wedges
- ½ pound apple, cored and cut into wedges
- Zest of 1 orange, grated
- Zest of 1 lemon, grated
- 2 cinnamon sticks

Directions:
1. Put the water, stevia, apples, pears, star anise, and cinnamon, orange and lemon zest in your slow cooker, cover, cook on High for 1 hour, divide into bowls and serve cold.

Nutrition: Calories 43, Fat 0.4g, Cholesterol 0mg, Sodium 6mg, Carbohydrate 14.3g, Fiber 2.7g, Sugars 5.9g, Protein 0.7g, Potassium 109mg

958. Mandarin Pudding

Preparation time: 10 minutes
Cooking time: 30 minutes
Servings: 8
Ingredients:
- 1 mandarin, peeled and sliced
- Juice of 2 mandarins
- 4 ounces low-fat butter, soft
- 2 eggs, whisked
- ¾ cup coconut sugar+ 2 tablespoons
- ¾ cup whole wheat flour
- ¾ cup almonds, ground

Directions:
1. Grease a loaf pan with some of the butter, sprinkle 2 tablespoons sugar on the bottom and arrange mandarin slices inside.
2. In a bowl, combine the butter with the rest of the sugar, eggs, almonds, flour and mandarin juice and whisk using a mixer.
3. Spoon mix over mandarin slices, introduce in the oven, bake at 350 degrees F for
4. 30 minutes, divide into bowls and serve
5. Enjoy!

Nutrition: Calories 202, Fat 3, Fiber 2, Carbs 12, Protein 6

959. Cherry Stew

Preparation time: 10 minutes
Cooking time: 10 minutes
Servings: 6
Ingredients:
- ½ cup cocoa powder
- 1 pound cherries, pitted
- ¼ cup coconut sugar
- 2 cups water

Directions:
1. In a pan, combine the cherries with the water, sugar and the cocoa powder, stir, cook over medium heat for 10 minutes, divide into bowls and serve cold. Enjoy!

Nutrition: Calories 207, Fat 1, Fiber 3, Carbs 8, Protein 6

960. Walnut Apple Mix

Preparation time: 10 minutes
Cooking time: 4 hours
Servings: 4
Ingredients:
- 6 big apples, roughly chopped
- Cooking spray
- ½ cup almond flour
- ½ cup walnuts, chopped
- ¼ cup coconut oil, melted
- 2 teaspoons lemon juice
- 3 tablespoons stevia
- ¼ teaspoon ginger, grated
- ¼ teaspoon cinnamon powder

Directions:
1. Spray your slow cooker with cooking spray.

2. In a bowl, mix stevia with lemon juice, ginger, apples and cinnamon, stir and pour into your slow cooker.
3. In another bowl, mix flour with walnuts and oil, stir, pour into the slow cooker, cover, and cook on Low for 4 hours.
4. Divide into bowls and serve.

Nutrition: Calories 474, Fat 30.3g, Cholesterol 0mg, Sodium 9mg, Carbohydrate 58.4g, Fiber 10.7g, Sugars 35g, Protein 7.7g, Potassium 444mg

961. Vanilla and Grapes Compote

Preparation time: 10 minutes
Cooking time: 2 hours
Servings: 4
Ingredients:
- 4 tablespoons coconut sugar
- 1 and ½ cups water
- 1 pound green grapes
- 1 teaspoon vanilla extract

Directions:
1. In your slow cooker, combine the grapes with the sugar and the other ingredients, put the lid on and cook on High for 2 hours, divide into bowls and serve.

Nutrition: Calories 227, Fat 1.5g, Cholesterol 0mg, Sodium 45mg, Carbohydrate 47.6g, Fiber 2.3g, Sugars 18.8g, Protein 3.6g, Potassium 271mg

962. Soft Pudding

Preparation time: 6 minutes
Cooking time: 1 hour
Servings: 4
Ingredients:
- ½ cup coconut water
- 2 teaspoons lime zest, grated
- 2 tablespoons green tea powder
- 1 and ½ cup avocado, pitted, peeled and chopped
- 1 tablespoon stevia

Directions:
1. In your slow cooker, mix coconut water with avocado, green tea powder, lime zest and stevia, stir, cover, cook on Low for 1 hour, divide into bowls and serve.

Nutrition: Calories 120, Fat 10.7g, Cholesterol 0mg, Sodium 35mg, Carbohydrate 8.5g, Fiber 4.4g, Sugars 1.1g, Protein 1.5g, Potassium 362mg

963. Green Pudding

Preparation time: 2 hours
Cooking time: 5 minutes
Servings: 6
Ingredients:
- 14 ounces almond milk
- 2 tablespoons green tea powder
- 14 ounces coconut cream
- 3 tablespoons coconut sugar

- 1 teaspoon gelatin powder

Directions:
1. Put the milk in a pan, add sugar, gelatin, coconut cream and green tea powder, stir, bring to a simmer, cook for 5 minutes, divide into cups and keep in the fridge for 2 hours before serving.
2. Enjoy!

Nutrition: Calories 170, Fat 3, Fiber 3, Carbs 7, Protein 4

964. Lemony Plum Cake

Preparation time: 1 hour and 20 minutes
Cooking time: 40 minutes
Servings: 8
Ingredients:
- 7 ounces whole wheat flour
- 1 teaspoon baking powder
- 1-ounce low-fat butter, soft
- 1 egg, whisked
- 5 tablespoons coconut sugar
- 3 ounces warm almond milk
- 1 and ¾ pounds plums, pitted and cut into quarters
- Zest of 1 lemon, grated
- 1-ounce almond flakes

Directions:
1. In a bowl, combine the flour with baking powder, butter, egg, sugar, milk and lemon zest, stir well, transfer dough to a lined cake pan, spread plums and almond flakes all over, introduce in the oven and bake at 350 degrees F for 40 minutes.
2. Slice and serve cold.
3. Enjoy

Nutrition: Calories 222, Fat 4, Fiber 2, Carbs 7, Protein 7

965. Lentils Sweet Bars

Preparation time: 10 minutes
Cooking time: 25 minutes
Servings: 14
Ingredients:
- 1 cup lentils, cooked, drained and rinsed
- 1 teaspoon cinnamon powder
- 2 cups whole wheat flour
- 1 teaspoon baking powder
- ½ teaspoon nutmeg, ground
- 1 cup low-fat butter
- 1 cup coconut sugar
- 1 egg
- 2 teaspoons almond extract
- 1 cup raisins
- 2 cups coconut, unsweetened and shredded

Directions:
1. Put the lentils in a bowl, mash them well using a fork, add cinnamon, flour, baking powder, nutmeg, butter, sugar, egg, almond extract, raisins and coconut, stir, spread on a lined baking sheet, introduce in the oven, bake at 350 degrees F for 25 minutes, cut into bars and serve cold.
2. Enjoy!

Nutrition: Calories 214, Fat 4, Fiber 2, Carbs 5, Protein 7

966. Lentils and Dates Brownies

Preparation time: 10 minutes
Cooking time: 15 minutes
Servings: 8
Ingredients:

- 28 ounces canned lentils, no-salt-added, rinsed and drained
- 12 dates
- 1 tablespoon coconut sugar
- 1 banana, peeled and chopped
- ½ teaspoon baking soda
- 4 tablespoons almond butter
- 2 tablespoons cocoa powder

Directions:

1. Put lentils in your food processor, pulse, add dates, sugar, banana, baking soda, almond butter and cocoa powder, pulse well, pour into a lined pan, spread, bake in the oven at 375 degrees F for 15 minutes, leave the mix aside to cool down a bit, cut into medium pieces and serve.
2. Enjoy!

Nutrition: Calories 202, Fat 4, Fiber 2, Carbs 12, Protein 6

967. Rose Lentils Ice Cream

Preparation time: 30 minutes
Cooking time: 1 hour and 20 minutes
Servings: 4
Ingredients:

- ½ cup red lentils, rinsed
- Juice of ½ lemon
- 1 cup coconut sugar
- 1 and ½ cups water
- 3 cups almond milk
- Juice of 2 limes
- 2 teaspoons cardamom powder
- 1 teaspoon rose water

Directions:

1. Heat up a pan over medium-high heat with the water, half of the sugar and lemon juice, stir, bring to a boil, add lentils, stir, reduce heat to medium-low and cook for 1 hour and 20 minutes.
2. Drain lentils, transfer them to a bowl, add coconut milk, the rest of the sugar, lime juice, cardamom and rose water, whisk everything, transfer to your ice cream machine, process for 30 minutes and serve.
3. Enjoy!

Nutrition: Calories 184, Fat 4, Fiber 3, Carbs 8, Protein 5

968. Coconut Figs

Preparation time: 6 minutes
Cooking time: 5 minutes
Servings: 4
Ingredients:

- 2 tablespoons coconut butter
- 12 figs, halved
- ¼ cup coconut sugar
- 1 cup almonds, toasted and chopped

Directions:

1. Put butter in a pot, heat up over medium heat, add sugar, whisk well, also add almonds and figs, toss, cook for 5 minutes, divide into small cups and serve cold.
2. Enjoy!

Nutrition: Calories 150, Fat 4, Fiber 5, Carbs 7, Protein 4

969. Lemony Banana Mix

Preparation time: 10 minutes
Cooking time: 0 minutes
Servings: 4
Ingredients:

- 4 bananas, peeled and chopped
- 5 strawberries, halved
- Juice of 2 lemons
- 4 tablespoons coconut sugar

Directions:

1. In a bowl, combine the bananas with the strawberries, lemon juice and sugar, toss and serve cold.
2. Enjoy!

Nutrition: Calories 172, Fat 7, Fiber 5, Carbs 5, Protein 5

970. Cocoa Banana Dessert Smoothie

Preparation time: 5 minutes
Cooking time: 0 minutes
Servings: 2
Ingredients:

- 2 medium bananas, peeled
- 2 teaspoons cocoa powder
- ½ big avocado, pitted, peeled and mashed
- ¾ cup almond milk

Directions:

1. In your blender, combine the bananas with the cocoa, avocado and milk, pulse well, divide into 2 glasses and serve.
2. Enjoy!

Nutrition: Calories 155, Fat 3, Fiber 4, Carbs 6, Protein 5

971. Kiwi Bars

Preparation time: 30 minutes
Cooking time: 0 minutes
Servings: 4
Ingredients:

- 1 cup olive oil
- 1 and ½ bananas, peeled and chopped
- 1/3 cup coconut sugar
- ¼ cup lemon juice
- 1 teaspoon lemon zest, grated
- 3 kiwis, peeled and chopped

Directions:

1. In your food processor, mix bananas with kiwis, almost all the oil, sugar, lemon juice and lemon zest and pulse well.

2. Grease a pan with the remaining oil, pour the kiwi mix, spread, keep in the fridge for 30 minutes, slice and serve,
3. Enjoy!

Nutrition: Calories 207, Fat 3, Fiber 3, Carbs 4, Protein 4

972. Black Tea Bars

Preparation time: 10 minutes
Cooking time: 35 minutes
Servings: 12
Ingredients:
- 6 tablespoons black tea powder
- 2 cups almond milk
- ½ cup low-fat butter
- 2 cups coconut sugar
- 4 eggs
- 2 teaspoons vanilla extract
- ½ cup olive oil
- 3 and ½ cups whole wheat flour
- 1 teaspoon baking soda
- 3 teaspoons baking powder

Directions:
1. Put the milk in a pot, heat it up over medium heat, add tea, stir, take off heat and cool down.
2. Add butter, sugar, eggs, vanilla, oil, flour, baking soda and baking powder, stir well, pour into a square pan, spread, introduce in the oven, bake at 350 degrees F for 35 minutes, cool down, slice and serve. Enjoy!

Nutrition: Calories 220, Fat 4, Fiber 4, Carbs 12, Protein 7

973. Lovely Faux Mac and Cheese

Preparation time: 15 minutes
Cooking Time: 45 minutes
Serving: 4
Ingredients:
- 5 cups cauliflower florets
- Salt and pepper to taste
- 1 cup coconut milk
- ½ cup vegetable broth
- 2 tablespoons coconut flour, sifted
- 1 organic egg, beaten
- 2 cups cheddar cheese

Directions:
1. Preheat your oven to 350 degrees F.
2. Season florets with salt and steam until firm.
3. Place florets in greased ovenproof dish.
4. Heat coconut milk over medium heat in a skillet, make sure to season the oil with salt and pepper.
5. Stir in broth and add coconut flour to the mix, stir.
6. Cook until the sauce begins to bubble.
7. Remove heat and add beaten egg.
8. Pour the thick sauce over cauliflower and mix in cheese.
9. Bake for 30-45 minutes.
10. Serve and enjoy!

Nutrition: Calories: 229; Fat: 14g; Carbohydrates: 9g; Protein: 15g

974. Beautiful Banana Custard

Preparation time: 10 minutes
Cooking Time: 25 minutes
Serving: 3
Ingredients:
- 2 ripe bananas, peeled and mashed finely
- ½ teaspoon of vanilla extract
- 14-ounce unsweetened almond milk
- 3 eggs

Directions:
1. Preheat your oven to 350 degrees F.
2. Grease 8 custard glasses lightly.
3. Arrange the glasses in a large baking dish.
4. Take a large bowl and mix all of the ingredients and mix them well until combined nicely.
5. Divide the mixture evenly between the glasses.
6. Pour water in the baking dish.
7. Bake for 25 minutes.
8. Take out and serve.
9. Enjoy!

Nutrition: Calories: 59; Fat: 2.4g; Carbohydrates: 7g; Protein: 3g otein: 2g

975. Summer Jam

Preparation time: 10 minutes
Cooking time: 3 hours
Servings: 6
Ingredients:
- 2 cups coconut sugar
- 4 cups cherries, pitted
- 2 tablespoons lemon juice
- 3 tablespoons gelatin

Directions:
1. In your slow cooker, mix lemon juice with gelatin, cherries and coconut sugar, stir, cover, cook on High for 3 hours, divide into bowls and serve cold.

Nutrition: Calories 171, Fat 0.1g, Cholesterol 0mg, Sodium 41mg, Carbohydrate 37.2g, Fiber 0.7g, Sugars 0.1g, Protein 3.8g, Potassium 122mg

976. Cinnamon Pudding

Preparation time: 10 minutes
Cooking time: 5 hours
Servings: 4
Ingredients:
- 2 cups white rice
- 1 cup coconut sugar
- 2 cinnamon sticks
- 6 and ½ cups water
- ½ cup coconut, shredded

Directions:
1. In your slow cooker, mix water with the rice, sugar, cinnamon and coconut, stir, cover, cook on High for 5 hours, discard cinnamon, divide pudding into bowls and serve warm.

Nutrition: Calories 400, Fat 4g, Cholesterol 0mg, Sodium 28mg, Carbohydrate 81.2g, Fiber 2.7g, Sugars 0.8g, Protein 7.2g, Potassium 151mg

977. Orange Compote

Preparation time: 10 minutes
Cooking time: 2 hours and 30 minutes
Servings: 4
Ingredients:
- ½ pound oranges, peeled and cut into segments
- ½ pound plums, pitted and halved
- 1 cup orange juice
- 3 tablespoons coconut sugar
- ½ cup water

Directions:
1. In the slow cooker, combine the oranges with the plums, orange juice and the other ingredients, put the lid on and cook on High for 2 hours and 30 minutes.
2. Stir, divide into bowls and serve cold.

Nutrition: Calories 130, Fat 0.2g, Cholesterol 0mg, Sodium 31mg, Carbohydrate 28.4g, Fiber 1.6g, Sugars 11.4g, Protein 1.8g, Potassium 240mg

978. Chocolate Bars

Preparation time: 10 minutes
Cooking time: 2 hours and 30 minutes
Servings: 12
Ingredients:
- 1 cup coconut sugar
- ½ cup dark chocolate chips
- 1 egg white
- ¼ cup coconut oil, melted
- ½ teaspoon vanilla extract
- 1 teaspoon baking powder
- 1 and ½ cups almond meal

Directions:
1. In a bowl, mix the oil with sugar, vanilla extract, egg white, baking powder and almond flour and whisk well
2. Fold in chocolate chips and stir gently.
3. Line your slow cooker with parchment paper, grease it, add cookie mix, press on the bottom, cover and cook on low for 2 hours and 30 minutes.
4. Take cookie sheet out of the slow cooker, cut into medium bars and serve.

Nutrition: Calories 141, Fat 11.8g, Cholesterol 0mg, Sodium 7mg, Carbohydrate 7.7g, Fiber 1.5g, Sugars 3.2g, Protein 3.2g, Potassium 134mg

979. Lemon Zest Pudding

Preparation time: 10 minutes
Cooking time: 5 hours
Servings: 4
Ingredients:
- 1 cup pineapple juice, natural
- Cooking spray
- 1 teaspoon baking powder

- 1 cup coconut flour
- 3 tablespoons avocado oil
- 3 tablespoons stevia
- ½ cup pineapple, chopped
- ½ cup lemon zest, grated
- ½ cup coconut milk
- ½ cup pecans, chopped

Directions:
1. Spray your slow cooker with cooking spray.
2. In a bowl, mix flour with stevia, baking powder, oil, milk, pecans, pineapple, lemon zest and pineapple juice, stir well, pour into your slow cooker greased with cooking spray, cover and cook on Low for 5 hours.
3. Divide into bowls and serve.

Nutrition: Calories 431, Fat 29.7g, Cholesterol 0mg, Sodium 8mg, Carbohydrate 47.1g, Fiber 17g, Sugars 10.9g, Protein 8.1g, Potassium 482mg

980. Maple Syrup Poached Pears

Preparation time: 10 minutes
Cooking time: 4 hours
Servings: 4
Ingredients:
- 2 cups grapefruit juice
- 4 pears, peeled and cored
- ¼ cup maple syrup
- 1 tablespoon ginger, grated
- 2 teaspoons cinnamon powder

Directions:
1. In your slow cooker, mix pears with grapefruit juice, maple syrup, cinnamon and ginger, cover, cook on Low for 4 hours, divide everything into bowls and serve.

Nutrition: Calories 214, Fat 0.5g, Cholesterol 0mg, Sodium 5mg, Carbohydrate 55.3g, Fiber 7.9g, Sugars 40.2g, Protein 1.6g, Potassium 461mg

981. Ginger and Pumpkin Pie

Preparation time: 10 minutes
Cooking time: 2 hours
Servings: 10
Ingredients:
- 2 cups almond flour
- 1 egg, whisked
- 1 cup pumpkin puree
- 1 and ½ teaspoons baking powder
- Cooking spray
- 1 tablespoon coconut oil, melted
- 1 tablespoon vanilla extract
- ½ teaspoon baking soda
- 1 and ½ teaspoons cinnamon powder
- ¼ teaspoon ginger, ground
- 1/3 cup maple syrup
- 1 teaspoon lemon juice

Directions:
1. In a bowl, flour with baking powder, baking soda, cinnamon, ginger, egg, oil, vanilla, pumpkin puree, maple

syrup and lemon juice, stir and pour in your slow cooker greased with cooking spray and lined with parchment paper, cover the pot and cook on Low for 2 hours and 20 minutes.

2. Leave the pie to cool down, slice and serve.

Nutrition: Calories 91, Fat 4.8g, Cholesterol 16mg, Sodium 74mg, Carbohydrate 10.8g, Fiber 1.3g, Sugars 7.5g, Protein 2g, Potassium 157mg

982. Cashew and Carrot Muffins

Preparation time: 10 minutes
Cooking time: 3 hours
Servings: 4
Ingredients:
- 4 tablespoons cashew butter, melted
- 4 eggs, whisked
- ½ cup coconut cream
- 1 cup carrots, peeled and grated
- 4 teaspoons maple syrup
- ¾ cup coconut flour
- ½ teaspoon baking soda

Directions:
1. In a bowl, mix the cashew butter with the eggs, cream and the other ingredients, whisk well and pour into a muffin pan that fits the slow cooker.
2. Put the lid on, cook the muffins on High for 3 hours, cool down and serve.

Nutrition: Calories 345, Fat 21.7g, Cholesterol 164mg, Sodium 247mg, Carbohydrate 28.6g, Fiber 10.7g, Sugars 6.7g, Protein 12.3g, Potassium 327mg

983. Lemon Custard

Preparation time: 10 minutes
Cooking time: 3 hours
Servings: 10
Ingredients:
- 2 pounds lemons, washed, peeled and sliced
- 2 pounds coconut sugar
- 1 tablespoon vinegar

Directions:
1. In your slow cooker, mix lemons with coconut sugar and vinegar, stir, cover, cook on High for 3 hours, blend using an immersion blender, divide into small bowls and serve.

Nutrition: Calories 46, Fat 0.3g, Cholesterol 0mg, Sodium 10mg, Carbohydrate 12.3g, Fiber 2.5g, Sugars 2.3g, Protein 1.2g, Potassium 126mg

984. Rhubarb Dip

Preparation time: 10 minutes
Cooking time: 3 hours
Servings: 8
Ingredients:
- 1 cup coconut sugar
- 1/3 cup water
- 4 pounds rhubarb, chopped

- 1 tablespoon mint, chopped

Directions:
1. In your slow cooker, mix water with rhubarb, sugar and mint, stir, cover, cook on High for 3 hours, blend using an immersion blender, divide into cups and serve cold.

Nutrition: Calories 60, Fat 0.5g, Cholesterol 0mg, Sodium 15mg, Carbohydrate 12.7g, Fiber 4.1g, Sugars 2.5g, Protein 2.2g, Potassium 657mg

985. Resilient Chocolate Cream

Preparation time: 10 minutes
Cooking time: 1 hour and 30 minutes
Servings: 4
Ingredients:
- 1 cup dark and unsweetened chocolate, chopped
- ½ pound cherries, pitted and halved
- 1 teaspoon vanilla extract
- ½ cup coconut cream
- 3 tablespoons coconut sugar
- 2 teaspoons gelatin

Directions:
1. In the slow cooker, combine the chocolate with the cherries and the other ingredients, toss, put the lid on and cook on Low for 1 hour and 30 minutes.
2. Stir the cream well, divide into bowls and serve.

Nutrition: Calories 526, Fat 39.9g, Cholesterol 0mg, Sodium 57mg, Carbohydrate 47.2g, Fiber 10.8g, Sugars 1.1g, Protein 13.4g, Potassium 141mg

986. Vanilla Poached Strawberries

Preparation time: 10 minutes
Cooking time: 3 hours
Servings: 10
Ingredients:
- 4 cups coconut sugar
- 2 tablespoons lemon juice
- 2 pounds strawberries
- 1 cup water
- 1 teaspoon vanilla extract
- 1 teaspoon cinnamon powder

Directions:
1. In your slow cooker, mix strawberries with water, coconut sugar, lemon juice, cinnamon and vanilla, stir, cover, cook on Low for 3 hours, divide into bowls and serve cold.

Nutrition: Calories 69, Fat 0.3g, Cholesterol 0mg, Sodium 18mg, Carbohydrate 14.7g, Fiber 1.8g, Sugars 4.6g, Protein 1g, Potassium 143mg

987. Lemon Bananas

Preparation time: 10 minutes
Cooking time: 2 hours
Servings: 4

Ingredients:
- 4 bananas, peeled and sliced
- Juice of ½ lemon
- 1 tablespoon coconut oil
- 3 tablespoons stevia
- ½ teaspoon cardamom seeds

Directions:
1. Arrange bananas in your slow cooker, add stevia, lemon juice, oil and cardamom, cover, cook on Low for 2 hours, divide everything into bowls and serve with.

Nutrition: Calories 137, Fat 3.9g, Cholesterol 0mg, Sodium 2mg, Carbohydrate 33.5g, Fiber 3.2g, Sugars 14.6g, Protein 1.4g, Potassium 433mg

988. Pecans Cake

Preparation time: 10 minutes
Cooking time: 5 hours
Servings: 4

Ingredients:
- Cooking spray
- 1 cup almond flour
- 1 cup orange juice
- 1 cup coconut sugar
- 3 tablespoons coconut oil, melted
- 1 teaspoon baking powder
- ½ teaspoon cinnamon powder
- ½ cup almond milk
- ½ cup pecans, chopped
- ¾ cup water
- ½ cup orange peel, grated

Directions:
1. In a bowl, mix flour with half of the sugar, baking powder, cinnamon, 2 tablespoons oil, milk and pecans, stir and pour this in your slow cooker greased with cooking spray.
2. Heat up a small pan over medium heat, add water, orange juice, orange peel, the rest of the oil and the rest of the sugar, stir, bring to a boil, pour over the mix in the slow cooker, cover and cook on Low for 5 hours.
3. Divide into bowls and serve cold.

Nutrition: Calories 565, Fat 48.8g, Cholesterol 0mg, Sodium 28mg, Carbohydrate 26g, Fiber 7.8g, Sugars 7.1g, Protein 10.2g, Potassium 459mg

989. Coconut Cream and Plums Cake

Preparation time: 10 minutes
Cooking time: 3 hours
Servings: 6

Ingredients:
- 2 cups whole wheat flour
- 1 teaspoon vanilla extract
- 1 and ½ cups plums, peeled and chopped
- ½ cup coconut cream
- 1 teaspoon baking powder
- ¾ cup coconut sugar
- 4 tablespoons avocado oil

Directions:
1. In the slow cooker lined with parchment paper, combine the flour with the plums and the other ingredients and whisk.
2. Put the lid on, cook on High for 3 hours, and leave the cake to cool down, slice and serve.

Nutrition: Calories 232, Fat 6.4g, Cholesterol 0mg, Sodium 10mg, Carbohydrate 38.3g, Fiber 2.2g, Sugars 2.7g, Protein 5.1g, Potassium 238mg

990. Pumpkin Pudding

Preparation time: 1 hour
Cooking time: 0 minutes
Servings: 4

Ingredients:
- 1 and ½ cups almond milk
- ½ cup pumpkin puree
- 2 tablespoons coconut sugar
- ½ teaspoon cinnamon powder
- ¼ teaspoon ginger, grated
- ¼ cup chia seeds

Directions:
1. In a bowl, combine the milk with pumpkin, sugar, cinnamon, ginger and chia seeds, toss well, divide into small cups and keep them in the fridge for 1 hour before serving.
2. Enjoy!

Nutrition: Calories 145, Fat 7, Fiber 7, Carbs 11, Protein 9

991. Cashew Lemon Fudge

Preparation time: 2 hours
Cooking time: 0 minutes
Servings: 4

Ingredients:
- 1/3 cup natural cashew butter
- 1 and ½ tablespoons coconut oil, melted
- 2 tablespoons coconut butter
- 5 tablespoons lemon juice
- ½ teaspoon lemon zest
- 1 tablespoons coconut sugar

Directions:
1. In a bowl, mix cashew butter with coconut butter, oil, lemon juice, lemon zest and sugar and stir well
2. Line a muffin tray with some parchment paper, scoop 1 tablespoon of lemon fudge mix in a lined muffin tray, keep in the fridge for 2 hours and serve
3. Enjoy!

Nutrition: Calories 142, Fat 4, Fiber 4, Carbs 8, Protein 5

992. Brown Cake

Preparation time: 10 minutes
Cooking time: 2 hours and 30 minutes
Servings: 8

Ingredients:
- 1 cup flour
- 1 and ½ cup stevia

- ½ cup chocolate almond milk
- 2 teaspoons baking powder
- 1 and ½ cups hot water
- ¼ cup cocoa powder+ 2 tablespoons
- 2 tablespoons canola oil
- 1 teaspoon vanilla extract
- Cooking spray

Directions:
1. In a bowl, mix flour with ¼-cup cocoa, baking powder, almond milk, oil and vanilla extract, whisk well and spread on the bottom of the slow cooker greased with cooking spray.
2. In a separate bowl, mix stevia with the water and the rest of the cocoa, whisk well, spread over the batter, cover, and cook your cake on High for 2 hours and 30 minutes.
3. Leave the cake to cool down, slice and serve.

Nutrition: Calories 150, Fat 7.6g, Cholesterol 1mg, Sodium 7mg, Carbohydrate 56.8g, Fiber 1.8g, Sugars 4.4g, Protein 2.9g, Potassium 185mg

993. Delicious Berry Pie

Preparation time: 10 minutes
Cooking time: 1 hour
Servings: 6
Ingredients:
- ½ cup whole wheat flour
- Cooking spray
- 1/3 cup almond milk
- ¼ teaspoon baking powder
- ¼ teaspoon stevia
- ¼ cup blueberries
- 1 teaspoon olive oil
- 1 teaspoon vanilla extract
- ½ teaspoon lemon zest, grated

Directions:
1. In a bowl, mix flour with baking powder, stevia, blueberries, milk, oil, lemon zest and vanilla extract, whisk, pour into your slow cooker lined with parchment paper and greased with the cooking spray, cover and cook on High for 1 hour.
2. Leave the pie to cool down, slice and serve.

Nutrition: Calories 82, Fat 4.2g, Cholesterol 0mg, Sodium 3mg, Carbohydrate 10.1g, Fiber 0.7g, Sugars 1.2g, Protein 1.4g, Potassium 74mg

994. Cinnamon Peach Cobbler

Preparation time: 10 minutes
Cooking time: 4 hours
Servings: 4
Ingredients:
- 4 cups peaches, peeled and sliced
- Cooking spray
- ¼ cup coconut sugar
- 1 and ½ cups whole wheat sweet crackers, crushed
- ½ cup almond milk
- ½ teaspoon cinnamon powder
- ¼ cup stevia
- 1 teaspoon vanilla extract

- ¼ teaspoon nutmeg, ground

Directions:
1. In a bowl, mix peaches with sugar, cinnamon, and stir.
2. In a separate bowl, mix crackers with stevia, nutmeg, almond milk and vanilla extract and stir.
3. Spray your slow cooker with cooking spray, spread peaches on the bottom, and add the crackers mix, spread, cover and cook on Low for 4 hours.
4. Divide into bowls and serve.

Nutrition: Calories 249, Fat 11.4g, Cholesterol 0mg, Sodium 179mg, Carbohydrate 42.7g, Fiber 3g, Sugars 15.2g, Protein 3.5g, Potassium 366mg

995. Cherry Stew

Preparation time: 10 minutes
Cooking time: 10 minutes
Servings: 6
Ingredients:
- ½ cup cocoa powder
- 1 pound cherries, pitted
- ¼ cup coconut sugar
- 2 cups water

Directions:
1. In a pan, combine the cherries with the water, sugar and the cocoa powder, stir, cook over medium heat for 10 minutes, divide into bowls and serve cold.
2. Enjoy!

Nutrition: Calories 207, Fat 1, Fiber 3, Carbs 8, Protein 6

996. Rice Pudding

Preparation time: 10 minutes
Cooking time: 45 minutes
Servings: 6
Ingredients:
- ½ cup basmati rice
- 4 cups almond milk
- ¼ cup raisins
- 3 tablespoons coconut sugar
- ½ teaspoon cardamom powder
- ¼ teaspoon cinnamon powder
- ¼ cup walnuts, chopped
- 1 tablespoon lemon zest, grated

Directions:
1. In a pan, mix sugar with milk, stir, bring to a boil over medium-high heat, add rice, raisins, cardamom, cinnamon, walnuts and lemon zest, stir, cover the pan, reduce heat to low, cook for 40 minutes, divide into bowls and serve cold.
2. Enjoy!

Nutrition: Calories 200, Fat 4, Fiber 5, Carbs 8, Protein 3

997. Apple Loaf

Preparation time: 10 minutes
Cooking time: 35 minutes
Servings: 6
Ingredients:

- 3 cups apples, cored and cubed
- 1 cup coconut sugar
- 1 tablespoon vanilla
- 2 eggs
- 1 tablespoon apple pie spice
- 2 cups almond flour
- 1 tablespoon baking powder
- 1 tablespoon coconut oil, melted

Directions
1. In a bowl, mix apples with coconut sugar, vanilla, eggs, apple pie spice, almond flour, baking powder and oil, whisk, pour into a loaf pan, introduce in the oven and bake at 350 degrees F for 35 minutes.
2. Serve cold.
3. Enjoy!

Nutrition: Calories 180, Fat 6, Fiber 5, Carbs 12, Protein 4

998. Cauliflower Cinnamon Pudding

Preparation time: 10 minutes
Cooking time: 20 minutes
Servings: 6
Ingredients:
- 1 tablespoon coconut oil, melted
- 7 ounces cauliflower rice
- 4 ounces water
- 16 ounces coconut milk
- 3 ounces coconut sugar
- 1 egg
- 1 teaspoon cinnamon powder
- 1 teaspoon vanilla extract

Directions:
1. In a pan, combine the oil with the rice, water, milk, sugar, egg, cinnamon and vanilla, whisk well, bring to a simmer, cook for 20 minutes over medium heat, divide into bowls and serve cold.
2. Enjoy!

Nutrition: Calories 202, Fat 2, Fiber 6, Carbs 8, Protein 7

999. Rhubarb Stew

Preparation time: 10 minutes
Cooking time: 5 minutes
Servings: 3
Ingredients:
- Juice of 1 lemon
- 1 teaspoon lemon zest, grated
- 1 and ½ cup coconut sugar
- 4 and ½ cups rhubarbs, roughly chopped
- 1 and ½ cups water

Directions:
1. In a pan, combine the rhubarb with the water, lemon juice, lemon zest and coconut sugar, toss, bring to a simmer over medium heat, cook for 5 minutes, and divide into bowls and serve cold.
2. Enjoy!

Nutrition: Calories 108, Fat 1, Fiber 4, Carbs 8, Protein 5

1000. Plum Cake

Preparation time: 1 hour and 20 minutes
Cooking time: 40 minutes
Servings: 8
Ingredients:
- 7 ounces whole wheat flour
- 1 teaspoon baking powder
- 1-ounce low-fat butter, soft
- 1 egg, whisked
- 5 tablespoons coconut sugar
- 3 ounces warm almond milk
- 1 and ¾ pounds plums, pitted and cut into quarters
- Zest of 1 lemon, grated
- 1-ounce almond flakes

Directions:
4. In a bowl, combine the flour with baking powder, butter, egg, sugar, milk and lemon zest, stir well, transfer dough to a lined cake pan, spread plums and almond flakes all over, introduce in the oven and bake at 350 degrees F for 40 minutes.
5. Slice and serve cold.
6. Enjoy!

Nutrition: Calories 222, Fat 4, Fiber 2, Carbs 7, Protein 7

1001. Lentils Sweet Bars

Preparation time: 10 minutes
Cooking time: 25 minutes
Servings: 14
Ingredients:
- 1 cup lentils, cooked, drained and rinsed
- 1 teaspoon cinnamon powder
- 2 cups whole wheat flour
- 1 teaspoon baking powder
- ½ teaspoon nutmeg, ground
- 1 cup low-fat butter
- 1 cup coconut sugar
- 1 egg
- 2 teaspoons almond extract
- 1 cup raisins
- 2 cups coconut, unsweetened and shredded

Directions:
4. Put the lentils in a bowl, mash them well using a fork, add cinnamon, flour, baking powder, nutmeg, butter, sugar, egg, almond extract, raisins and coconut, stir, spread on a lined baking sheet, introduce in the oven, bake at 350 degrees F for 25 minutes, cut into bars and serve cold.
5. Enjoy!

Nutrition: Calories 214, Fat 4, Fiber 2, Carbs 5, Protein 7

1002. Dates Brownies

Preparation time: 10 minutes
Cooking time: 15 minutes
Servings: 8
Ingredients:
- 28 ounces canned lentils, no-salt-added, rinsed and drained
- 12 dates

- 1 tablespoon coconut sugar
- 1 banana, peeled and chopped
- ½ teaspoon baking soda
- 4 tablespoons almond butter
- 2 tablespoons cocoa powder

Directions:
4. Put lentils in your food processor, pulse, add dates, sugar, banana, baking soda, almond butter and cocoa powder, pulse well, pour into a lined pan, spread, bake in the oven at 375 degrees F for 15 minutes, leave the mix aside to cool down a bit, cut into medium pieces and serve.
5. Enjoy!

Nutrition: Calories 202, Fat 4, Fiber 2, Carbs 12, Protein 6

1003. Rose Lentils Ice Cream

Preparation time: 30 minutes
Cooking time: 1 hour and 20 minutes
Servings: 4

Ingredients:
- ½ cup red lentils, rinsed
- Juice of ½ lemon
- 1 cup coconut sugar
- 1 and ½ cups water
- 3 cups almond milk
- Juice of 2 limes
- 2 teaspoons cardamom powder
- 1 teaspoon rose water

Directions:
2. Heat up a pan over medium-high heat with the water, half of the sugar and lemon juice, stir, bring to a boil, add lentils, stir, reduce heat to medium-low and cook for 1 hour and 20 minutes.
3. Drain lentils, transfer them to a bowl, add coconut milk, the rest of the sugar, lime juice, cardamom and rose water, whisk everything, transfer to your ice cream machine, process for 30 minutes and serve.
4. Enjoy!

Nutrition: Calories 184, Fat 4, Fiber 3, Carbs 8, Protein 5

1004. Mandarin Almond Pudding

Preparation time: 10 minutes
Cooking time: 30 minutes
Servings: 8

Ingredients:
- 1 mandarin, peeled and sliced
- Juice of 2 mandarins
- 4 ounces low-fat butter, soft
- 2 eggs, whisked
- ¾ cup coconut sugar+ 2 tablespoons
- ¾ cup whole wheat flour
- ¾ cup almonds, ground

Directions:
1. Grease a loaf pan with some of the butter, sprinkle 2 tablespoons sugar on the bottom and arrange mandarin slices inside.

2. In a bowl, combine the butter with the rest of the sugar, eggs, almonds, flour and mandarin juice and whisk using a mixer.
3. Spoon mix over mandarin slices, introduce in the oven, bake at 350 degrees F for 30 minutes, divide into bowls and serve
4. Enjoy!

Nutrition: Calories 202, Fat 3, Fiber 2, Carbs 12, Protein 6

1005. Green tea and Banana Sweetening Mix

Preparation time: 10 minutes
Cooking time: 5 minutes
Servings: 3-4

Ingredients:
- cups pitted avocados, chopped
- 1 cup coconut cream
- 2 peeled and chopped bananas
- 2 tablespoons green tea powder
- 1 tablespoon palm sugar
- 2 tablespoons grated lime zest

Directions:
1. Take all of the ingredients in the instant pot.
2. Toss this, cover, and then cook on low for 5 minutes manual, natural pressure release, and then divide and serve it cold.

Nutrition: Calories: 207, Fat: 2g, Carbs: 11g, Net Carbs: 8g, Protein: 3g, Fiber: 8g

1006. Cheesecake Made Easy!

Preparation time: 10 minutes
Cooking Time: 50 minutes
Servings: 8-10

Ingredients:
- 10 oz. crushed whole wheat crackers
- 16 oz., fat-free cream cheeses
- 2 teaspoons vanilla extract
- 5 tablespoons fat-free butter
- 1 cup coconut sugar
- 2 large eggs
- ¼ cup coconut cream
- 8 oz. sugar-free chocolate, melted
- 2 cups water
- cooking spray
- 2 tablespoons whole wheat flour

Directions:
1. In one bowl, mix crackers with butter and stir, then grease a cooking tin and push crackers into bottom.
2. Mix the rest of the ingredients into another bowl, and then put it over the crust, then cover pan with foil.
3. Put it in instant pot and cook on manual high for 45 minutes.
4. Chill cheesecake in fridge before you serve it.

Nutrition: Calories: 265, Fat: 9g, Carbs: 15g, net Carbs: 12g, Protein: 4g, Fiber: 3g

1007.   Grapefruit Compote

Preparation time: 5 minutes
Cooking Time: 8 minutes
Servings: 4
Ingredients:
- 1 cup palm sugar
- 64 oz. Sugar-free red grapefruit juice
- ½ cup chopped mint
- 2 peeled and cubed grapefruits

Directions:
1. Take all ingredients and combine them into instant pot.
2. Cook on low for 8 minutes, then divide into bowls and serve!

Nutrition: Calories: 131, Fat: 1g, Carbs: 12g, Net Carbs: 11g, Protein: 2g, Fiber: 2g

1008.   Instant Pot Applesauce

Preparation time: 10 minutes
Cooking Time: 10 minutes
Servings: 8
Ingredients:
- 3 pounds of apples
- ½ cup water

Directions:
1. Core and peel the apples and then put them at the bottom of the instant pot and then secure the lid and seal the vent. Let it cook for 10 minutes, then natural pressure release.
2. From there, when it's safe to remove the lid, take the apples and juices and blend this till smooth.
3. Stores these in jars or serve immediately.

Nutrition: Calories: 88, Fat: 0g, Carbs: 23g, Net Carbs: 19g, Protein: 0g, Fiber: 4g

1009.   Green Pudding

Preparation time: 2 hours
Cooking time: 5 minutes
Servings: 6
Ingredients:
- 14 ounces almond milk
- 2 tablespoons green tea powder
- 14 ounces coconut cream
- 3 tablespoons coconut sugar
- 1 teaspoon gelatin powder

Directions:
1. Put the milk in a pan, add sugar, gelatin, coconut cream and green tea powder, stir, bring to a simmer, cook for 5

minutes, divide into cups and keep in the fridge for 2 hours before serving.
2. Enjoy!
Nutrition: Calories 170, Fat 3, Fiber 3, Carbs 7, Protein 4

1010.   Healthy Tahini Buns

Preparation time: 10 minutes
Cooking Time: 15-20 minutes
Servings: 3 buns
Ingredients:
- 1 whole egg
- 5 tablespoons Tahini paste
- ½ teaspoon baking soda
- 1 teaspoon lemon juice
- 1 pinch salt

Directions:
1. Preheat your oven to 350 degrees F.
2. Line a baking sheet with parchment paper and keep it on the side.
3. Add the listed ingredients to a blender and blend until you have a smooth batter.
4. Scoop batter onto prepared sheet forming buns.
5. Bake for 15-20 minutes.
6. Once done, remove from oven and let them cool.
7. Serve and enjoy!

Nutrition: Total Carbs: 7g Fiber: 2g Protein: 6g Fat: 14g Calories: 172

1011.   Spicy Pecan Bowl

Preparation time: 10 minutes
Cooking Time: 120 minutes
Serving: 3
Ingredients:
- 1 pound pecans, halved
- 2 tablespoons olive oil
- 1 teaspoon basil, dried
- 1 tablespoon chili powder
- 1 teaspoon oregano, dried
- ¼ teaspoon garlic powder
- 1 teaspoon rosemary, dried
- ½ teaspoon onion powder

Directions:
1. Add pecans, oil, basil, chili powder, oregano, garlic powder, onion powder, rosemary and toss well.
2. Transfer to Slow Cooker and cook on LOW for 2 hours.
3. Divide between bowls and serve.
4. Enjoy!

Nutrition: Calories: 152; Fat: 3g; Carbohydrates: 11g; Protein 4

CONCLUSION

The Dash Diet is designed to help ladies lose weight and stay healthy. There are many useful tips and easy recipes in this cookbook that can help you better understand the Dash Diet and make healthy food choices.

Even if you aren't following the Dash Diet, this cookbook can help you need a well-made, delicious meal. At Dash Diet, we understand that our products' quality is just as important as the quality of our products. That is why Dash Diet uses hardened steel components for its ratchets.

Our ratchets are made with hardened steel that is hand polished and handcrafted by experts in the USA. This ensures a long life for your new tool. Each part is made with precision to ensure a strong bond between the ratchet tool's male and female heads. Most people don't use their kitchen knives for cooking. Most people don't know that you should always wash them after cutting something, primarily if you've used a grinder on them.

The Dash Diet Cookbook will have you hacking out your cutlery in no time so you can finally become a healthier human being! It's all about being healthy and learning to enjoy the foods you eat again. We have concluded that Dash Diet Cookbook is an excellent way of losing weight and following a healthy, balanced diet. Our editors and team are hard at work putting together another fantastic Dash Diet cookbook that will be available in December. Keep checking back for exclusive Dash Diet products that will be sold only at Dash Diet! The Dash Diet Cookbook is a collection of simple recipes that are easy to prepare and incredibly tasty. Many different styles of cooking are featured, so you can find something that works for you. The Dash Diet Cookbook is perfect for anyone who wants to eat better and feel great while saving money and time.

If you're ready to get started, the Dash Diet Cookbook is here to help. There's something for everyone in this book, from breakfast items like oatmeal and French toast to dinner side dishes like zucchini noodles and ranch dressing. Feel great about what you eat with the Dash Diet Cookbook!

This guide is your guide to the Dash Diet Cookbook. If you have been following the diet for any amount of time, you will appreciate the information in this guide. Take advantage of the resources that was provided in this guide to ensure that you succeed on a diet.

After reviewing the Dash Diet Cookbook, it appears that some people have expressed concern about the lack of a portion specified in the diet. While there are no food requirements listed in the diet, it does teach you how to make healthy meals and snacks from the foods listed in the recipes. After learning how to cook Dash recipes, anyone can create a healthy and delicious meal with the right ingredients. The Dash Diet Cookbook teaches you how to plan, so you don't have to stress over making your meals before you get home from work.

Made in the USA
Monee, IL
09 January 2022